ANNUAL REVIEW OF WOMEN'S HEALTH

ANNUAL REVIEW OF WOMEN'S HEALTH

Edited by
Beverly J. McElmurry
and
Randy Spreen Parker

National League for Nursing Press • New York
Pub. No. 19-2546

ISBN 0-88737-598-7

Cover illustration: *Seasons of Life,* by Maxine Noel-Ioyan Mani.

This book was set in Aster and Trump by Publications Development Company. The editor and designer was Nancy Jeffries. The cover was designed by Lauren Stevens.

Printed in the United States of America

Contents

Preface

As the purview of women's health has moved in the last three decades from gynecology, synonymous more or less with women's plumbing, to GYN-ecology, encompassing all aspects of the relationship between women and their environments (McBride, 1993), it has become increasingly important that major efforts aimed at synthesizing the rapid expansion of the field proceed apace. This *Annual Review of Women's Health* accomplishes that purpose because it covers both topics of traditional interest to women with fresh information (e.g., sexuality, PMS, contraception, childbearing) and subjects traditionally considered to be the primary concern of men with an appreciation of how they play out differently in women's lives (e.g., heart disease, occupational health, alcohol/addiction). The resulting chapters collectively make the case that women's health is concerned about the overall well being of women as women, their dis-eases and not just their diseases (Stevenson, 1977). Because the contents substantively address the issues that concern most women in a readable manner, this volume should be of interest to both professional and lay audiences. Indeed, this book's emphasis on the information that women need to make good choices should have both an empowering effect on individuals reading it for their own benefit and serve to remind all health care professionals that their obligation is to help women make such informed choices.

Women's health scholarship is in the process of undergoing a major shift of emphasis. What began as a critique of patriarchal practices (e.g., not including women as subjects in health care research, minimizing the extent to which sociocultural factors shape women's experience, regarding male behavior as normative, ignoring women's special concerns) is evolving into a positive statement of new values (McBride & McBride, 1993). That shift from critique to assertion is evident in this volume's recognition of morbidity as a particular concern of women, as opposed to the traditional medical focus on mortality outcomes. Women's health problems are discussed not only with an appreciation of the gravity and urgency of chronic conditions, but with the perspective that matters of health must be understood within the overall context of quality of life. That approach broadens the mandate of the health delivery system to mean every effort must be made to help women feel as vital as possible within the limitations imposed by any disease process.

As this book reviews the health care problems that concern many women, it also conveys an overall sense of the beliefs and assumptions undergirding women's health at this point in time: Women should not be regarded as a monolithic group for their experiences may differ by age, race and ethnic origin, class, sexual preference, and so forth. Patients' perceptions of what health means to them must be the starting-off point for designing suitable interventions, for the objective of the professional is neither to do what she or he thinks is good (patriarchal ethics) nor to treat others as one would wish to be treated (the golden rule), but to help patients achieve what they think will benefit them (feminist ethics). In this process, special attention is paid to developing non-invasive treatments, to avoiding the iatrogenic consequences of massive technology and hyper-pharmacy, and to monitoring cost effectiveness as well as benefits.

Because the contributors are all actively involved in women's health research themselves, the information provided is state of the science. As a group, these authors remind us of the inroads women scientists have made in reformulating our nation's practice-research agenda, because their analyses of women's issues and problems go far beyond the biomedical model. It is this reach that ultimately makes the book so satisfying.

REFERENCES

McBride, A. B. (1993). From gynecology to gyn-ecology: Developing a practice-research agenda for women's health. *Health Care for Women International, 14*, 316–325.

McBride, A. B., & McBride, W. L. (1993). Women's health scholarship: From critique to assertion. *Journal of Women's Health, 2*, 43–47.

Stevenson, J. S. (1977). Women's health research. Why, what and so what? *CMR Voice* (Ohio State University School of Nursing), *21*, 1–2.

Angela Barron McBride

Contributors

Linda A. Bernhard, PhD, RN
Associate Professor
Department of Adult Health and Illness Nursing, and Center
  for Women's Studies
The Ohio State University

Catherine Ingram Fogel, PhD, RN
Associate Professor
School of Nursing
University of North Carolina at Chapel Hill

Patricia A. Geary, EdD, RN
Associate Dean Undergraduate Academic Affairs
School of Nursing
University of Pittsburgh

Marie Hastings-Tolsma, PhD, RN, C
Assistant Professor
University of Southern Main
School of Nursing

Jeanne Beauchamp Hewitt, PhD, RN
Assistant Professor
School of Nursing
University of Wisconsin at Milwaukee

Karyn Holm, PhD, FAAN,
Professor and Chair
School of Nursing
Loyola University, Chicago

Tonda L. Hughes, PhD, RN
Assistant Professor
Department of Psychiatric Nursing
College of Nursing
University of Illinois, Chicago

Susan R. Johnson, MD
Associate Professor
Department of Obstetrics and Gynecology
College of Medicine
University of Iowa

Pamela Fox Levin, MS, RN
Doctoral Candidate
College of Nursing
University of Illinois at Chicago

Angela Barron McBride, PhD, RN, FAAN
Distinguished Professor and University Dean
School of Nursing
Indiana University

Theresa Lawlor McDonald, MA, PA, NP
Clinical Director
Hillcrest Family Services
Dubuque, Iowa

Beverly J. McElmurry, EdD, RN, FAAN
Professor
College of Nursing
University of Illinois at Chicago

Susan Terry Misner, MS, RN
Research Specialist
College of Nursing
University of Illinois at Chicago

Amy C. Olson, PhD, RD
Associate Professor of Nutrition
College of Saint Benedict

Randy Spreen Parker, MSN, RN, C
Doctoral Candidate
College of Nursing
University of Illinois at Chicago

Thelma Patrick, PhD
Assistant Professor
School of Nursing
University of Pittsburgh

Sue M. Penckofer, PhD, RN
Assistant Professor
School of Nursing
Loyola University, Chicago

Dianne Voytko, PhD, RN
Assistant Professor of Nursing
School of Nursing
University of Pittsburgh

Amgad Wahba, PhD, RN
Associate Professor of Nursing
School of Nursing
Clarion University

Denise C. Webster, PhD, RN, CS
Associate Professor
School of Nursing
University of Colorado

Nancy Fugate Woods, PhD, RN, FAAN
Professor, Parent Child Nursing
Director, Center for Women's Health Research
University of Washington

Introduction

Beverly J. McElmurry

The idea for an annual review of perspectives in women's health began in the mid 1980s as graduate faculty and students at the University of Illinois in Chicago launched the graduate concentration in women's health. Our interest in fostering knowledge development about the health of women was built on the desire for a critical examination of the existing knowledge base to determine nursing interventions that promoted and enhanced the well being of women. To this end there was an interest in understanding women as capable of determining what interventions were acceptable to them and accurately reflected the biopsychosocial context of their lived experience.

Our work was built on a consensus about certain assumptions regarding the health care of women. These assumptions are:

1. The human body, mind, and spirit form a whole.
2. Women have the capacity for self-care and self-healing.
3. Events and interactions in the family, community, and world affect and shape the health of women.
4. Health care is a shared responsibility.
5. Health reflects integrity, flexibility, capacity to develop, and capacity to creatively transcend difficult situations.
6. Control over one's body is a basic right.
7. Lived experiences are the starting point for future action.
8. Women's health settings vary.
9. The health of all is improved by focusing on women's health.

McElmurry & Huddleston (1991, p. 16)

In order to enhance our capacity for critical thinking about women's health, we used the above assumptions about women's health as we examined the words found in the literature to describe women's health. As we initially sorted the existing literature in women's health, it became obvious that the usual terms for literature retrieval were driven by an emphasis on illness. Through a laborious process of retrieving literature from multiple databases, the key words for hundreds of references were identified and then grouped in related categories by women's health scholars.

Carol Leppa was a doctoral student at the time that the categorization format was developed and a key leader in this effort. This process of "taking control" of the women's health literature was akin to our assumption about the importance of women having control over their bodies. At the same time, we learned many lessons about the social construction of knowledge and the often unrecognized influences on our thinking about women's health. The importance of words in shaping individual and societal views of women was recognized by our shift from "key words" to the use of "access words" to sort references. Overall, we tried to identify "women friendly" words and accepted the reality that articles pertinent to women's health might reflect: (1) opinions, (2) conceptual/theoretical positions, (3) research, (4) insights based on personal observation, (5) practice experience, and (6) educational synthesis of diverse knowledge areas.

The categories were eventually labeled and then used to organize the literature in women's health. For many years we used the categories and access words to index the literature included in the *Women's Health Nursing Scan* bimonthly publication of the J. B. Lippincott Company and later the Nursecom-owned Scan.

The categories derived as well as the access words included in each category are presented in Table 1. In our experience any one women's health publication may cover more than one category of concern in women's health and combine a mix of personal and scholarly insights on a given topic.

The predecessors to this women's health review were the three volumes on *Women's Health Perspectives,* published by Oryx Press, (Leppa, Miller, 1988; Leppa, 1989; Leppa, 1990). Those early volumes established the criteria for selection of topics and content. For example, each author collects and evaluates the information published during a given time period and offers ideas on areas that need additional attention. Likewise, the literature is selected for review because it concerns women only or effects them differently (Leppa & Miller, 1988). We urged the authors of the women's health reviews to consider our assumptions about women's health as they wrote. For example, does the article reviewed depict women as active participants in health care? The authors of each review were encouraged to think about entering into an exchange with the reader. In this regard, what we concluded about the area of women's health is shared with the readers and they in turn will further inform our understanding through a process of validation or challenge.

Overall, the chapters included in this review illustrate the categories identified in Table 1. Most of the authors incorporate information about the characteristics of women, research/theoretical issues, and policy/ethics/economic/ legislative concerns of importance to a particular topic. Development across the life cycle is a category covering the chapters in midlife women's health and sexuality. Health promotion and maintenance describes the concern about weight control. The inclusion of a chapter on occupational health issues illustrates the categories of women as providers of health care and health and work. The discussion of childbearing represents the reproductive health category and contraceptive products are categorized in the area of drugs/devices/therapeutic interventions. The mental health category is covered by one chapter along with separate chapters on the health problems of

**Table 1. Categories and Access Words
for Women's Health**

Characteristics of Women	**Physical Diseases and Health Problems**
Development Across the Life Cycle	substance abuse/addiction
menstrual cycle	osteoporosis
sexuality	STD
physiology	gynecological issues
child-rearing/	cancer
parenting	
relationships	**Mental Health/Illness**
family	violence/abuse
	body image
Health Promotion and Maintenance	eating disorders
nutrition	
lifestyles	**Drugs, Devices, Therapeutic Interventions**
risk factors	
screening	**Economics, Ethics, Policy, Legislation**
status/assessment	
environmental health	**Research/Theoretical Issues**
	methods
Women as Providers of Health Care	theories
professional providers	scales/instruments
non-professional	lived experience
providers	feminism
work of the nurse	
	Additional/Alternative Access Words:
Delivery of Health Care to Women	
	_____
Health and Work	_____
Reproductive Health	_____
maternal-fetal	_____
health/illness	
intrapartum	
postpartum	

alcohol, sexually transmitted diseases, and cardiovascular disease. Attention to acute care highlights considerations of health care delivery for women. The following paragraphs offer brief highlights of the content covered in each chapter of this review.

The choice of materials covered by Denise Webster focuses on selected review articles, books, audiotapes, and pamphlets that capture trends in literature on women's mental health. While depression, overmedication, and overdiagnosis are still prevalent concerns in the consideration of mental illness, this review recognizes that trauma and violence have emerged as significant issues for women. The interaction of socio-politico-economic factors is noted as a continuation of historical mental health influences.

The social construction of women's mental health reality is recognized by the author.

The literature on women's health contains limited current and comprehensive information about occupational issues in women's health. Therefore, the chapter by Susan T. Misner, Pamela Fox Levin, and Jeanne Beauchamp Hewitt offers a substantive contribution to the review of occupational concerns in women's health. The phenomenal change in women's roles over the past 20 years has enhanced access to equitable employment in workplaces. However, the inadequate, conflicting, and often unscientific knowledge of the occupational factors affecting women has a negative impact on women's health that must be addressed. Women continue to work in settings where many have lower pay, power, and autonomy than their male colleagues. Although acknowledged, the stress for women who juggle home responsibilities with work has not resulted in adequate implementation of family leave policies, worksite child care, and flexible scheduling. The workplace hazards discussed by the authors of this chapter are grouped according to physical, biological, chemical, and psychological dimensions. There is growing consumer recognition and concern about the violence and homicide women (e.g., checkout clerks and nurses in emergency rooms or psychiatric settings) face when they work. The lack of attention to chemical exposure such as pesticides and pharmaceuticals is another area highlighted in this chapter. In addition, there are policy areas and methodological issues that the authors note for further occupational health research. Overall, the articles included in this review represent a goldmine of information on the scientific basis for workplace health.

Control over reproductive activity remains a women's health concern. Theresa McDonald and Susan Johnson remind us that, in the 1980s, the oppressive climate for investment in contraceptive products resulted in a lost generation of research and progress toward improving the health of childbearing women in the United States. An assessment of the fertility rates of women across the world, by age and education, highlights the need for a global perspective on contraception. Between the overview and the abstracted articles, the authors cover contraceptive alternatives from abstinence to drugs, vaccines, and mechanical devices.

The discussion of literature on childbearing by Patricia Geary, Marie Hastings-Tolsma, Diane Voytko, Amgad Wahba, and Thelma Patrick has a pivotal focus: what care promotes the health of childbearing women, their infants, and their families? Giving women control and choices over childbearing decisions frames the authors' discussion and provides a lens for examining the dilemmas of cost containment and the use of new technologies. In our society, mothers and families are becoming increasingly responsible for postpartum care in the home, and this change is identified as an important policy issue in the debate on reimbursement systems needed in health care reform. Overall, the diversity of women and their experiences with childbearing is celebrated by these authors in their discussion of research, services, professional issues such as legal and ethical dimensions of reproductive health care, as well as intrapartum, after birth, cesarean sections and breastfeeding experiences of women, illnesses during pregnancy, women with special needs, and teen pregnancy. This chapter offers valuable insights from caregivers with expertise in childbearing and women's health.

Nancy Fugate Woods' chapter emphasizes that considerations in the health of women at midlife must include more than menopause. In her scholarly review, covering the 12 years from 1980 through 1992, she notes that regardless of various definitions used to define midlife health a pivotal point remains: to try to understand the context for the experience of a particular group born at the same time. The need for contemporary studies of midlife women is urged as a means to integrate existing knowledge with the current complexity of women's lives and the multiple dimensions of their health. Overall, Woods cites the recommendations of others to urge future work that: (1) establishes priorities for health care research reflecting women's experiences as well as the findings from social, behavioral, and medical sciences; (2) establishes an information base considering precursors of health at midlife, for example, nutrition and exercise; (3) redefines research priorities to include nonclinical populations and prospective studies about women's experiences; (4) presents a more realistic view of midlife women to health professionals in their training; and (5) supports environments in which women can develop realistic expectations about midlife health issues.

Linda A. Bernhard's discussion of women's sexuality covers multidisciplinary literature published from 1988 through 1992. Bernhard makes the important point that our understanding of "normal" women's sexuality lags because of the traditional emphasis on problems. The five-year trends discerned from this review include: descriptors of sexual behaviors for purposes of AIDS prevention; emphasis on the diversity of women; the predominance of male medical models for defining sexuality; and growth in women-oriented definitions and descriptions of sexuality. The author encourages the development of models which incorporate a biopsychosocial approach to the study of women's sexuality across the lifespan and within diverse social and cultural contexts.

Tonda Hughes' review and update of research on alcohol and other drug use among women indicates that some progress is being made in this area of women's health. However, special populations are identified and discussed in terms of existing and further needs for research. The lifestyle aspects of alcohol and associated problems such as violence, AIDS, and other drug abuse are part of the framework used in this chapter along with physiologic consequences and implications for treatment.

The problems in addressing sexually transmitted diseases (STDs) have been highlighted by the emergence of the AIDS epidemic. Catherine Fogel's discussion of the topic of STDs emphasizes that "no sexually active person is without risk of infection." Furthermore, it is well-recognized that STDs are often associated with women's increased incidence of AIDS. Women need information on STDs to prevent them, recognize them when they occur, and judge the adequacy of treatment.

Karyn Holm and Sue Penckofer have been concerned for some time about the inadequate attention paid to the cardiovascular health of women. In their introduction, it is noted that as recently as 1964 women were invited to statewide conferences to learn how to protect their husbands against heart disease. Never mind that more women die each year from cardiovascular disease then all forms of cancers. An important emphasis in this chapter is the discussion of risk factors for women and the risk assessment information women require in order to make informed decisions. The authors achieve their aim by increasing the readers understanding of heart disease in women, emphasizing the continuing bias in diagnosis and treatment of heart disease in women, and identifying effective interventions. The information in this chapter is important to the current and future health of women.

Patricia Geary's chapter on acute care of women touches upon the emerging concern for attention to the cancers and heart diseases that kill women. The national interest in increased funding for women's health research has been fueled by the increasing recognition that many areas of research have inadequate samples of women and clinical trials including women. This is a brief review of a very important area and one which is ripe for further development.

Amy Olson presents a formidable review of women and weight control. Her background in biochemistry, nutrition, and clinical dietetics is brought to the full service of the reader in this review and organization of information on weight control. The overview covers normal nutrition, obesity, the biochemical dynamics in dieting, and various radical surgeries for the treatment of obesity. This is an important topic for women since the majority of people consuming weight loss products and services are women of middle or higher incomes between the ages of 18 and 49 years. In this chapter, there is information for women of all ages and weights.

Given the preceding review of chapters and reflection on roughly 15 years of work to advance women's health research as an acceptable focus in nursing science, what conclusions can be made? There are more scholars who identify with a women's health focus, numerous research agenda have been published, the literature is exploding and the boundaries have expanded to an international focus and recognition of the pivotal relationship of women's health to the development of society, families, and individuals (McElmurry, Norr, & Parker, 1993).

Considering all of the possible developments that could be cited, are there areas needing attention? Of course. The increased funding for women's health research and the inclusion of women's health objectives/ goals in the statements of various professional associations is primarily a professionally driven agenda. We have yet to find adequate means for low-income women to influence or participate in "clinical trials" or setting research agenda and funding priorities. Likewise, concern for women's health requires that we accommodate a feminist agenda for the nursing profession. Yet as Joan Mulligan (1992) noted in her retrospective 20-year review of nursing and feminism, the mainstream nursing response to feminist scholarship has been to ignore it (p. 175). Unlike other disciplines, Mulligan makes it very clear that in nursing, with the possible exception of nursing research, it is difficult to locate the nursing scholarship that has been stimulated by a feminist analysis of nursing and health care.

The recent emergence of caring as a focus for nursing is consistent with a concern for relationships and participatory engagement with patients, clients, and research participants. Being able to care for others is consistent with caring for self and enabling action. We are pleased to have the National League for Nursing (NLN) assist with this publication as the NLN's vision for health care reform will result in a realignment of nursing accountability to the populations and communities we serve. If we realize the reorientation of nursing education and practice and achieve a community-based response to the health of the public, it will be possible to trace the impact of feminism on the health of providers, as well as patient/client participants.

In closing, I want to acknowledge the special contribution that Randy S. Parker made to the preparation of this book. As each author submitted a manuscript, she critically read the material and noted editorial suggestions. Then, I critically read the manuscript and together we determined whether further correspondence with the author and/or publisher was merited. Randy's special gifts in writing and helping others tell their stories facilitated the work of everyone associated with this publication.

REFERENCES

McElmurry, B. J., & Huddleston, D. (1991). Self-care and menopause: Critical review of research. *Health Care for Women International*, 12:15–26.

McElmurry, B. J., Norr, K., & Parker, R. S. (1993). *Women's health and development: A Global challenge*. Boston: Jones and Bartlett Publications.

Leppa, C. J., & Miller, C. (1988). *Women's Health Perspectives: An Annual Review*, Vol. I. Phoenix: Oryx Press.

Leppa, C. J. (1988). *Women's Health Perspectives: An Annual Review*, Vol. II. Phoenix: Oryx Press.

Leppa, C. J. (1990). *Women's Health Perspectives: An Annual Review*, Vol. III. Phoenix: Oryx Press.

Mulligan, J. (1992). Nursing and feminism: Caring and curing. In C. Kramarac and D. Spender (Eds.), *The Knowledge explosion: Generations of feminist scholarship*, 172–180. New York: Teachers College Press.

National League for Nursing (1993). A Vision for nursing education. New York: National League for Nursing Press.

Chapter 1

Women and Mental Health

Denise C. Webster

INTRODUCTION

Choosing representative offerings for the years 1989 through 1992 presents several challenges. The sheer number of books, articles, and audiotapes related to women and mental health is daunting. Resources vary in theoretical perspective, focus, and intended audience. Because articles appearing in academic journals are more readily accessible through computerized literature searches, this chapter, with the exception of selected review articles, will be limited to books, audiotapes, and selected pamphlets.

Several trends noted in this review have been in evidence for many years. The "Decade of the Brain" was ushered in by Congress on January 1, 1990. Major mental illness, stroke, addictions, toxins, perinatal, and other traumas were targeted for increased research, treatment, and rehabilitation (Buckwalter, 1990). The advances in pharmacotherapy in the previous decade had been impressive, so many hoped that it would be possible to identify the etiologic sources of mental health problems and to prevent, eradicate, or reduce symptoms by manipulating neurotransmitters or other biologic phenomena. The greater prevalence of depression among women would suggest that the specter of a rapid cure would be welcomed by women's health advocates. However, there has been an impressive and ongoing history of concern that women are overdiagnosed with mental problems conceptualized as personal inadequacies and overmedicated for any signs of rebellion against the social status quo (McGrath, Keita, Strickland, & Russo, 1990; Unger & Crawford, 1992). While maintaining the importance of a holistic model of health, many feminist therapists have argued that the social antecedents of women's mental health problems have been underdiagnosed and undertreated (Chesler, 1989).

Against these contemporary and historical trends it appears that all of the above perspectives may be converging as we learn more about the immediate and long-term effects of trauma (Herman, 1991; Courtois, 1988). The rapprochement noted in recent years between feminists and psychoanalytic theorists has accelerated as both groups struggle to understand the place of gender, sexuality, and safety in the development of psychological problems. Retrieval of Freud's original "seduction theory" has emerged as one powerful explanatory factor for women's problems that have been labelled, among other diagnoses as "hysteria," "borderline personality disorder," "somatization disorder," "dysthymia," and "dissociation" (Herman, 1992; Arnold & Saunders, 1992). At the juncture of the intrapsychic response to trauma and the social institutions which have ignored, denied, and distorted the existence of the actual trauma events looms an epistemologic void which has been filled with many different and competing explanations (Hare-Mustin & Marecek, 1990; Unger & Crawford, 1992; Kaschak, 1992; Tavris, 1992). The question "how can this happen?" then becomes many questions: "Did it really happen?", "Why didn't her mother protect her?", "Why didn't she tell anyone?", "Why hasn't this been talked about?" are some questions addressed by seeking intrapersonal and selective intrafamilial answers. "How can a society ignore this?", "How does this replicate power differences in the general society?" are among the questions that frame social explanations for the etiology of interpersonal violence. The reemergence of the diagnosis of "Multiple Personality Disorder" has polarized the mental health community in many directions; those who don't believe it exists and those who believe there may be systemic intrapersonal, social, and/or transpersonal forces at work intent on destruction of children, family values, and/or society.

While the sequelae of sexual abuse of children, and particularly girls, has become the source of an unending stream of books, articles, and self-help groups for victims/survivors, others have pointed at the larger arena of domestic violence as an additional powerful explanatory factor for women's problems, such as depression, eating disorders, agoraphobia, substance abuse, and psychotic presentations (Herman, 1992; Courtois, 1988; Walker, 1989; Koss, 1990). As evidence mounts that it may be impossible to separate intrapsychic (and physiologic) from social and political explanations for various acute and chronic manifestations of psychological distress, the DSM-III-R diagnosis of Post Traumatic Stress Disorder is becoming a catch-all category that may more accurately describe the social origins of many psychological problems and modify earlier tendencies to automatically "blame the victim." The arena of debate, for many, has shifted now to definitions: "What constitutes trauma?" and "What constitutes abuse?" Included here as well are treatment concerns such as "What are the biologic consequences of chronic stress?", "What diagnoses would be appropriate?", and "How do you help trauma victims/survivors/transcenders heal?"

Out of the latter question have come a plethora of individual, group, and family interventions including therapies based on cognitive, behavioral, psychoanalytic, feminist, and spiritual models, with and without psychotropic pharmacologic therapy. The books and articles reviewed here reflect the tensions between competing epistemologies as evidenced by continuing debates around diagnostic, etiologic, and dynamic formulations (Laidlow & Malmo, 1980; Dolan, 1991; Courtois, 1988; Herman, 1992). Several books address the concepts of knowledge development itself, representing a wave of interest in critical theory, postmodern, deconstructivist, and social constructivist approaches to understanding (Hare-Mustin & Marecek, 1990; Squire, 1989). New understandings of the mother-daughter relationship and the role of power and gender in families and in women's lives reflect other related trends (Firman & Firman, 1989; Hancock, 1989; Mercer, Nichols, & Doyle, 1989; Kantor & Okun, 1989; Goodrich, 1991). The shift by many to a theory of traumatic response has led to questions about use of pejorative diagnostic labels, such as "borderline," "codependent," "self-defeating personality disorders" to describe behaviors which may have been essential to survival at one time (Walters, 1990; Arnold & Saunders, 1992; Herman, 1992; Dolan, 1991). New diagnostic categories for women's psychological distress have been suggested by many of the authors reviewed here (Brown & Ballou, 1992; Herman, 1992; Tavris, 1992; Chesler, 1989; Courtois, 1988; Kaschak, 1992), along with matching suggested diagnoses for the male counterpart behaviors, for example, "Sadistic Personality Disorder" and "Delusional Dominating Personality Disorder" (Tavris, 1992). It is too early to tell what parts the decade of the brain, the recognition of traumatic phenomena, and the rapidly shifting political climate will play between now and the new century. In some ways, women's problems described today are no different from those described a century and more ago.

REFERENCES

Arnold, F., & Saunders, E. (1986–1992). *Borderline personality disorder and childhood abuse: Revisions in clinical thinking and treatment approach.* The Stone Center, Wellesley College, Wellesley, Massachusetts.

Brown, L., & Ballou, M. (Eds.) (1992). *Personality and psychopathology: Feminist reappraisals.* New York: Guilford Press.

Buckwalter, K. (1990). The decade of the brain and psychiatric nursing. *Archives of Psychiatric Nursing, 4*(5), 283.

Chesler, P. (1989). *Women and madness.* San Diego: Harcourt, Brace.

Courtois, C. (1988). *Healing the incest wound: Adult survivors in therapy.* New York: W. W. Norton.

Dolan, Y. (1991). *Resolving sexual abuse.* New York: W. W. Norton.

Firman, J., & Firman, D. (1989). *Daughters and mothers: Healing the relationship.* New York: Continuum.

Goodrich, T. (Ed.) (1991). *Women and power: Perspectives for family therapy.* New York: W. W. Norton.

Hancock, E. (1989). *The girl within.* New York: Dutton.

Hare-Mustin, R., & Marecek, J. (Eds.) (1990). *Making a difference: Psychology and the construction of gender.* New Haven: Yale University Press.

Herman, J. (1992). *Trauma and recovery.* New York: Basic Books.

Kantor, D., & Okun, B. (Eds.) (1989). *Intimate environments: Sex, intimacy and gender in families.* New York: Guilford Press.

Kaschak, E. (1992). *Engendered lives: A new psychology of women's experience.* New York: Basic Books.

Koss, M. (1990). The women's mental health research agenda: Violence against women. *American Psychologist, 45*(3), 374–380.

Laidlow, T., Malmo, C., et al. (1990). *Healing voices: Feminist approaches to therapy with women.* San Francisco: Jossey-Bass.

McGrath, E., Keita, G., Strickland, B., & Russo, N. (1990). *Women and depression: Risk factors and treatment issues: Final report of the American Psychological Association's National Task Force on Women and Depression.* Washington, DC: American Psychological Association.

Mercer, R., Nichols, E., & Doyle, G. (1989). *Transitions in a woman's life: Major life events in developmental context.* New York: Springer.

Squire, C. (1989). *Significant differences.* New York: Routledge.

Tavris, C. (1992). *The mismeasure of woman.* New York: Touchstone.

Unger, R., & Crawford, M. (1992). *Women and gender: A feminist psychology.* Philadelphia: Temple University Press.

Walker, L. (1989). *Psychology and violence against women. American Psychologist, 44*(4), 695–702.

Walters, M. (1990). The codependent Cinderella who loves too much . . . fights back. *The Family Therapy Networker* (July/August), 53–57.

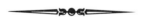

BOOKS

Anderson, S., & Hopkins, P. (1991). *The feminist face of God: The unfolding of the sacred in women.* New York: Bantam Books.

The merging of psychological and spiritual is an implicit but powerful thread running through this book's descriptions of the feminine experience of spirituality. In her foreword, Jean Shinoda Bolen notes that most of the more than 100 notable women interviewed by Anderson and Hopkins found it difficult to maintain a spiritual path as well as a long-term relationship with a man. The spiritual paths described by these women bear limited resemblance to the patriarchal religions which many found they could no longer support. For women who believe their pain is related to loss of spirit or destruction of their souls, these women's stories and the themes that connect them may be more healing than traditional or feminist psychotherapies.

Bernay, T., & Cantor D. (Eds.) (1989). *The psychology of today's woman: New psychoanalytic visions.* Cambridge: Harvard University Press. (Reprinted from hardcover 1986 Analytic press).

The 1989 paperback version of *The Psychology of Today's Woman: New Psychoanalytic Visions* might be the best introductory choice for readers who may be minimally familiar with psychoanalytic concepts. The editors present a variety of traditional and newly formulated ideas about women's development. The introductory chapter, entitled "Is Freud an Enemy of Women's Liberation? Some Historical Considerations," provides a clear overview of some of the criticisms of traditional Freudian theory as androcentric and sexist analytic formulations of women's ubiquitous inadequacies, in contrast with other psychoanalytic perspectives. Many of the chapters demonstrate a greater commitment to "explaining" why women are inadequate than presenting models for helping to deal with women's problems. Two chapters on "Anger in the Mother-Daughter Relationship" and "The

Self-in-Relation: Empathy and the Mother-Daughter Relationship" are particularly well-written and demonstrate again, the mother-daughter relationship is a potentially positive resource throughout women's lives. The last section of the book considers the relationships between the analyst and the client in a changing world.

Brody, C. (Ed.) (1987). *Women's therapy groups: Paradigms of feminist treatment.* New York: Springer.

One of the Springer *Focus on Women* Series, this edited volume is a mixture of previously published and newer contributions to the literature on group therapy with women. Since the beginning of the second wave of feminism there has been a general acceptance that group approaches, including consciousness-raising and self-help groups, are the modality of choice for women. The major themes of shared female experience and learning to value the support of other women are found throughout the chapters. The first section of the book deals with how women's groups may be different from all-male or mixed gender groups and some trends in group approaches during the past two decades. The second section contains writings on consciousness-raising groups and group interventions with women who are in abusive relationships or suffer from agoraphobia. A third section covers group models for mixed cultural groups, black women, lesbian couples, along with two examples of cognitive and behavioral theoretical approaches for work with women, while the last section is concerned with group treatment for homeless women and chronic alcoholic women, adult survivors of incest, depressed women, as well as women with bulimia or sexual dysfunctions. As might be expected, the quality of the chapters varies considerably.

Of special interest to the therapist is the chapter by Marsha Linehan describing a group approach called Dialectical Behavior Therapy for treating Borderline Personality Disorder and parasuicidal behaviors. In sharp contrast to most of the literature on treatment of women with these diagnoses which describe individual long-term psychoanalytic therapies, this model has a clear outline of behavioral and didactic sessions, each lasting three hours, for a period of one year. Each participant experiences the three modules at least twice. The author provides a clear description of the syndromes the women may experience, the rationales for the topics discussed, and the learning approaches used. Particularly impressive is the emphasis on helping the women develop mutually-supportive relationships with each other and the inherent opportunities for them to "debrief" during breaks and after sessions by having time together without the therapists being present.

Brown, L., & Ballou, M. (Eds.) (1992). *Personality and psychopathology: Feminist reappraisals.* New York: Guilford Press.

In most feminist critiques of psychological theory, a few schools of thought are discussed (and often dismissed) in one or two paragraphs. At the other extreme are books, such as Prozan's *Feminist Psychoanalytic Psychotherapy* (1992), which are dense, detailed dissections comparing feminist theory with a particular theoretical tradition. This book devotes four chapters to mid-level critiques of the feminist therapy potential of Humanistic Personality Theory, Object Relations and Self Psychology, Jungian therapy and Cognitive-Behavioral Therapy. A chapter on ethnicity, race, class, and gender concludes the first section by suggesting that a social construction perspective provides a viable and valuable alternative for interpreting women's experiences. The second section offers feminist perspectives on selected issues of psychopathology, including depression, psychosis, and agoraphobia. Of particular interest are Brown's feminist critique of personality disorders and her proposed category of "Abuse/Oppression Artifact Disorders." This chapter and Root's chapter on the impact of trauma take a different but congruent view of trauma from that taken by Herman in *Trauma and Recovery* (1992).

Butler, S., & Wintram, C. (1991). *Feminist groupwork.* London: Sage.

The authors, two English social workers, describe their work with women from both inner city and rural environments. Impressed with the degree of isolation and fear experienced by these "family caretakers," they set up two community-based women's groups. This well-organized text outlines in detail their approach to setting up and maintaining groups, based on feminist principles. It will be particularly helpful to the beginning group therapist trying to translate feminist philosophy into practice. Examples of the women's experiences are artfully woven into the structure to enhance understanding of women's anger, losses, and identities. The final chapter, appropriately, describes some termination issues which must be anticipated as well as some ways to link local experience to the larger female experience, socially, politically, and historically.

Cantor, D. (Ed.) (1990). *Women as therapists: A multitheoretical casebook.* Northvale, NJ: Jason Aronson.

As the title suggests, this book compares and contrasts the problem formulations and treatment approaches brought to the therapy situation as a reflection of the therapists' theoretical orientation. The first chapters provide a context for the later case study by providing brief overviews of research on factors affecting therapeutic outcome, including gender of the therapist and therapists' theoretical orientation. Other chapters describe a study exploring how women choose their therapists and a review of information about how therapists choose their theoretical positions. The two case studies refer to individual clients, Mary and Rick. Each case is then formulated and discussed by four female therapists representing one of the following perspectives: psychoanalytic, feminist, family systems, and cognitive-behavioral. A final chapter, by Laura Brown, notes the similarities among the therapies, primarily in relation to the therapeutic process in working with women. Foremost is the capacity for creating with clients a relationship characterized by empathy and flexibility of the therapist's ego boundaries, as well as the related capacity to personally tolerate ambiguity and powerlessness both as a therapist and in relation to clients' vulnerability. Finally, whatever the theoretical

orientation, she believes the role of the therapist in empowering clients remains a constant. While one might question whether there is "a" feminist (or any other) theoretical position, the book would act as a catalyst for discussion among graduate students in therapy-related fields and, potentially, facilitate interdisciplinary understanding among members of therapy teams.

Caplan, P. (1989). *Don't blame mother: Mending the mother-daughter relationship.* New York: Harper & Row.

This book and the Firman book (on healing the mother-daughter relationship) are similar to each other in their attempt to do more than merely explain the difficulties evident in these relationships. Oriented for the lay reader, both utilize social, historical, and political analyses for understanding the interpersonal dynamics women experience. Both books were also written to incorporate the material and experiences the authors had developed in teaching courses on mothers and mother-daughter relationships. In contrast to the greater emphasis on development and intrapsychic explanations in the psychoanalytic readings, they encourage women to actively work on the relationship—not in therapy but in contact with mothers when possible. This book has guidelines for "expressive training" (similar to psychodrama role-playing) and for "interviewing" one's mother. The explanatory notes, complete references, and pointed critique of mother-blaming and double-binding of mothers in the culture and in the theories and practice of psychotherapy make this book the preferable choice for more academically-inclined readers.

Chesler, P. (1989). *Women and madness.* San Diego: Harcourt Brace.

Many credit this book, reissued with a new introduction, with the beginning of public awareness of the dangerous and hidden dimensions of gender bias in the mental health system. In the nearly twenty years since the original version, the author notes there have been both many and not enough changes. In contrast to previous views of expertise, based on abstract theories and therapist objectivity, mental health systems have been challenged by grass-roots movements to redress problems of battering, sexual abuse, and other problems more likely to affect women. The belief that women are the best authorities on women has been heard, but not always heeded. Although there are more women therapists, and women patients are more likely to ask to see women therapists, institutions have not greatly changed their stereotypical views of women.

Perhaps most remarkable about this book is the author's ability, twenty years after we all "know this," to engage the reader in a contagious passion about women who have suffered in a society which constrains female passion and punishes its expression in men or women. Even on re-reading the classic myths of Demeter and her four daughters, the power of the stories remains. Against this background of ancient history and myth, Chesler weaves the recent stories of Elizabeth Packard, Sylvia Plath, Zelda Fitzgerald, and Edith West. Later chapters integrate interviews with 60 women who have experienced the reality of life in various mental institutions. The appendix, which has figures to support the preponderance of female patients in certain categories, has not been updated and has been challenged by earlier critics. Recognizing the many changes in the mental health system since 1969, the author notes in the introduction that the inability to receive needed hospitalization is perhaps as serious a problem now as the overuse of such treatments has been in earlier eras.

Chodorow, N. (1989). *Feminism and psychoanalytic theory*. New Haven: Yale University Press.

Readers unfamiliar with the specialized languages of the various schools of Lacanian, Foucauldian, Derridian, Self-Psychology, Object Relations (as well as Freudian, Kleinian, and Hornian) psychoanalytic thought would best avoid many of the recent selections. However, this book is made somewhat easier to read by Chodorow's presentation of her personal views, and her explanation of the language and politics of each given view, as well as the relationship (or

lack thereof) of these views to gender-related issues. The introduction to this collection of writings, which spans the years 1971 to the present, documents not only her thinking about the importance of mothering and gender relations but her own journey from anthropology, sociology, and personality studies to becoming an object relations psychoanalyst. For those who seek a more personal, rather than theoretical perspective, the last chapter includes findings from a study in which she interviewed female psychoanalysts who trained during the 1920s and 1930s. She argues that not only does psychoanalysis have much to offer in developing the multiple theories needed to understand gender inequality, but that there is a value in studying "psychoanalysis-for-itself" to understand the role of the unconscious as developing out of contributing to the social realms of reality.

Chrisler, J., & Howard, D. (Eds.) (1992). *New directions in feminist psychology: Practice, theory, and research*. New York: Springer.

This collection of papers presented at the 1988 meeting of the Association for Women in Psychology reflects the diversity of ideas and experiences to which a feminist perspective can be brought. Some chapters draw our attention to ongoing concerns of feminist therapists such as inclusion of the African-American perspective, gender issues in couple and family therapy, and specific clinical problems such as bulimia. More unusual chapters describe feminist therapy with severely disturbed clients and with family caretakers of brain-injured patients. The theory chapters provide feminist critiques of sex research, the role of the female graduate psychology student, campus rape prevention programs, and women with cancer. The chapter comparing psychoanalytic and social constructivist theories of lesbianism seems unfortunately brief to adequately address the social constructivist perspective and the consequent changes in therapeutic practice which would follow.

A final section covering new directions in feminist research explores several unusual topics, including gender dimensions of jury instructions, white male biases against black female job applicants, college students' perceptions of how to avoid date rape, and a study of gender differences in response to personal ads for dating. The range of topics presented will both broaden the understanding of the role of feminist theory in research, theory, and practice and probably limit the number of readers who would find the text, as a whole, useful.

Courtois, C. (1988). *Healing the incest wound: Adult survivors in therapy.* New York: W. W. Norton.

Among the recent compilations of facts, figures, and theories about incest, Courtois's book stands out as scholarly, sensitive, and thorough. Section one provides descriptions of the different forms of incest and related family dynamics while section two covers the range of symptoms, aftereffects, and diagnoses associated with the incest experiences. Courtois agrees with Briere that an Axis II diagnosis of Borderline Personality Disorder is probably more usefully conceptualized and treated as Post Traumatic Stress Disorder. The last section covers the spectrum of available treatments (including individual, group and family interventions) for aftermath symptoms of incest. The Incest History Questionnaire used in her own research is included, along with an extensive list of educational resource materials on the topic.

Dolan, Y. (1991). *Resolving sexual abuse.* New York: W. W. Norton.

In a growing market of "incest survivor" books, Dolan's book stands out for its clarity and integrity. Directed at the therapist who wishes to help incest survivors but, understandably, worries about how fast and how far to go, Dolan focuses on careful and respectful progress guided by cooperation with the client's unconscious. Individual work is emphasized via Ericksonian hypnosis and Solution-Focused dialogue. Utilizing survivors' skills at dissociation, Dolan seldom finds it necessary to use formal inductions to access hypnotic responses, which makes the approach less threatening to client and therapist alike. This is a well-written, gentle map which includes a section addressing the need for

therapists to care for themselves and to recognize their own potential vulnerability to Post Traumatic Stress Disorder associated with constant exposure to stories of violence and abuse.

Dutton-Douglas, M., & Walker, L. (Eds.) (1988). *Feminist psychotherapies: Integration of therapeutic and feminist systems.* Norwood, NJ: Ablex.

A recent addition to the growing number of books that provide therapists with a variety of ways to conceptualize women's problems and conduct therapy consistent with feminist values, this volume describes an historical context and guidelines for specific interventions with several target populations. Part One traces the development of feminist therapies. Fodor's chapter on cognitive-behavioral therapy for addressing women's issues is particularly well-written and provides a balanced discussion of the treatment along with a feminist critique of the strengths and weaknesses of the model. The author provides a strong argument for expanding the focus of therapy beyond the symptoms and "irrational thinking" clients present in order to empower clients to recognize their own patterns of behavior and identify the relationships between society, personality, temperament, conflict, and socialization.

Part Two features articles with therapy approaches for divorced, single, female parents, male clients, lesbians and gay men, blacks, Hispanics, and the elderly. Brief overviews of major issues for each group are well-referenced. The final chapter, on future directions in development, application, and training, authored by the editors, might have provided a better introduction to the book than an epilogue. The authors discuss "First Generation" feminist therapy theory as providing some mutual understandings for therapists who came from many different schools of thought. Second generation feminist therapy, which sought to revise the theories and training for therapists working with women, is presented as beginning during the 1980s as a response to earlier criticisms of mainstream theories. The third generation has just begun, and will eventually result in a theory of the psychological development of women. Furthermore, the authors argue, there is a need for a feminist theory of male behavior if therapists are to be effective in helping women and men grow and change. A "Feminist Self-Analysis Test for Psychotherapists" is included for use in graduate training programs.

Estes, C. (1992). *Women who run with the wolves: Myths and stories of the wild woman archetype.* New York: Ballantine Books.

In travels in several areas of the country and among many different groups of women, the question seems universal: "Have you read the book?" "Have you heard the tapes?" A self-described poet, artist, and cantadora (storyteller) as well as Jungian analyst, Estes plies her art by entertaining her readers with fairytales most of us never heard as children—myths with women at the center, and no assurance of "happily ever after" endings. Life is not like that, Estes tells us. Nor are women like what they have been told they are or should be. Drawing images from many cultures, we learn that women can be wise, brave, strong, beautiful, ugly, and mean-spirited. All of this and more comes through in stories of the "wild woman archetype" through her initiation, the retrieval of gifts, her search for companionship and community, independence, and joy in the physical. The oral tradition which has carried these stories and their lessons remains a powerful source of a culture's truth. Women's culture and female experience are delightfully celebrated in taped versions of many of the stories. The growing list includes *The House of the Riddle Mother*, on archetypal images in women's dreams, *The Red Shoes*, which describes common threats to women's self-preservation instincts, and *Women Who Run with the Wolves* (the title story), revealing the lost stories of women's wild natures. Tapes are available from Sounds True, 735 Walnut St., Dept. FC5, Boulder, Colorado 80302.

Firman, J., & Firman, D. (1989). *Daughters and mothers: Healing the relationship.* New York: Continuum.

Written in a workbook style by a mother and daughter, this book appears to be based in Transactional Analysis and Gestalt. In contrast to the Caplan book (1989), the book presents a wider variety of experiential exercises drawn from

workshops the authors have facilitated. The research and theory basis for this book is much less developed than is found in the Caplan book, but may be more accessible to readers who wish to explore their own dynamics as well as their mothers'.

Goodrich, T. (Ed.) (1991). *Women and power: Perspectives for family therapy.* New York: W. W. Norton.

This book is similar to Kantor and Okun's (1989) offering in moving the recognition of feminist concerns about family therapy beyond theoretical critique to a focus on particular concepts. It also includes male contributors. Early chapters by Goodrich, Jean Baker Miller, and Linda Webb-Watson provide the theoretical social and psychological context for the remaining chapters concerning particular issues in family therapy. The awareness of power, both within the family and within the therapy session is discussed (e.g., use of language, choice of metaphors, gender of therapists). The collection of short (often 2–3 pages) clinical practice issues would be particularly useful for stimulating dialogue among therapists and therapists-in-training. The editors acknowledge that power differences exist in violence against women and children; however, it is disturbing that the editors do not address this issue in the clinical practice chapters nor provide adequate theoretical explanations.

Hancock, E. (1989). *The girl within.* New York: Dutton.

Taking a different emphasis from Mercer, Nichols, and Doyle (1989) and starting from different questions, *The Girl Within* reports a study of adult development in women. Where the Mercer, Nichols, and Doyle study assumed that all women could identify "turning points" in their lives, and found that many women could not describe such phenomena, this study screened its subjects for a high degree of "emotional maturity" and self-reflectiveness before they were chosen for interview. Perhaps as a consequence, the descriptions of identity development in adult life are rich and focused on process rather than identifiable points in time. The manner in which this study is written also reflects the more personal repeated interviews with subjects. The final chapter describes the research approach and theoretical framework. The most interesting story may be the author's own rendition of the reanalysis of her data after several years and her discovery that for most of her informants the rediscovery of the girl they had been from ages eight through ten often provided a map for a conscious development of an adult identity, often needed at midlife. In contrast to the burgeoning literature about the vulnerable and frightened "child within," the latency-aged girl is usually described as adventurous, open to experience, feeling considerable power, and having active hopes for her future. The author's description of rediscovering her own "girl within" provides the reader with a positive model of self-disclosure that impressively avoids the ever-present charge of sentimental confession.

Hare-Mustin, R., & Marecek, J. (Eds.) (1990). *Making a difference: Psychology and the construction of gender.* New Haven: Yale University Press.

Hare-Mustin and Marecek published an important paper in 1988, "The Meaning of Difference: Gender Theory, Postmodernism, and Psychology" (American Psychologist, 43(6), 455–464), describing gender theories in terms of alpha bias (exaggerating gender differences) or beta bias (minimizing/ignoring gender differences). This edited book extends that work and explores epistemologic perspectives on gender with a particular emphasis on the gendered meanings embedded in language. The metatheoretical perspective offered will also make this book useful to graduate students in women's studies whether or not they are students of psychology. As a guide to feminist therapy practice or an introduction to the psychology of women, the focus is probably too narrow and academic to be a first choice.

Herman, J. (1992). *Trauma and recovery.* New York: Basic Books.

Subtitled "The aftermath of violence—from domestic abuse to political terror," Herman takes the issue of trauma out of the gender battle by providing a scholarly description of the experience of trauma across many situations, from "shell shock" and combat-related traumas suffered by concentration-camp survivors, hostages, and prisoners (more frequently experienced by men) to the "combat neurosis of the sex war." The latter category includes survivors of domestic battering, childhood sexual and physical abuse, rape, and "organized sexual exploitation." Building on original observations of Freud and Charcot, Herman uses multiple sources to develop her argument for a new Diagnostic and Statistical Manual of Mental Disorders (DSM) diagnosis of "Complex Post-Traumatic Stress Disorder." In addition, she outlines similarities in trauma response and trauma recovery patterns as guidelines for expected stages of recovery from these traumas. Written in an accessible academic style, this book is a valuable resource for survivors and their loved ones, as well as for therapists and theorists.

Jack, D. (1991). *Silencing the self: Women and depression.* Cambridge, MA: Harvard University Press.

Based on the Stone Center's perspectives on women's development, the author describes a study of 12 clinically depressed women. Ranging from 19 to 55 years old, the sample is very limited: all were Caucasian women, though from differing socioeconomic backgrounds. The research participants were interviewed while they were actively depressed and again, two years later. Semistructured interviews were used along with The Silencing the Self Scale (SSS) to measure women's beliefs about self in intimate relationship. As a phenomenological study, the metaphor of the depressed women's "having a voice" is matched by the necessity for others (researchers, partners, society) to have a "preparedness to listen." This is not an easy book to read because these are not easy stories to hear. The women's stories reflect all too painfully the relational (social and interpersonal) basis for their depressions. In this "Decade of the Brain," these stories provide a powerful reminder that physiologic measures of depression are not necessarily the sources of depression.

Johnson, K., & Ferguson, T. (1990). *Trusting ourselves: The sourcebook on psychology for women.* New York: The Atlantic Monthly Press.

Ferguson has edited the magazine *Medical Self-Care* for over a decade, with frequent contributions from Johnson in relation to women's issues, and particularly psychological issues. Written in the style of self-help books, an overview of historical and contemporary perspectives on women's psychology is followed by information about relationships (following the Stone Center acceptance of relationships as central in women's lives). The last two sections describe the signs and symptoms of common psychological concerns for women such as low self-esteem, depression, anxiety, sexuality, alcohol, body image, abuse, and violence. A final section includes a form for taking a self-history covering biological, social and psychological questions, as well as advice and information to help women choose professional help. Each chapter contains a list of resources providing further information, along with community resources and self-help groups which may be available to women. This is a down-to-earth resource for consumers who are less interested in epistemology and politics than in obtaining relief for symptoms.

Jordan, J., Kaplan, A., Miller, J., Stiver, I., & Surrey, J. (1991). *Women's growth in connection: Writings from the Stone Center.* New York: Guilford Press.

The Stone Center Works in Progress, a series of working papers on women's development, have been reviewed throughout this series on women's health. Originally called the "self-in-relation" perspective, the authors now refer to the "relational approach to psychological understanding." As practicing psychotherapists, researchers, and theorists, with differing clinical backgrounds, the authors grapple with the intricacies of concept development (including concepts such as mutuality, empathy, dependency, power) and therapeutic relationship more than

technique. In seeking to describe women's experience from the perspective of women, their clinical practice provides the basis for questions which are then delineated and checked against practice. This paperback collection of papers developed between 1981 and 1986 makes the group's work far more financially and geographically accessible. However, some of the more theoretical papers, those less obviously grounded in the practice of therapy with women, may be less accessible to readers unfamiliar with psychoanalytic reasoning. The authors' continued emphasis on the centrality of relationship in women's lives remains the focus of an ongoing debate in women's psychology. [See Hare-Mustin and Maracek, Prozan, Tavris and others reviewed here.]

Kantor, D., & Okun, B. (Eds.) (1989). *Intimate environments: Sex, intimacy and gender in families.* New York: Guilford Press.

It is not clear how to classify this book except as a possible clue that the rapprochement with former enemies in the battle to redefine female experience may be accelerating. The mixture of writings from psychoanalytic, family systems, as well as feminist views of sex, gender, and intimacy is unique. Perhaps equally noteworthy is that the text has eight female and eleven male writers who were asked to provide personal information about themselves with respect to their own socialization around these issues and how their experiences may have affected their current views on the topic. The range of writers includes Carl Whitaker and Karl Tomm discussing the topic from experiential and cybernetic-systemic positions, respectively. Feminist family therapists Virginia Goldner and Michele Bograd both address passion (of clients and therapists) as an element in family therapy.

A middle section of the book includes selected text from three focus groups of male, female, and mixed gender groupings of the following therapists: David Kantor, Barbara Okun, Donald Bloch, Peggy Penn, and Maggie Scarf. Major themes included definitions of intimacy, the relationship between intimacy and sexuality, therapist neutrality, and differences between males and females, and between male and female therapists. In this section, the dialogue is highly charged, interspersed with random "comments" by various members who reflected on the material and the process. Of particular interest is the outrage the women expressed at the idea of therapist-client sexual involvement in contrast to the men's views. More research into the different ways men and women think about such issues as abandonment, autonomy, love, and commitment is necessary if the culture is to continue to expect nonviolent cohabitation between the genders.

Kaschak, E. (1992). *Engendered lives: A new psychology of women's experience.* New York: Basic Books.

As a feminist therapist and chairperson of a marriage, family, and child counseling program, Kaschak provides a somewhat different perspective on women's psychology and the inclusion of gender in family therapy. Using examples from literature and mythology, as well as contemporary research and theories of feminist therapy and mainstream psychology, the tone is academic while retaining a charming personal sense. Kaschak describes the pervasiveness of gender in explaining every aspect of life, in particular the cultural and developmental contexts in which language and meanings are embedded. Extending Freud's use of the Oedipus myth to include the stories that provided context for his Oedipal conflict, we learn about Antigone, the daughter/sister of Oedipus and her experience, much as Virginia Woolf described the imagined life of Shakespeare's sister in the short story "A Room of One's Own." This book may have most appeal for articulate readers, not necessarily therapists, who are interested in a scholarly understanding of "women's issues," women's problems and feminist approaches to helping women.

Kasl, C. (1992). *Many roads, one journey.* New York: HarperCollins.

Intended primarily for the educated consumer of 12-step self-help therapy groups, Kasl's book provides a bridge between some feminists' despair over the burgeoning codependency movement and the fact that many women report finding these self-help programs valuable—up to a point. Carefully basing her argument for different kinds of "recovery" programs for women, Kasl traces the history of the development of Alcoholics Anonymous as well as contemporary information about a range of addictions. Kasl critiques the limitations of 12-step programs for meeting women's needs to define their own experiences. Her range of alternative practices for self-care includes nutrition, mandala work, and energy balancing through awareness of body chakras. Based on her own research and experiences in workshops and 12-step groups, Kasl eventually developed a 16-step program, with more open language and flexibility than traditional 12-step programs.

Laidlow, T., Malmo, C., et al. (1990). *Healing voices: Feminist approaches to therapy with women.* San Francisco: Jossey-Bass.

Another book directed primarily at therapists who work with women in healing from experiences of interpersonal violence, the balance of therapist and client views provides a clear example of feminist philosophy in action. Individual and group interventions are described by therapists from different backgrounds along with voices of participants/clients, heard from their own perspectives, as coauthors of each chapter. The range of approaches includes experiential exercises to access "whole person" participation for identifying both needs and healing resources. Phototherapy (use of photography—this definition differs from other uses of the same word, see McGrath reference), dream analysis, hypnosis, and imagery are described along with several examples of "touch therapies." Many of the therapist and client authors describe interventions congruent with their own Native American culture, such as storytelling. Therapists working with groups of women will find these examples particularly helpful in designing personalized, creative approaches to working *with* women.

Lerner, H. (1989). *The dance of intimacy.* New York: Harper and Row.

This book builds on some of the concepts presented by Lerner in *The Dance of Anger* (1985). Both books use Bowen's theory of multigenerational family dynamics. While Bowen's theory is often criticized for its male bias (valuing "differentiation/separate sense of self" over connectedness/relatedness), Lerner presents a more balanced view in her examples of intimacy problems in relationships. With refreshing transparency, Lerner tells of her own family and foibles, while presenting the reader (or listener to abridged audiotape versions) with clear examples of how to deal effectively and consistently with the "triangles" that Bowen described in all intimate relationships. The book is directed to lay people, but references and appendix notes are helpful for professionals too. One section contains instructions for doing a genogram of your own family, while another addresses systems theory for understanding families. The last chapter, though very brief, provides an overtly feminist analysis of the social context in which relationships in families and between people are embedded. The book is one of those rare presentations which will probably appeal to women who would not usually choose to be political bedsisters.

McGrath, E., Keita, G., Strickland, B., & Russo, N. (1990). *Women and depression: Risk factors and treatment issues: Final report of the American Psychological Associations' National Task Force on Women and Depression.* Washington, DC: American Psychological Association.

This small report is a valuable resource for researchers and therapists seeking to understand, study, or treat depression in women. The first section covers risk factors and research issues, describing the need for a biopsychosocial context of understanding. The factors covered include reproductive-related events, personality traits, and other psychological factors as well as women's roles and status, with particular attention to victimization and poverty as risk factors for depression in women. In contrast to the 1991 Jack book on women's depression, the stories related here are drawn from facts and figures. The second section provides an overview of different theories and treatments of depression, along with some of the methodologic constraints involved in studying treatments for depression. Five forms of psychotherapy are compared (interpersonal, cognitive-behavioral, behavioral, psychodynamic, and feminist) as well as phototherapy (exposure to light), pharmacotherapy, and combined therapies. The last section covers the risk factors and treatment issues related to selected ethnic minority women: African American/black, Hispanic/Latina, Asian American, and Native American women. Issues specific to developmental categories (female adolescents, older women), and social/identity categories (professional women and lesbians) are briefly reviewed along with problem-oriented categories: physical abuse, poverty, eating disorders, and substance abuse. The wide-ranging recommendations provide some direction for training therapists, matching clients and therapists, and identifying special needs. Conspicuously absent are recommendations to change the social contexts that allow poverty and victimization to be a growing problem. Individually-oriented therapy, medications, and shelters are necessary, but not sufficient to deal with the enormity of the social risk factors for depression.

Mercer, R., Nichols, E., & Doyle, G. (1989). *Transitions in a woman's life: Major life events in developmental context.* New York: Springer.

The most recent in the Springer Series on Women, *Transitions in a Woman's Life* contributes to the new literature on female development through the life cycle. The authors questioned the prevailing assumption that motherhood is the major transition in women's lives. They interviewed 80 adult Caucasian women to determine what events and transitions characterized the reports of women who had never married, those who had married and, in each category, those who did or did not have children. The findings are reported in several ways taking into consideration the political and historical influences during each woman's lifetime. Geographic moves, losses, and inter-personal relationships are discussed in separate chapters as factors affecting women's psycho-social development. A separate chapter dis-cusses the emergence of creativity later in women's lives. Of particular interest is the con-clusion that being a mother is reported to be of less importance to the women than the moth-ering they received. Women who were married with children seemed to develop a sense of in-dependence as they entered their forties, and women who never married were more likely to develop their sense of "integrity"— peace with their lives. This text would probably be a provocative choice for introductory courses on development and useful to therapists who are seeking data to "normalize" clients' experi-ences.

Prozan, C. (1992). *Feminist psychoanalytic psychotherapy.* Northvale, NJ: Jason Aronson.

Most critiques of psychoanalysis reviewed in this series of books (particularly Volume I) have been by those finding fault with psychoana-lytic formulations of female development. In more recent years, we have seen a rapprochement between the psychoanalytic view and feminism, with many feminists honoring the psychoana-lytic insistence on addressing sexuality as im-portant. In Prozan's book we see a psychoanalyst who lays out both the issues and the critiques of the issues in an impressive review which covers influences of culture, history, and literature, as well as reviews of some Neo-Freudians' battles with traditional psychoanalysis (e.g., Horney, Klein, Thompson). Contemporary psychoana-lytic views are addressed, especially with regard to the concept of penis envy. The work of the Stone Center and its affiliates is also reviewed along with selected family systems approaches and selected feminist psychotherapy perspec-tives. Female orgasm, as it has been addressed by psychoanalysis, feminism, and sex researchers, seems to be of particular interest to the author, as is the topic of homosexuality. This book raises many controversial points as it demonstrates a level of maturity in these decades-old debates. The final chapter seeks to integrate some of the positions of feminism and psychoanalysis with examples of work by contemporary femi-nists and psychoanalysts to support the au-thor's view that new psychoanalytic theories have eliminated the distortions created by pa-triarchal bias.

Squire, C. (1989). *Significant differences— Feminism in psychology.* New York: Routledge.

Among several British publications, *Signifi-cant Differences—Feminism in Psychology,* is also fairly difficult to interpret for several rea-sons. The first confusion relates to the cover photo of a busty young blond woman who looks somewhat guilty as she removes a book, *The Sex-ual Dialogue,* from the shelf far above her head. The hint of something slightly improper is also apparent in the defensive language used in the book to justify the need for psychology to be aware of feminism and feminists and to be more open to psychological, rather than social, expla-nations for gender inequalities. Another area of confusion seems related to the terminology used in Britain to describe different feminist perspec-tives. What we call Liberal Feminists appear to be called "egalitarian feminists," radical femi-nists are called "woman-centered," although many authors seem to be mentioned under both categories. The author describes a "more com-plex" feminist perspective called "associative" feminism which creates helpful associations with alternative sources of knowledge—primary here are the psychoanalytic perspectives of La-can, Foucault, and the deconstructionists. Al-though the discussion of the tensions of each of these positions is potentially engaging, the au-thor seems to assume that the reader has an understanding of the specialized terminology used—few definitions or explanations are pro-vided to support the points and counterpoints made. The notes at the end of the book are more helpful, but greater integration of the informa-tion into the text would make it considerably more accessible to people unfamiliar with the intricacies of British feminism, British schools of psychology, or current European psychoana-lytic debates.

Sullivan, B. (1989). *Psychotherapy grounded in the feminine principle.* Wilmette, IL: Chiron Publications.

The Jungian perspective has often been seen by some feminists to be less inclined toward gender biases than other analytic traditions. The balanced valuing of the masculine and feminine principles seemed similar to the concept of androgyny and the attraction for female, as well as male, archetypes has been equally appealing. However, the potential for gender-biased interpretation of some basic concepts has been questioned in recent years. In response, the author of this very academic text laments the relative devaluing of the feminine principle in working with male and female clients, as well as the therapists' own process in the therapy. While oriented toward depth work, the author does not see a useful discrimination between analysis and therapy and prefers to compare some of the ideas in Winicott, Kohut, Balint, and Jungian therapy in terms of their contributions to reclaiming the feminine principle. The case studies and the genuine attempt of the author to communicate to a broader audience make the book both interesting and challenging.

Tavris, C. (1989). *Anger: The Misunderstood emotion (rev. ed.).* New York: Simon & Schuster.

The reissue of this book, with many updated revisions, should be required reading for anyone concerned with the mental health of women or men. Unfortunately, Tavris's wisdom has been slow to permeate the cultures of pop psychology and mainstream therapy. For several decades women were socialized that they needed to be properly feminine by never showing anger, followed by a period which stressed training on how to be assertive ("not aggressive"). In between and subsequently there has continued to be considerable confusion about the often unquestioned desirability of emotional catharsis and the ventilation of pent-up feelings. This book covers a vast array of research about when anger is, and isn't likely to be helpful to an individual, a relationship or a cause. The book's updated areas address new research on some of the physiology of emotions, along with discussion of the use of legal defenses based on claims of "uncontrollable" urges. The similarities between the genders in relation to anger experience and expression are addressed, and a discussion of family systems approaches to anger in family situations was added. Another addition is a listing of conditions in which catharsis is likely to be helpful. The chapter on the women's movement as a form of anger directed toward justice has been revised to include a too-brief discussion of the political realities of the 1980s. A new, final chapter includes some guidelines for getting through or living with the kinds of situations that are likely to incite anger but remain unrelieved by the expression of it. This highly readable book is one of the sanest explications to be found of feeling less than sane in a world in which the old rules for raising children, solving disputes, and starting wars are all under revision.

Tavris, C. (1992). *The mismeasure of woman.* New York: Touchstone.

The Mismeasure of Woman will come as welcome relief to those who are tired of reading about "women who (fill-in-the-blank)." Tavris writes passionately and clearly when describing the flaws in defining men and women as opposites, similar, or differentially representative of any universal quality. Eschewing reductionist explanations of gender difference (biologic or otherwise), Tavris reviews evidence for similarities and differences before wrestling with the myths, diagnoses, and economics of gender. Never afraid of controversy, she questions popular acceptance of women's "codependency" and proposes a diagnostic classification recognizing the problem of "Delusional Dominating Personality Disorder," a problem best addressed by Independency self-help groups. Similarly, she questions the assumption that a sexual abuse history constitutes a satisfactory explanation for all of a woman's subsequent life difficulties, or that "survivor groups" are inherently therapeutic. Covering much of the territory that Hare-Mustin and Maracek explore, this often refreshingly amusing book would appeal to academics and non-academics.

Unger, R., & Crawford, M. (1992). *Women and gender: A feminist psychology.* Philadelphia: Temple University Press.

Clearly intended as a textbook for psychology of women courses, this collection of facts, figures, and theories provides a solid introduction for undergraduates unfamiliar with women's issues or why male theories and research developed by white middle-class European-North Americans can't apply to everyone. It would also be a useful resource for graduate students in psychology, sociology, or women's studies. Topics covered include data on gender differences, the images of women, developmental and socialization perspectives, role and relationship experiences, violence against women, and the role of gender in psychological disorders.

Wehr, D. (1987). *Jung and feminism: Liberating archetypes.* Boston: Beacon Press.

Although this book predates the current review period, it is a counterpart to the collection of Freud's writings on women, edited by Young-Bruehl (1990). Both of these books would enlighten the serious student of therapy and could provide helpful background reading for appreciating the chapter on Jungian therapy in Brown and Ballou's *Personality and Psychopathology* (1992) or Prozan's review of psychoanalytic theories on women in *Feminist Psychoanalytic Psychotherapy* (1992). Wehr's short and readable book draws on three fields: Jung and Jungian psychology, feminism, and religion. The explicit connection between psychology and religion stands in contrast to the development of slowly growing connections between psychology and spirituality. The literature in women's spirituality has tended to revalue the historic worship of goddesses by cultivating women's culture, women's rituals, and a gynecentric perspective. In contrast, the Jungian perspective seeks balance within each person between anima and animus, the known and the unknown of the self. Wehr argues that Jung's psychology is also a religion, a theology, and an ontology. The reader interested in the potential for Jungian psychology

to liberate women will probably find this book easier to tackle than many Jungian texts.

Worell, J., & Remer, P. (1992). *Feminist perspectives in therapy: An empowerment model for women.* Chichester: John Wiley & Sons.

An unusual combination of theory, research, and practice in feminist therapy, this book would be a good choice for therapy programs implementing or integrating a feminist approach. Squarely located in psychology traditions, there are many self-assessment tools covering beliefs and knowledge about women and men, gender roles in society and sex-role socialization. Other self-assessments cover counseling values, personal theoretical positions, assessment of clients, beliefs, and facts about depression, and beliefs about abuse in close relationships and rape. Career development, cross-cultural counseling skills, and ethical issues are also assessed. Graphs, visual models, charts, and lists will delight the learner who seeks highly-organized information. A final section describes a training model in feminist therapy and includes, naturally, a self-assessment of one's current educational program.

Young-Bruehl, P. (Ed.) (1990). *Freud on women: A reader.* New York: W. W. Norton.

Young-Bruehl, a professor of Letters with connections to psychiatry and humanities, was a Freud Fellow from 1987–1988. How this role affects the perspective she takes in her introduction is not addressed. This first collection of Freud's papers on women will appeal to those who prefer to read from the original, rather than through others' interpretations. Obviously, the volume is an English translation. It contains some abbreviated notes originally included in the *Standard Edition of the Complete Psychological Works of Freud,* edited by James Strachey. The 21 papers include selected letters between Freud and Fleiss and abridged versions of papers on masochism, the theory of sexuality essays, sexual morality, and modern nervous illness. While

Young-Bruehl's introduction addresses the feminist critiques of Freud's work, and particularly the case of Dora, conspicuously absent is any reference to Jeffrey Masson's 1984 book, *The Assault on Truth: Freud's Suppression of the Seduction Theory*, a scathing criticism of the integrity of Freud and the contemporary protectors of the papers and keepers of the flame. Given the oversight, one might consider that any "released" versions of papers may selectively represent the original documents.

PAPERS AND TAPES

The following papers and audiotapes are available from the Stone Center, Wellesley College, Wellesley, Massachusetts, 02181. Papers which are also available as tapes are marked with an asterisk (*). The working papers and tapes describe the ongoing development of a clinical and research-based theory of women's psychology. These recent papers focus less on abstract concepts, such as mutuality and anger, and specify the social factors underlying the dynamics of women's mental health. Building on a growing conviction that disconnection is a major source of pain in women's lives, these papers elaborate the traumatic sequelae of disconnection in all relationships, including the therapeutic relationship. Because clinical practice has been both a source of theory development and a testing ground for their evolving concepts, the more recent papers have begun to address specific contemporary concerns of clients. Issues of diagnosis and etiology are developed and discussed using a contextual understanding of women's development. In many cases, the papers include discussion with members of the audiences at Stone Center presentations.

Arnold, F., & Saunders, E. (1986–1992). *Borderline personality disorder and childhood abuse: Revisions in clinical thinking and treatment approach*. The Stone Center, Wellesley College, Wellesley, Massachusetts.(*)

Fedele, N., & Harrington, E. (1989). *Women's groups: How connections heal*. The Stone Center, Wellesley College, Wellesley, Massachusetts.(*)

Heyward, C. (1989). *Coming out and relationship empowerment: A lesbian feminist theological perspective*. The Stone Center, Wellesley College, Wellesley, Massachusetts.(*)

Jordan, J. (1989). *Relational development: Therapeutic implications of empathy and shame*. The Stone Center, Wellesley College, Wellesley, Massachusetts.(*)

Kaplan, A. (1991). *Surviving incest: One woman's struggle for connection*. The Stone Center, Wellesley College, Wellesley, Massachusetts.(*)

Kaplan, A., & Klein, R. (1989). *Women and suicide: A cry for connection*. The Stone Center, Wellesley College, Wellesley, Massachusetts.(*)

Kilbourne, J., & Surrey, J. (1986–1991). *Women, addiction and codependency*. The Stone Center, Wellesley College, Wellesley, Massachusetts.(*)

Miller, J. & Stiver, I. (1986–1991). *A relational reframing of psychotherapy*. The Stone Center, Wellesley College, Wellesley, Massachusetts.(*)

Stiver, I. (1989). *Dysfunctional families and wounded relationships*. The Stone Center, Wellesley College, Wellesley, Massachusetts.(*)

Surrey, J. (1989). *The mother-daughter relationship themes in psychotherapy*. The Stone Center, Wellesley College, Wellesley, Massachusetts.(*)

ARTICLES

The following overview articles stand out as excellent resources covering recent research findings related to women's mental health. All identify the trends in findings and recommend directions for future research. The Russo article presents the five priority areas for a women's mental health research agenda: poverty, elderly women's needs, violence against women, multiple roles for women, and diagnosis and treatment of mental disorders in women. Koss and McBride call for more complex models to capture the multiple feedback loops involved in the biopsychosocial experiences of women. Koss reveals the appalling dearth of information and awareness about the extent of intimate violence, while McBride calls attention to the need for greater understanding of the physiologic factors associated with chronic stress. The interrelatedness of poverty, femaleness, old age, and violence will challenge clinicians and researchers who can no longer naively pursue "the" causes for women's mental illness.

Belle, D. (1990). Poverty and women's mental health. *American Psychologist, 45*(3), 385–389.

Koss, M. (1990). The women's mental health research agenda: Violence against women. *American Psychologist, 45*(3), 374–380.

McBride, A. (1990). Mental health effects of women's multiple roles. *American psychologist, 45*(3), 381–384.

Russo, N. (1990). Overview. Forging research priorities for women's mental health. *American Psychologist, 45*(3), 368–373.

Walker, L. (1989). Psychology and violence against women. *American Psychologist, 44*(4), 695–702.

Chapter 2

Occupational Issues in Women's Health

Susan Terry Misner
Pamela Fox Levin
Jeanne Beauchamp Hewitt

INTRODUCTION

In recent years, employment roles and the work environment have changed dramatically for many women. These changes have led to increasing concern regarding the interrelationship between women's employment and their health. Nevertheless, women must have access to equitable employment opportunities, *while still protecting* the right to a safe and healthful workplace. At the same time, there exist outmoded traditions, conflicting priorities, and limited scientific knowledge regarding women's occupational health risks. These complex issues have prompted labor, management, and governmental agencies to consider social policy changes and further research on occupational issues for women. The aim in this paper is to broadly review current occupational issues and workplace hazards affecting women's health.

The age old misperception that "women's work is safe" has persisted. Consequently, the health and safety of women workers have long been neglected. Current occupational issues affecting women's health stem from events occurring over the past century. Historically, policies were first instituted during the industrial revolution to protect and ultimately discriminate against women workers (Hunt, 1979). The British Mines Act of 1842 forbade the employment of female mine workers (Collins, 1990). This act may have set the stage for the continuing practice of removing selected groups of workers from unsafe conditions instead of improving the safety of the worksite.

Although there was little concern with the health and safety of workers until the early 20th century, women benefitted when the United States Department of Labor gained a Women's Bureau in 1920 (Department of Labor, 1944). During the 1920s and 1930s, the Women's Bureau was directed by Alice Hamilton, one of America's first occupational health physicians; nevertheless, it was limited to generating reproductive research related to maternal employment. Together with the Children's Bureau of the Department of Labor, the Women's Bureau published extensive epidemiological studies on the effect of mothers' employment on infant mortality. Acknowledged toxins were lead, carbon monoxide, tobacco, benzene, carbon disulfide, and nitrobenzene (Hunt, 1979). During this time, concern for the health of female workers exposed to these toxins seemed to be limited to reproductive issues only. As an example, the New York Department of Labor published a special bulletin in 1927 warning against the effects of lead and benzol on pregnant workers. Special protection was needed only if women were known to be pregnant (Hunt, 1979).

Despite a decade of data gathering, in 1934 the Women's Bureau identified a lack of information regarding the number of women exposed to hazardous occupations and the sparsity of data to develop control programs (Department of Labor, 1944). As a result of the Bureau's efforts, the United States Public Health Service planned to investigate the health of workers;

gender and pregnancy were to be included as variables (Department of Health, Education, and Welfare, 1940). However, the plans were never carried through, probably due to the start of World War II. The health and safety of women were major concerns during World War II as they constituted the majority of the workforce. The Women's Bureau was active in generating research and pamphlets concerning women in "traditional male" factory, mining, and construction jobs (Department of Labor, 1944). Recommendations to industry from the Bureau included: provision of appropriately sized protective clothing; adjustment of factory equipment to women's strength and build; and installation of mechanical devices for heavy lifting (International Labour Office, 1946). Post World War II, as men returned to their previous employment, the health and safety of working women was no longer at the forefront.

Although the labor and feminist movements continued to fight for worker health and safety, the hazards identified and the issues raised by the Women's Bureau still menace employed women today. Not until the Occupational Health and Safety Act (OSHAct) was passed in 1970 was there another government agency responsible for the health of women workers. Between 1890 and 1970, when the OSHAct was passed, the percentage of women ages 20 to 64 in the workforce increased from 19.2 percent to 49.2 percent (Foster, Siegel, & Jacobs, 1988). The number of women in the civilian workforce more than tripled between 1948 and 1988 (Bureau of Labor Statistics, 1989). In 1988, women constituted 66.9 percent of the workforce (Department of Labor, 1988), but with the budget cuts of the 1980s, few Occupational Health and Safety (OSHA) inspections occurred in female-dominated industries (Klitzman, Silverstein, Punnett, & Mack, 1990). Research and programs on women's occupational health have begun to move forward substantively in recent years only.

CURRENT ISSUES IN WOMEN'S OCCUPATIONAL HEALTH

Today, social forces, including demographic changes, increase the need for women's occupational health programs and research, while many political and legal forces impede the ability to provide these services. Because women now live longer than men, the United States has an increasing proportion of women in the general population (National Center for Health Statistics, 1989a). The number of employed women with infants and children under six years of age is steadily increasing. Between 1960 and 1991, the civilian labor force participation rate for married women with children under six years of age increased from 18.6 percent to 59.9 percent (U.S. Bureau of the Census, 1992). As women themselves are aging, they are also increasingly responsible for the care of their elderly parents (Brody, Kleban, Johnsen, Hoffman, & Schoonover, 1987).

Although the percentage of working women has grown, their salaries have not kept pace with this increased representation. In 1991, the median weekly earnings of full-time wages for women was 26 percent less than men's weekly wages (U.S. Bureau of Census, 1992). This reflects differences in the distribution of men's and women's employment status by occupation and industry, where women hold positions with lower pay, lower power, and lower autonomy (LaRosa, 1988).

These economic and power differences between men and women adversely affect the health status of employed women. Between 1983 and 1985, women in the labor force were less likely to assess their health status as excellent (37.8%) as compared to men (43.7%) (National Center for Health Statistics, 1989b).

Employment status has been investigated as a potential risk factor for women's mental and physical health. Employment status as a risk factor has not been clearly demonstrated to impair women's health (Kotler & Wingard, 1989; Repetti, Matthews, & Waldron, 1989). One exception is the Framingham Study in which Haynes and Feinleib (1980) found an increased risk of coronary heart disease among female clerical workers who had children and were married to blue collar workers. Although employment has been shown to improve women's economic status and access to health care, health status itself does affect entry into the workforce (Waldron & Jacobs, 1988).

Women often fill multiple roles associated with work, family, and community; these multiple roles are often considered a stress factor. However, a number of studies have indicated that multiple roles themselves do not contribute to the perceived stress of working women (Waldron & Jacobs, 1989; Baruch, Biener, & Barnett, 1987; Repetti et al., 1989). Some factors do increase the stress that women report: lack of supportive workplace policies, such as flextime and onsite day care, and lack of social support at work and home.

Unlike men, U.S. women workers report that they experience stress, not from work as such, but from their home responsibilities. This role conflict often springs from rigid or unsupportive workplace policies and cultural expectations. However, previous studies have shown that with supportive workplace policies and shared home responsibilities, women's perception of stress does not differ between home and work (Freedman & Bisesi, 1988; Matthews & Rodin, 1989; Baruch et al., 1987). In addition, recent attention to issues of sexual harassment in the workplace may redefine perceptions of women's workplace stress (Riger, 1991).

Family leave, worksite child care, and flexible scheduling are some policies designed to decrease stress and thereby improve the health of workers. Previously, women have carried disproportionate responsibility for family caregiving (Rexroat & Sherhan, 1987). Because of this imbalance in family caregiving, issues regarding these workplace policies differentially impact on women's well-being. The ease of making adequate childcare arrangements has been associated with employed mothers' psychological well-being (Ross & Mirowsky, 1988). Worksite childcare has been reported to have a beneficial effect on employee productivity, absenteeism, and turnover (Wayne & Burud, 1986). Yet, between 1980 and 1986, direct federal funding for childcare programs was estimated to have decreased by 18 percent in real dollars (Kahn & Kamerman, 1987). Also, it has been estimated that less than half of employed women received maternity leave with partial pay and a job guarantee (Schroeder, 1989). After being vetoed by President Bush, national support finally led to President Clinton's signing of the Family and Medical Leave Act in 1993 (Public Law No. 103-3). Grassroots and well organized movements continue to build toward supportive policies for paid family leave, child care, security in retirement, and minimal health coverage (Berry, 1993).

Klitzman and colleagues (1990) outlined several legislative proposals for more specific worker protection. These proposals include: minimum employee benefits, dependent care, and the elimination of the use of electronic surveillance in computer equipment to monitor employee productivity.

WORKPLACE HAZARDS

Certainly, some women are exposed to specific occupational hazards. The differences in impact of these hazards on men's and women's health may be significant due to exposure levels, occupational risks, and biological variability. However, gender differences in reported symptom levels have been shown to diminish when working conditions for men and women are similar (Mergler, Brabant, Vezina, & Messing, 1987). Recent areas of concern include: physical hazards (e.g., radiation, thermal stress, noise, repetitive motion); biological hazards (e.g., human immunodeficiency virus, hepatitis B, cytomegalovirus); and chemical hazards (e.g., lead, mercury, solvents, pesticides, pharmaceuticals). Psychological hazards such as stress and violence also are of concern.

Excessive exposure to ionizing radiation (such as X-rays) is a commonly recognized physical hazard associated with cancer, birth defects, and other genetically based problems (Voelz, 1988). Exposure to radiation has been of concern for health care workers, some laboratory workers, and some workers in the manufacturing sector. Video display terminals (VDTs), which are a source of non-ionizing radiation, have raised public concern regarding possible health effects. Although most studies of the health effects of VDTs have not measured radiation emissions, even those studies which have measured exposure demonstrate conflicting findings.

In addition to the concerns regarding possible radiation hazard, VDTs are associated with worker complaints including muscular fatigue, visual discomfort, and stress. In one study reviewed, frequent short breaks were beneficial for data entry workers when taken at the user's discretion. However, use of short breaks is likely to be influenced by workplace policies such as incentive pay (Henning, Sauter, Salvendy, & Krieg, 1989). Also, women in manufacturing, offices, and other service sector work are at risk for work related musculoskeletal strain, especially of the neck, shoulder, or upper extremity. This is likely to be associated with performing repetitive tasks.

Although occupational noise exposure is more commonly known to be related to hearing loss, some research has been conducted on the nonauditory health effects of chronic occupational exposure to noise. The health effects of noise exposure on pregnancy outcome and its mediating effects in conjunction with shift work have been investigated. In addition, noise may be an inducer of stress through psychophysiological mechanisms. The effects of noise have been studied in critical care nurses and found to be positively related to the chronic stress of work, or so-called, burnout. Also, evidence has suggested that there are gender-based physiological differences in response to thermal stress. The use of engineering controls, such as ventilation, as well as acclimatization to heat or cold are likely to override physiological differences between men and women. Questions have been raised regarding fetotoxicity of excessive heat, yet very little recent research in this area was found.

Sources of biological hazards are humans, animals, and plant products. There were relatively few reports of biological hazards to women found in the literature. Risk of human immunodeficiency virus (HIV) and hepatitis B (HBV) exposure has dominated the literature, both of which are major threats to women workers in the health care field. Tuberculosis is re-emerging as a public health concern. Cytomegalovirus (CMV) and rubella have been shown to be reproductive toxins and hazards for women working with young children in day care facilities and health care settings.

Industrial dusts may be physical, chemical, or biological agents, or a combination of these. Previous research has shown that women as well as men are at risk for lung diseases as a result of dust exposures such as asbestos, grain, cotton, and hemp.

There is a plethora of chemical hazards in the workplace. Health effects of various chemicals include both acute and chronic health effects. Acute conditions can range from an annoying contact dermatitis to a life threatening allergic reaction. Chronic health effects include cancer, hypertension, cardiovascular diseases, neurological disorders, as well as target organ dysfunction (e.g., liver or kidney failure). Reproductive problems include infertility, spontaneous abortions, birth defects, and perinatal mortality, which can be mediated by toxic exposures to either parent, whereas low birth weight and altered period of gestation most likely would be attributable to maternal exposure.

A primary psychological work hazard is stress. Work is commonly believed to be the principal source of stress for employed working women. However, research reviewed here indicated that when multiple roles and family/home issues were included, the home rather than the worksite was more stressful for employed women. Although there has been a great deal of research recently on worksite stress that investigates gender, there is no generally consistent operational definition for stress. Care must be taken in comparing results between studies when multiple roles and family/home issues are not addressed.

In addition to health hazards, there are safety issues that pose a serious threat to the well-being of women workers. In the United States, homicide is the leading cause of mortality from occupational injuries for women (Levin, Hewitt, & Misner, 1992). Forty-two percent of all fatal occupational injuries for women were due to homicide compared to only 11 percent for men (Centers for Disease Control, 1987). In one study, after homicide, motor vehicle accidents were the second leading cause of fatal injuries for employed women in Texas (Davis, Honchar, & Suarez, 1987).

The impact on women's health from these safety issues is clear. However, the effects from health hazards may be less obvious due to a time lag between exposure and health effects. Reproductive studies dominate women's occupational health literature, whereas other acute and chronic health problems have been studied less thoroughly. For instance, relatively few studies by comparison to men could be found in a computer search of the literature from 1967 to the present for cancer and chronic pulmonary disease in occupationally exposed women (Andjelkovich, Mathew, Richardson, & Levine, 1990; Andjelkovich, Taulbee, & Blum, 1978; Armstrong, DeKlerk, Musk, & Hobbs, 1988; Comba et al., 1992a; Comba et al., 1992b; Finkelstein, 1989; Gardner, Coggon, Pannett, & Harris, 1989; Giarelli, Bianchi, & Grandi, 1992; Hansen, Hasle, & Lander, 1992; Jones, Smith, & Thomas, 1988; Monson & Nakano, 1976; Paci et al., 1989; Park, Silverstein, Green, & Mirer, 1990; Polednak, Steheney, & Rowland, 1978; Wignall & Fox, 1982; Yin et al., 1989).

There have been a number of studies on nurses (Cohen, Bellville, & Brown, 1971; Hemminki, Mutanen, Saloniemi, Niemi, & Vainio, 1982; Selevan, Lindbohm, Hornung, & Hemminki, 1985; Shortridge, 1988) and clerical workers (Bryant & Love, 1989; Henning, Sauter, Salvendy, & Krieg, 1989; LaMarte, Merchant, & Casale, 1988; Lindbohm et al., 1992) as female-dominated occupational groups. There is a paucity of research on other occupational groups. As more women enter traditionally male-dominated occupations, research will be needed to identify potential health risks (Blue, 1993).

POLICY MAKING

A number of agencies at the federal and state levels are responsible for identifying and regulating hazards in the workplace. The Occupational Safety and Health Administration (OSHA) carries the major responsibility for worksite inspections and enforcement of standards for various chemical, biological, and physical hazards (Robbins, 1988). The exception is the mining industry, which is regulated by the Mine Safety and Health Administration. Other agencies that have specific areas of responsibilities for occupational health are: the Environmental Protection Agency, the Nuclear Regulatory Commission, and the Food and Drug Administration (Robbins, 1988). The National Institute for Occupational Safety and Health (NIOSH) is responsible for research, hazard evaluation, and training of health and safety personnel.

Policy making also occurs at the workplace. These policies can have a major impact on the well-being of workers. At this level of policy making, the so-called "fetal protection policies" have been controversial. Previously, although reproductive risks occur for both men and women, corporate policies have excluded women, but not men (U.S. Congress, Office of Technology Assessment, 1985). Of 189 firms surveyed in one study, with one exception, exclusions for reproductive risks applied solely to women (Paul, Daniels, & Rosofsky, 1989).

In 1991, a U.S. Supreme Court decision was given in the case of the *International Union, United Automobile, Aerospace and Agricultural Workers of America v. Johnson Controls*, a sex discrimination suit related to a fetal protection policy. The court ruled that limiting a woman's right to employment may be done only when her gender or pregnancy interferes with job performance. This decision supports a consensus statement issued by a World Health Organization (1985) conference panel which concluded that there is no research basis for such exclusionary policies.

METHODOLOGICAL ISSUES

In the future, it will be important to determine women's occupational health risks as well as to focus on the methodological issues for research performed in this area. Various epidemiological study designs have been used to study occupationally related adverse health outcomes. These study designs include cluster (outbreak) investigations, as well as cross-sectional, proportional mortality ratio (PMR), case-control, and cohort studies. One type of cohort study design, the standard mortality ratio (SMR) study, is widely used in occupational epidemiology (Checkoway, Pearce, & Crawford-Brown, 1989).

Many of the women's occupational epidemiological studies reported in the literature are of poor quality and/or suffer from an inadequate number of subjects. These limitations adversely affect conclusions that can be drawn from the reported findings. Another factor that has affected the quality of studies has been the use of unstandardized methods to design or analyze data, which seems to have occurred most often in cluster investigations. Investigators only recently have described standardized methods to study clusters of acute or chronic diseases and adverse reproductive outcomes that occur in the workplace (Abenhaim & Lert, 1991; Fleming, Ducatman, & Shalat, 1992).

Occupational epidemiological study designs vary in their ability to be used to decide if an exposure is causally associated with a given disease or injury. Cluster investigations and PMR studies are more useful for generating hypotheses than for testing them. In cross-sectional or case-control designs, rates of disease among exposed groups and the temporal pattern between exposure and disease or injury are not generally available. Consequently, these study designs are primarily useful for studying associations. Standard mortality ratio (SMR) studies, which use the general population for comparison, may underestimate the association between exposure and disease/injury. This underestimate is due to the "healthy worker effect" in which healthier people are selected into the workforce and compared to the health of the general population (Checkoway et al., 1989). This is because the general population includes ill, disabled, and retired, as well as healthy people.

The cohort study design is the most robust design for elucidating causal associations, particularly when measures of exposure are well documented. Cohort studies may be either prospective or historical. In prospective cohort studies, workers who are disease/injury free, but who have an occupational exposure in common, are followed over time to determine if there is an increased risk for adverse health effects. In historical cohort studies, exposures have occurred in the past and disease/injury may also have occurred prior to the beginning of the study. In occupational epidemiology, historical designs are much more common. Although cohort studies are more robust than other designs, many occupational health studies, including those of women, have used weaker designs (e.g., PMR, cross-sectional). Weaker designs limit the usefulness of these studies for drawing conclusions about occupational risks.

Judgments about causality are made sequentially. First, appropriateness of the study design, analytic methods, sample size, and precision of exposure and disease measurements must be demonstrated (Checkoway et al., 1989). Next, chance and sources of bias, such as selection, information, or confounding, need to be ruled out as explanations for the findings. Finally, causality would be judged on the basis of: (a) the strength of the association between exposure and disease/injury; (b) the consistency of this association among studies; (c) temporality (exposure precedes disease); (d) biological plausibility; and (e) a dose response relationship (Mausner & Kramer, 1985).

Several measurement problems are common in occupational epidemiological studies. Disease status may be subject to either random or biased misclassification. Exposure also may be subject to misclassification due to a lack of reliable and valid measures (Checkoway et al., 1989). When random misclassification of either disease or exposure occurs, the effect is to bias the estimate of risk toward unity (no association). Biased (nonrandom) misclassification may over- or underestimate the true risk. Measurement of exposures with regard to women may be especially problematic for several reasons: (a) interruption of work due to childbearing/childrearing and other family responsibilities; (b) a lack of record keeping due to the assumption that traditional women's occupations are safe; and (c) multiple jobs and/or workplaces over a lifespan. Any of these factors may minimize the ability to estimate risks.

A pervasive problem in occupational epidemiological studies has been the lack of power to detect a true association due to inadequate sample size in relation to the magnitude of effect (risk) (Rothman, 1986). When "no association" results are reported, a power analysis should be included in the report (Schlesselman, 1982). However, a power analysis is seldom provided. The reader frequently concludes that no association is synonymous with no effect, when in fact, no conclusion can reasonably be drawn unless there is adequate (generally 80–90%) power.

Several other problems are specific for occupational reproductive studies. Both partners may contribute to risk, yet few studies consider occupational, environmental, genetic, and lifestyle factors of both partners. There is a lack of statistical independence among reproductive outcomes in the same woman (Butler & Kalasinski, 1989), which frequently is not addressed in the study design or analysis.

A dose-response may not be observable due to a shift in the type of adverse reproductive outcome at different levels of exposure (Selevan & Lemasters, 1987). For instance, a given reproductive toxic agent may produce subfertility and spontaneous abortions at high doses, birth defects at moderate doses, and prematurity at low doses. Unless the entire range of reproductive responses are studied concurrently, a dose-response may not be observed. In contrast to other occupational studies, even when a dose-response is not detected, there still may be a causal association between exposure and adverse pregnancy outcome(s).

Unless all possible reproductive outcomes are investigated simultaneously, the presence or absence of an observed effect in one reproductive outcome should not be generalized to other outcomes. An example of an unwarranted generalization is: if agent A is not significantly associated with congenital malformations, then agent A is safe with respect to other reproductive outcomes (e.g., fertility, spontaneous abortions, or other types of birth defects).

Exposure models are much more complicated in studies of reproductive outcomes than in other occupational health studies. In particular, exposure must be linked to a specific outcome (Lemasters & Selevan, 1984). For example, the window of vulnerability for congenital malformations is narrow. Exposure must be linked to the period during organogenesis when the structural integrity of the affected organs could be altered (Kline, Levin, Stein, Susser, & Warburton, 1981). By contrast, the window of vulnerability for altered chromosomal numbers (e.g., Down syndrome) attributable to the woman is wide, most often occurring during meiosis, which begins during the fetal development of the woman and continues through the time of fertilization of the ovum (Kline et al., 1981).

DIRECTIONS FOR FUTURE RESEARCH AND RESEARCH UTILIZATION

Research funding needs to be allocated for cost-effective cohort studies on women in various workplace settings. In 1992, only about 11 percent of the National Institutes of Health's (NIH's) over $10 billion budget was awarded for women's health research (P. Wexler, personal communication, July 13, 1993). The Office of Research on Women's Health, established by the NIH in 1990, has a mandate to ensure that research funded through NIH adequately addresses women's health issues. However, health hazards for women in female-dominated occupations continue to need fuller investigation, as do hazards for women in currently male-dominated occupations.

Certain research issues must be addressed before occupational health care for women can progress optimally. First, researchers must be able to track occupational exposures to women throughout the course of worklife, including interruptions in work activities. Therefore, it is important that mechanisms be developed to monitor their lifetime occupational exposures. Without the existence in the United States of a national registry system such as exists in Finland, employees, both men and women, should be encouraged to retain a personal health history over the course of their lifetime. This health history should include, among other data, information regarding occupational exposures, illnesses, and injuries.

As previously mentioned, much of the current research on occupational risks to women's health examines reproductive outcomes. In addition to reproductive outcomes, more studies are needed to investigate other physiological and psychological effects of occupational exposures on women.

Several concerns identified by the Women's Bureau have not been adequately studied more than fifty years later. Research is needed on the adequacy and availability of appropriately designed personal protective equipment. Research also is needed in the area of environmental control of occupational exposures. For example, improved designs are needed for ventilation systems, hazard containment, and ergonomically sound work stations. Known measures of hazard control should be instituted instead of selectively excluding women from the worksite.

Other issues that need to be considered for future research include: (a) the effects of multiple exposures and mediating factors, (b) the comparison of genders on exposure and health effects, and (c) the study of women's health throughout their employment lifespan. Information from basic research (e.g., physiological effects of thermal stress), could be used more frequently to guide the direction of occupational health research on women.

Greater emphasis is needed on creating and testing innovative prevention strategies and incorporating successful strategies into worksite programs. Finally, for research to have an impact, researchers need to disseminate and interpret their findings to policy makers.

CONCLUDING REMARKS

We reviewed for commentary English language journal articles from the years 1967 to 1992. We selected from current and classic literature in the field. The reviews were primarily focused on four occupational hazard classifications and related issues. The four hazard classifications were physical, chemical, biological, and psychological. Within these classifications, articles were selected on the basis of the range of health effects on women workers and workers in female-dominated occupations. Articles also were selected on the basis of diversity of occupations, cultural differences, and unique contributions to the literature in women's occupational health.

Although we tried to focus our review for commentary to articles published in the past few years, our efforts were hampered by an apparent clustering effect. For example, there has been recent interest in ergonomic issues and health effects of video display terminals (VDTs). This interest has generated a number of studies in the areas of ergonomics and reproductive effects of VDTs. By contrast, we were surprised to find few published studies of health effects of biological agents on working women, despite a renewed interest in infectious agents. Reports of chemical hazards seem to follow cycles. Unfortunately, there is a relative dearth of recently published studies for the four chemical classifications that we think are particularly relevant for women's health: heavy metals, solvents, pharmaceuticals and pesticides and other halogenated hydrocarbons.

While this essay discussion of occupational health issues has addressed the state of the art in women's health, we have attempted to summarize the state of the science in the commentaries.

REFERENCES

Abenhaim, L., & Lert, F. (1991). Methodological issues for the assessment of clusters of adverse pregnancy outcomes in the workplace: The case of video display terminal users. *Journal of Occupational Medicine, 33,* 1091–1096.

Andjelkovich, D. A., Mathew, R. M., Richardson, R. B., & Levine, R. J. (1990). Mortality of iron foundry workers: I. Overall findings. *Journal of Occupational Medicine, 32,* 529–540.

Andjelkovich, D. A., Taulbee, J., & Blum, S. (1978). Mortality of female workers in rubber manufacturing plant. *Journal of Occupational Medicine, 20,* 823–824.

Armstrong, B. K., DeKlerk, N. H., Musk, A. W., & Hobbs, M. S. T. (1988). Mortality in miners and millers of crocidolite in Western Australia. *British Journal of Industrial Medicine, 45,* 5–13.

Baruch, G. K., Biener, L., & Barnett, R. C. (1987). Women gender in research on work and family stress. *American Psychologist, 42*, 130–136.

Berry, M. F. (1993). *The politics of parenthood: Child care, women's rights, and the myth of the good mother.* New York: Viking Penguin.

Blue, C. L. (1993). Women in nontraditional jobs: Is there a risk for musculoskeletal injury? *AAOHN Journal, 41*, 235–240.

Brody, E. M., Kleban, M. H., Johnsen, P. T., Hoffman, C., & Schoonover, C. B. (1987). Work status and parent care: A comparison of four groups of women. *Gerontologist, 27*, 201–208.

Bryant, H. E., & Love, E. J. (1989). Video display terminal use and spontaneous abortion risk. *International Journal of Epidemiology, 18*, 132–138.

Bureau of Labor Statistics. (1989). *Handbook of Labor Statistics.* Washington, DC: U.S. Government Printing Office.

Butler, W. J., & Kalasinski, L. A. (1989). Statistical analysis of epidemiological data of pregnancy. *Environmental Health Perspectives, 79*, 223–227.

Centers for Disease Control. (1987). Traumatic occupational fatalities. *Morbidity and Mortality Weekly Report, 36*, 461–470.

Checkoway, H., Pearce, N. E., Crawford-Brown, D. J. (1989). *Research methods in occupational epidemiology.* New York: Oxford University Press.

Comba, P., Barbieri, P. G., Battista, G., Belli, S., Ponterio, F., Zanetti, D., & Axelson, O. (1992a). Cancer of the nose and paranasal sinuses in the metal industry: A case-control study. *British Journal of Industrial Medicine, 49*, 193–196.

Comba, P., Battista, G., Belli, S., de Capua, B., Merler, E., Orsi, D., Rodella, S., Vidigni, C., & Axelson, O. (1992b). A case-control study of cancer of the nose and paranasal sinuses and occupational exposures. *American Journal of Industrial Medicine, 22*, 511–520.

Cohen, E. N., Bellville, J. W., & Brown, B. W. (1971). Anesthesia, pregnancy, and miscarriage: A study of operating room nurses and anesthetists. *Anesthesiology, 35*, 343–347.

Collins, J. (1990). Health care of women in the workplace. *Health Care for Women International, 11*, 21–32.

Davis, H., Honchar, P. A., & Suarez, L. (1987). Fatal occupational injuries of women, Texas, 1975–1984. *American Journal of Public Health, 77*, 1524–1527.

Department of Health, Education and Welfare. (1940). *A preliminary survey of the industrial hygiene problem in the United States.* Washington, DC: Department of Health, Education and Welfare.

Department of Labor. (1944). *The industrial nurse and the woman worker.* Washington, DC: Women's Bureau.

Department of Labor. (1988). *Employment and earnings.* Washington, DC: Bureau of Labor Statistics.

Family and Medical Leave Act of 1993, Pub. L. No. 103-3.

Finkelstein, M. M. (1989). Mortality rates among employees potentially exposed to chrysotile asbestos at two automotive plants. *Canadian Medical Association Journal, 141,* 125–130.

Fleming, L. E., Ducatman, A. M., & Shalat, S. L. (1992). Disease clusters in occupational medicine: A protocol for their investigation in the workplace. *American Journal of Industrial Medicine, 22,* 33–47.

Foster, C. D., Siegel, M. A., & Jacobs, N. R. (1988). *Women's changing roles.* Wylie, TX: Information Aids.

Freedman, S. M., & Bisesi, M. (1988). Women and workplace stress. *AAOHN Journal, 36,* 271–275.

Gardner, M. J., Coggon, D., Pannett, B., & Harris, E. C. (1989). Workers exposed to ethylene oxide: A follow up study. *British Journal of Industrial Medicine, 46,* 860–865.

Giarelli, L., Bianchi, C., & Grandi, G. (1992). Malignant mesothelioma of the pleura in Trieste, Italy. *American Journal of Industrial Medicine, 22,* 521–530.

Hansen, E. S., Hasle, H., & Lander, F. (1992). A cohort study on cancer incidence among Danish gardeners. *American Journal of Industrial Medicine, 21,* 651–660.

Haynes, S. G., & Feinleib, M. (1980). Women, work, and coronary heart disease: Prospective finding from the Framingham Heart Study. *American Journal of Public Health, 70,* 133–141.

Hemminki, K., Mutanen, P., Saloniemi, I., Niemi, M.-L., & Vainio, H. (1982). Spontaneous abortions in hospital staff engaged in sterilizing instruments with chemical agents. *British Medical Journal, 285,* 1461–1463.

Henning, R., Sauter, S., Salvendy, G., & Krieg, C. (1989). Microbreak length, performance, and stress in a data entry task. *Ergonomics, 32,* 855–864.

Hunt, V. (1979). *Work and the health of women.* Boca Raton, FL: CRC Press.

International Labour Office. (1946). *The war and women's employment: The experience of the United Kingdom and the United States.* Montreal: International Labour Office.

International Union, United Automobile, Aerospace and Agricultural Implements Workers of America v. Johnson Controls, 111 S.Ct. 1196 (1991).

Jones, R. D., Smith, D. M., & Thomas, P. G. (1988). Mesothelioma in Great Britain in 1968–1983. *Scandinavian Journal of Work and Environmental Health, 14,* 145–152.

Kahn, A. J., & Kamerman, S. D. (1987). *Child care: Facing the hard choices.* Dover, MA: Auburn House.

Kline, J., Levin, B., Stein, Z., Susser, M., & Warburton, D. (1981). Epidemiologic detection of low-dose effects on the developing fetus. *Environmental Health Perspectives, 42,* 119–126.

Klitzman, S., Silverstein, B., Punnett, L., & Mock, A. (1990). A women's occupational health agenda for the 1990's. *New Solutions, 1*(1), 7–17.

Kotler, P., & Wingard, D. (1989). The effect of occupational, marital, and parental roles on mortality: The Alameda County study. *American Journal of Public Health, 79,* 607–612.

LaMarte, F. P., Merchant, J. A., & Casale, T. B. (1988). Acute systemic reactions to carbonless copy paper associated with histamine release. *Journal of the American Medical Association, 260,* 242–243.

LaRosa, J. H. (1988). Women, work, and health: Employment as a risk factor for coronary heart disease. *American Journal of Obstetrics and Gynecology, 158,* 1597–1602.

Lemasters, G. K., & Selevan, S. G. (1984). Types of exposure models and advantages and disadvantages of sources of exposure data for use in occupational reproductive studies. *Progress in Clinical and Biological Research, 160,* 67–79.

Levin, P. F., Hewitt, J. B., Misner, S. T. (1992). Female workplace homicides: An integrative research review. *AAOHN Journal, 40,* 229–241.

Lindbohm, M.-L., Taskinen, H., Kyyronen, P., Sallmen, M., Anttila, A., & Hemminki, K. (1992). Effects of parental occupational exposure to solvents and lead on spontaneous abortion. *Scandinavian Journal of Work and Environment and Health, 18*(Suppl. 2), 37–39.

Matthews, K. A., & Rodin, J. (1989). Women's changing work roles: Impact on health, family, and public policy. *American Psychologist, 44,* 1389–1393.

Mausner, J. S., & Kramer, S. (1985). *Mausner and Bahn epidemiology, an introductory text* (2nd ed.). Philadelphia: W. B. Saunders.

Mergler, D., Brabant, C., Vezina, N., & Messing, K. (1987). The weaker sex? Men in women's working conditions report similar health symptoms. *Journal of Occupational Medicine, 29,* 417–421.

Monson, R. R., & Nakano, K. K. (1976). Mortality among rubber workers. II. Other employees. *American Journal of Epidemiology, 103,* 297–303.

National Center for Health Statistics (1989a). *Health United States, 1988.* Washington, DC: Government Printing Office.

National Center for Health Statistics (1989b). *Vital and health statistics, health characteristics by occupation and industry: United States, 1983–1985.* Hyattsville, MD: National Center for Health Statistics.

Paci, E., Bulatti, E., Costantini, A. S., Miligi, L., Pucci, N., Scarpelli, A., Petrioli, G., Simonato, L., Winkelmann, R., & Kaldor, J. M. (1989). Aplastic anemia, leukemia and other cancer mortality in a cohort of shoe workers exposed to benzene. *Scandinavian Journal of Work and Environmental Health, 15,* 313–318.

Park, R. M., Silverstein, M. A., Green, M. A., & Mirer, F. E. (1990). Brain cancer mortality at a manufacturer of aerospace electromechanical systems. *American Journal of Industrial Medicine, 17,* 537–552.

Paul, M., Daniels, C., & Rosofsky, R. (1989). Corporate response to reproductive hazards in the workplace: Results of family, work and health survey. *American Journal of Industrial Medicine, 16,* 267–280.

Polednak, A. P., Stehney, A. F., & Rowland, R. E. (1978). Mortality among women first employed before 1930 in the U.S. radium dial-painting industry. *American Journal of Epidemiology, 107,* 179–195.

Repetti, R. L., Matthews, K. A., & Waldron, I. (1989). Employment and women's health: Effects of paid employment on women's mental and physical health. *American Psychologist, 44,* 1394–1401.

Rexroat, C., & Sherhan, C. (1987). The family life cycle and spouses' time in housework. *Journal of Marriage and the Family, 49,* 737–750.

Riger, S. (1991). Gender dilemmas in sexual harassment policies and procedures. *American Psychologist, 46,* 497–505.

Robbins, M. C. (1988). Governmental regulations. In B. A. Plog (Ed.), *Fundamentals of industrial hygiene* (3rd ed.) (pp. 677–689). Chicago: National Safety Council.

Ross, C. E., & Mirowsky, J. (1988). Child care and emotional adjustment to wives' employment. *Journal of Health and Social Behavior, 29,* 127–138.

Rothman, K. J. (1986). *Modern epidemiology.* Boston: Little Brown.

Schlesselman, J. J. (1982). *Case-control studies design, conduct, analysis.* New York: Oxford University Press.

Schroeder, P. (1989). Toward a national family policy. *American Psychologist, 44,* 1410–1413.

Selevan, S. G., & Lemasters, G. K. (1987). The dose-response fallacy in human reproductive studies of toxic exposures. *Journal of Occupational Medicine, 29,* 451–454.

Selevan, S. G., Lindbohm, M.-L., Hornung, R. W., & Hemminki, K. (1985). A study of occupational exposure to antineoplastic drugs and fetal loss in nurses. *New England Journal of Medicine, 313,* 1173–1177.

Shortridge, L. A. (1988). *The effects of menstrual function associated with occupational exposure to antineoplastic drugs.* Unpublished doctoral dissertation. University of Cincinnati, Cincinnati, OH.

U.S. Bureau of the Census. (1992). *Statistical abstract of the United States: 1992* (112th ed.) (pp. 388, 412). Washington, DC: U.S. Government Printing Office.

U.S. Congress, Office of Technology Assessment. (1985). *Reproductive health hazards in the workplace.* OTA-BA-266. Washington, DC: U.S. Government Printing Office.

Voelz, G. L. (1988). Ionizing radiation. In C. Zenz (Ed.), *Occupational medicine: Priniciple and practical applications* (pp. 426–462). Chicago: Year Book Medical Publishers.

Waldron, I., & Jacobs, J. A. (1988). Effects of labor force participation on women's health: New evidence from a longitudinal study. *Journal of Occupational Medicine, 30,* 977–983.

Waldron, I., & Jacobs, J. A. (1989). Effects of multiple roles on women's health: Evidence from a national longitudinal study. *Women and Health, 15*(1), 3–19.

Wayne, W., & Burud, S. L. (1986). A hospital's on-site child care center proves to make business sense. *Health Care Management Review, 11,* 81–87.

Wignall, B. K., & Fox, A. J. (1982). Mortality of female gas mask assemblers. *British Journal of Industrial Medicine, 39,* 34–38.

World Health Organization. (1985). Women should not be banned from any type of employment. *World Health,* (July), 30.

Yin, S.-N., Li, G.-L., Tain, F.-D., Fu, Z.-I., Jin, C., Chen, Y.-J., Luo, S.-J., Ye, P.-Z., Zhang, J.-Z., Wang, G.-C., Zhang, X.-C., Wu, H.-N., & Zhong, Q.-C. (1989). A retrospective cohort study of leukemia and other cancers in benzene workers. *Environmental Health Perspectives, 82,* 207–213.

BOOKS AND JOURNALS

Pregnancy and Work

Mamelle, N., Bertucat, I., & Munoz, F. (1989). Pregnant women at work: Rest periods to prevent preterm birth? *Paediatric and Perinatal Epidemiology, 3,* 19–28.

McDonald, A. D., McDonald, J. C., Armstrong, B., Cherry, N., Delorme, C., Nolin, A. D., & Robert, D. (1987). Occupation and pregnancy outcome. *British Journal of Industrial Medicine, 44,* 521–526.

Saurel-Cubizolles, M. J., & Kaminski, M. (1987). Pregnant women's working conditions and their changes in pregnancy. A national study in France. *British Journal of Industrial Medicine, 44,* 236–243.

Savitz, D. A., Whelan, E. A., Rowland, A. S., & Kleckner, R. C. (1990). Maternal employment and reproductive risk factors. *American Journal of Epidemiology, 132,* 933–945.

This series of articles provides a broad overview of the continued debate on the potential benefits and/or risks of employment during pregnancy. Much of the research in this area to date has focused on the relationship of occupational activity to the outcome of pregnancy. Commonly, these studies investigate four types of adverse outcomes: congenital birth defects, stillbirth, spontaneous abortion, and low birth weight, such as those described by Saurel-Cubizolles and Kaminski in their review of epidemiological studies. As Mamelle and colleagues report, employment during pregnancy may not be a risk factor for adverse pregnancy outcomes, but heavy workloads may be of concern. However, as McDonald et al. have shown in their Montreal Study, subgroups of women by occupation may be at risk. Some of these are women in agriculture, leatherwork, sales, manufacturing, health care, and cleaning services. Yet, good evidence is presented that for most pregnant women, employment itself carries little or no risk of adverse pregnancy outcome and may indeed provide some benefit. Using the U.S. National Natality Study, Savitz et al. found that when compared to unemployed married women, employed women had more favorable health indicators (e.g., optimal age at pregnancy [20–34 years], earlier prenatal care, adequate weight gain, fewer cigarettes smoked). Nonetheless, these employed women were more likely than their unemployed counterparts to have a history of spontaneous abortions, stillbirths, and induced abortions. At the same time, few studies have investigated the combined effects of employment and pregnancy on women's health and life experiences. Also, few studies comparing employed and nonemployed women's health consider the nature of women's work done at home or in a nonemployment setting. The nature of work at home may differ substantially and needs to be considered in future comparisons.

PHYSICAL HAZARDS

Ionizing Radiation

Boice, J. D., Mandel, J. S., Doody, M. M., Yoder, R. C., & McGowan, R. (1992). A health survey of radiologic technologists. *Cancer, 69,* 586–588.

Boice and colleagues (1992) present the initial findings from a cohort study of low-dose radiation effects on radiologic technologists. A total of 143,517 technologists who were certified between 1926 and 1982 are being traced for mortality outcomes and followed for reproductive and cancer outcomes. The majority are female (73%). Most (97.5%) of the cohort members had been monitored for radiation exposure at some time in their careers. Nearly three-fourths of the female technologists and spouses of male technologists had ever been pregnant. In female technologists, the adverse pregnancy outcome rates were: 20.2 percent for spontaneous abortions, 1.4 percent for stillbirths, and 8.9 percent for birth defects. In wives of male technologists, the adverse pregnancy outcome rates were: 18.1 percent for spontaneous abortions, 1.9 percent for stillbirths, and 7.9 percent for birth defects. The researchers identified the most prevalent cancer sites among respondents as skin (31.9%), cervix (15.3%), breast (14.0%), uterus (5.1%), and thyroid (4.5%). Among the 9,282 deaths in the cohort, 1,850 were attributed to cancer. For mortality, the most frequently coded cancer sites were: breast (358), lung (350), and leukemia (85). Preliminary analysis of proportionate mortality ratios (PMRs) revealed slightly elevated but unstable risks for breast cancer (PMR = 1.38) and leukemia (PMR = 1.2). The risk for lung cancer was not elevated (PMR = 1.0). This is the first study known to the authors in which female workers exposed to low levels of radiation have been studied for reproductive and cancer risks. Because dosimetry is available for most respondents, this study will ultimately allow the evaluation of a dose-response. Important analytical findings are anticipated from subsequent reports.

Non-Ionizing Radiation

Lindbohm, M.-L., Hietanen, M., Kyyronen, P., Sallmen, M., vonNandelstadh, P., Taskinen, H., Pekkarinen, M., Ylikoski, M., & Hemminki, K. (1992). Magnetic fields of video display terminals and spontaneous abortion. *American Journal of Epidemiology, 136,* 1041–1051.

Schnorr, T. M., Grajewski, B. A., Hornung, R. W., Thun, M. J., Egeland, G. M., Murray, W. E., Conover, D. L., & Halperin, W. E. (1991). Video display terminals and the risk of spontaneous abortion. *New England Journal of Medicine, 324,* 727–733.

Lindbohm and colleagues (1992) conducted a case-control study of video display terminal (VDT) exposure and risk of spontaneous abortion in females who were predominantly employed as bank clerks or as other clerical workers. Employment records from 1975 through 1985 were linked to pregnancy outcomes through national data from hospital discharge and polyclinic records. Women were selected as cases if treatment for a spontaneous abortion occurred in the hospital. For each case, three controls were chosen from among women who had given birth during the same time period. Controls were not eligible for selection if registry data indicated that they had a spontaneous abortion or a child born with a birth defect during the study period. Matching was done on year of pregnancy and age (±1 year) at conception. Exposure was measured by self-reported use of VDTs during the first trimester, the number of hours worked per week, VDT model (confirmed by company records), and measurement of magnetic fields associated with 17 VDT models that had been used by these women during the study period. For each of these models, a total of 12 measurements were taken at the approximate position of a fetus (50cm directly in front, 25 cm straight down). In the adjusted analysis, there was no increased risk for spontaneous abortion associated with use of a VDT during the first trimester (OR = 1.1, 95% CI = 0.7, 1.6). However, when compared to those who used VDTs 10 hours or less per week, risks were elevated for women exposed to VDTs for 11–20 hours per week (OR = 1.7, 95% CI = 0.9, 3.4) and for women exposed to VDTs for more than 20 hours per week (OR = 1.7, 95% CI = 0.8, 3.7). Exposure levels were grouped according to an exposure index and classified as very low frequency (VLF) emission or extremely low frequency (ELF) emission then linked to each woman according to the model they used. The odds ratio for spontaneous abortion was significantly elevated in relation to the VLF range (OR = 2.7, 95% CI = 1.2, 6.1) and the ELF range (OR = 3.8, 95% CI = 1.6, 8.8).

Schnorr and colleagues (1991) examined the risk of spontaneous abortion among a cohort of women employed as directory assistance operators (n = 2,118) who worked with VDTs and a similar cohort of general telephone operators (n = 2,128) who did not work with VDTs at the time of the study. Pregnancies were included in the study if they terminated with a livebirth or stillbirth (fetal loss after 28 weeks gestation) between May 1, 1983 and December 31, 1986 or if spontaneous abortion that was reported to a physician occured (fetal loss at ≤ 28 weeks gestation) between January 1, 1983 and December 31, 1986. Self-reported pregnancy outcomes were validated by comparing them with vital records for live births, which also include data on previous fetal loss and stillbirths. Both personnel records and self-reported exposure to VDTs were used in the analysis. For general assistance operators, two indices of VDT use were calculated: one for first trimester exposure and one for exposure during the first 28 weeks of gestation.

General operators had no occupational exposure to VDTs. Only two models of VDTs were used during the study period. These differed significantly in VLF and ELF emmissions for measurements taken at several frontal positions as well as at the level of the abdomen. In the multivariate analyses, use of VDTs during the first trimester was not associated with spontaneous abortion (OR = 0.9, 95% CI = 0.6, 1.4). The odds ratios remained near unity when VDT use was measured as 1–25 hours per week or more than 25 hours per week. Similarly, no elevated risk of stillbirth was found in any analyses that used 28 weeks of exposure to VDTs (dicotomous, 1–25 hours/week, or more than 25 hours/week). The investigators also used the two types of VDT models to examine if risk was increased with these models; no increased risk was found. It is interesting to note that the investigators did not create an index of exposure for each subject using VDT emissions and the number of cumulative hours worked during the first trimester. Such an index then could have been used to link exposure to outcome. It is also important to note that the use of the 28 weeks of exposure is only valid when stillbirths are compared to live births since many spontaneous abortions would actually terminate before the 28th week. The studies by Schnorr et al. (1991) and Lindbohm et al. (1992) illustrate two very different methodologies used for studying the effects of occupational exposures on reproductive outcomes. Although Lindbohm et al. (1992) demonstrated an increased risk associated with VDT exposure, like Schnorr et al. (1991), most studies do not show an increased risk for adverse reproductive outcomes. Consequently, controversy remains about the reproductive effect of VDT exposure.

Council on Scientific Affairs. (1987). Health effects of video display terminals. *Journal of the American Medical Association, 257,* 1508–1512.

In this concise, yet comprehensive report from the Council on Scientific Affairs of the American Medical Association, a review is presented of research and reports regarding potential adverse health effects of video display terminals (VDTs). Public debate regarding these potential health effects continues. Labor and special interest groups have proposed that legislation be enacted for standards regarding equipment design and labor conditions. The concerns about the potential hazards of VDTs have ranged from eye strain to birth defects. Some complaints have been based on the possibility that VDTs emit radiation, both ionizing (low energy X-rays) and non-ionizing (electromagnetic radiation and ultrasound). The Council concluded upon review of the literature that no association had been found to date between VDT radiation emissions and any adverse health effect. Thus far, any emission levels have been considered to be well below accepted exposure standards. The report includes important recommendations for continued research, especially of ergonomic issues associated with many VDT complaints. The report proposes that corporate management policies address work environment issues related to VDTs. Cohort studies of VDT exposure and health effects are in progress. Results from these studies may resolve the current conflict over the safety of VDTs.

Ergonomics

Kilbom, A., & Broberg, E. (1988). Health hazards related to ergonomic work conditions. *Women and Health, 13*(3–4), 81–93.

Sweden has been viewed as a model system for preventive health care in the work environment due to a high degree of employee health service coverage and a good system for reporting work-related exposures, injuries, and illnesses. In this excellent review article, Kilbom and Broberg discussed work-related factors that affected female workers' risks of musculoskeletal injuries in Sweden. In light of the relative paucity of studies that adequately address the relative risk for specific strain injuries by both gender and occupational work factors, this well-written article provides an important overview of the literature. The authors raise several pertinent issues regarding work-related musculoskeletal injuries in women. These include organizational and work related factors such as monotony and repetitiveness, as well as more traditional ergonomic factors, such as equipment design. Another important point addressed is the difference between men and women by the distribution of injuries. Analysis of data from the Swedish occupational injuries registry indicated that women sustained 50 percent of all musculoskeletal injuries to the shoulder, arm, or neck, compared to 36 percent in men. The authors attributed these gender differences to workload characteristics such as repetitive tasks. Although many women are working in the service sector, an increasing percentage of women are seeking non-traditional female occupations, such as manufacturing. The authors suggest that this redistribution of women in the workforce may result in an increase in musculoskeletal morbidity unless changes are made in the work environment.

Henning, R., Sauter, S., Salvendy, G., & Krieg, C. (1989). Microbreak length, performance, and stress in a data entry task. *Ergonomics, 32,* 855–864.

Statham, A., & Bravo, E. (1990). The introduction of new technology: Health implications for workers. *Women & Health, 16*(2), 105–129.

The concerns regarding the possible health hazards of video display terminals (VDTs) include ergonomic factors such as fatigue and musculoskeletal strain and stress effects of equipment use. It has been proposed that short, frequent work breaks might prevent problems of strain and fatigue. In Henning et al.'s novel experimental study, 20 female subjects participated by performing data entry skills in a National Institute of Occupational Safety and Health (NIOSH) laboratory, which simulated an office environment. The purpose of this investigation was to determine whether short pauses (microbreaks) in a repetitive, computer-based task would be effective in controlling fatigue. There were three morning and three afternoon sessions, each of 40 minutes duration. Each session was interrupted by the computer program after 20 minutes to initiate the microbreak. The subjects terminated the microbreak at their own discretion by resuming data entry. The investigators obtained computer-generated measurements for microbreak length; performance, as

measured by keystrokes per minute and percentage of errors and corrections; and electrocardiographic heartbeat. The mean microbreak length as reported in the text was 27.4 seconds. The authors concluded that data entry workers controlled discretionary microbreaks according to fatigue perception, but that subjects demonstrated a tendency to end the break before performance recovery was complete. Further examination of this issue, perhaps using one or more comparison groups with fixed microbreak length(s), would be helpful to determine optimal microbreak lengths for preventing fatigue. The results and conclusions in Henning et al.'s study raise several issues applicable to the worksite including: performance pressures, both internal and external to the employee; performance appraisal; and incentive pay. Workplace policies will need to support any measure, including microbreaks, designed to alleviate strain and increase performance for workers engaged in these repetitive tasks. Statham and Bravo's study examined the hypothesis that planning deficiencies (not involving workers in planning and/or unrealistic expectations from worker's equipment) would result in symptoms of stress from VDT operators. Survey results from 162 secretaries, 96.6 percent of whom were female, suggest that workers should be involved in planning for changes in technology. At least for some worker groups, this personal control may improve worker satisfaction with and reaction to new technology, thereby minimizing stress.

Noise

Nurminen, T., & Kurppa, K. (1989). Occupational noise exposure and course of pregnancy. *Scandinavian Journal of Work, Environment, and Health, 15,* 117–124.

This case-control study is important because relatively little attention has been given to the effect of occupational noise on non-auditory health outcomes to date. Under investigation here were threatened abortion, pregnancy induced hypertension, length of gestation, and birth weight. The sample consisted of 1,190 infants without structural birth defects who served as controls (referents) for the Finnish Register of Congenital Malformations. Threatened abortion was associated with noise exposure, as estimated by two industrial hygienists, adjusted for shift work and nonagricultural manual labor. Paradoxically, self-reported use of hearing protection among shift workers was significantly associated with threatened abortion and pregnancy induced hypertension. For women in non-agricultural manual occupations and in the manufacturing sector, the odds ratios were significantly elevated for giving birth to babies small for gestational age. This study provides groundwork for further investigation of the effects of noise and shift work in women.

Topf, M., & Dillon, E. (1988). Noise-induced stress as a predictor of burnout in critical care nurses. *Heart & Lung, 17,* 567–573.

Of all the traditionally female-dominated occupational groups, nurses are perhaps the most frequently studied in regard to work-related health issues. For many nurses, the work environment contributes to their risk of hazardous exposure, ranging from blood borne disease to sources of stress. In terms of stress, noise can become particularly hazardous. In this unique study, noise induced stress is investigated in a sample of 100 critical care nurses (91% women). Perceived noise induced stress was measured using self-report questionnaires, then positively correlated with emotional exhaustion. Topf and Dillon reported that nurses with intrinsic sensitivity to noise had no higher risk for burnout than less sensitive nurses. However, the authors caution that this correlational data analysis does not demonstrate a causal relationship. Yet, this study constitutes an important effort to describe noise as a possible source of stress for nurses, one of the largest occupational groups of women.

Thermal Hazards

Solter, M., Brkic, K., Petek, M., Posavec, L., & Sekso, M. (1989). Thyroid hormone economy in response to extreme cold in healthy factory workers. *Journal of Clinical Endocrinology and Metabolism, 68,* 168–172.

Carpenter, A. J., & Nunneley, S. A. (1988). Endogenous hormones subtly alter women's response to heat stress. *Journal of Applied Physiology, 65,* 2313–2317.

For employees who are exposed to extremes of cold and heat, risks may be increased for hypothermia and heat stroke, respectively. Women are now seeking employment more frequently where these thermal hazards exist such as food handling services and fire fighting. Yet, upon review of the literature, few studies are found that examine gender as a variable in human responses to heat and cold stress. The two studies cited here are important because consideration is given to the effects of either heat or cold stress on the physiologic responses of women. Carpenter and Nunneley (1988) concluded that the menstrual cycle may subtly alter temperature regulation without obvious changes in output of sweat. However, these changes in thermoregulation were considered minimal and not sufficient to diminish a woman's ability to work in dry heat. Solter et al. (1989) compared the role of the thyroid in adaption to extreme cold in men and women. In a group of meat cutters and canners, these investigators reported a significant post exposure decrease in serum T4-binding globulin for women ($n = 9$), but not in men ($n = 38$). The investigators reported that the role of gender in the effects of cold exposure on thyroid function was difficult to interpret. These studies are examples of research with implications for future occupational health investigations. Researchers in this area must address the concerns of women experiencing work-related exposures to heat and cold. In addition to thermoregulation, other topics need further exploration of gender as a factor in physiological responses to work-related exposures. These topics might also include muscle strength, equilibrium, and reaction time.

CHEMICAL HAZARDS

Heavy Metals

Hemminki, K., Niemi, M.-L., Koskinen, K., & Vainio, H. (1980). Spontaneous abortions among women employed in the metal industry in Finland. *International Archives of Occupational and Environmental Health, 47,* 53–60.

Women who are engaged in various manufacturing processes may be exposed to heavy metals such as lead, mercury, and cadmium. In addition, some women employed in the service sector, such as dentists and laboratory workers, also may be potentially exposed to heavy metals. Many of the heavy metals are neurotoxic, nephrotoxic, fetotoxic, and teratogenic, making evaluation of health effects in occupationally exposed workers very important. In this study, Hemminki and colleagues compared the spontaneous abortion rates (spontaneous abortions/pregnancies) and the spontaneous abortion ratios (spontaneous abortions/births) of women working in various metal industries with those rates and ratios of the general population of Finnish women. They adjusted for differing age distributions using the direct standardization procedure. Women were identified from files of the Union of Metal Workers ($n = 35,000$). From that group of women, 195 spontaneous abortions were identified from the national hospital discharge registry from 1973–1979. Statistically non-significant elevated proportions were observed for women employed in the manufacturing of household machinery, steel, and precious metal (e.g., gold and silver) objects. Using an internal comparison, both the rate and the ratio were significantly elevated for pregnancies occurring after joining the Union than for pregnancies occurring before Union membership began. Women working in the production of radios and televisions were at increased risk of spontaneous abortions and this risk was tentatively attributed to exposure to soldering fumes. Although these rates and ratios were age adjusted, the investigators did not take into account the lack of statistical independence among reproductive events in the same woman. Potential confounders other than age were not adjusted for in the analysis, nor were increased levels of cumulative exposure with each subsequent pregnancy taken into consideration. Despite these limitations, this study is important because it suggests a process (soldering) that may increase the risk of spontaneous abortion. Further studies of specific metals and processes is warranted using cohort or case-control study designs.

Sikorski, R., Juszkiewicz, T., Paszkowski, T., & Szprengier-Juszkiewicz, T. (1987). Women in dental surgeries: Reproductive hazards in occupational exposure to metallic mercury. *International Archives of Occupational and Environmental Health, 59,* 551–557.

Several large scale environmental disasters have clearly demonstrated that mercury is highly toxic, that it readily crosses the placenta, and that it is excreted in human milk. Studies of occupational exposures, therefore, are of considerable importance. This cross-sectional study was conducted to evaluate mercury exposure of women in the dental profession and reproductive outcomes. Hair samples were used to measure long-term exposure to mercury in the manufacture and placement of dental amalgams. Samples were analyzed using cold vapor atomic absorption spectrometry. Women dentists ($n = 45$) and dental assistants ($n = 36$) were compared to a group of women not occupationally exposed to mercury ($n = 34$). Levels of mercury in scalp and pubic hair were both significantly higher in the exposed group than in the control group. Levels of mercury in both types of hair samples were highly correlated with years of working in the dental profession and with the number of amalgam fillings prepared or placed per week. Fifty-seven of the women occupationally exposed to mercury had one or more pregnancies in which they worked during the pregnancy (including the first trimester). Of the 117 exposed pregnancies, 23.9 percent ended in adverse outcomes (spontaneous abortion, stillbirth, or major congenital malformations) compared to 11.1 percent of the 63 pregnancies in the unexposed women. The adverse pregnancy outcomes in the exposed women were significantly associated with mercury levels in scalp and pubic hair samples, but not for unexposed women. Menstrual disorders (irregular, painful, or hemorrhagic menses) were significantly associated with mercury levels in scalp hair, but not with pubic hair. These analyses were not adjusted for age or other potential confounders, nor was the lack of independence of multiple pregnancy outcomes in the same woman taken into account. The use of a physical detection measure strengthens the validity of the study and the findings are consistent with animal and human studies. This study provides useful information regarding several reproductive hazards associated with occupational exposure of women and conceptuses to mercury. This study design could be replicated with modifications using appropriate physical detection measures for studying mercury, lead, cadmium, and other heavy metal exposures.

Pesticides and Other Halogenated Hydrocarbons

Kimbrough, R. D. (1985). Laboratory and human studies on polychlorinated biphenyls (PCBs) and related compounds. *Environmental Health Perspectives, 59,* 99–106.

This is a very good review article on occupational and environmental epidemiological studies and animal toxicology studies for halogenated aromatic compounds, which include polychlorinated biphenyls (PCBs), polybrominated biphenyls (PBBs), naphthalenes, dibenzodioxins, and dibenzofurans. Women occupationally exposed to PCBs were at increased risk for cancer of the rectum and from all causes of deaths in two studies cited by Kimbrough. Other studies cited are of males or have too little follow-up time for evaluating chronic health problems (e.g., cancer and cardiovascular diseases), which have long latency periods between exposure and the development of disease. The issues related to absorption and excretion of these chemicals and the relevance of animal toxicology studies for understanding human health effects is particularly valuable. The limited number of occupational epidemiological studies, especially of women, persists. Nonetheless, this somewhat dated review is still valuable.

Kundiev, Y. I., Krasnyuk, E. P., & Viter, V. P. H. (1986). Specific features of the changes in the health status of female workers exposed to pesticides in greenhouses. *Toxicology Letters, 33,* 85–89.

Women who engage in farming (including migrant workers), horticultural and forestry work, commercial pesticide spraying, and home gardening are likely to have direct exposure to pesticides. Others workers such as roadside crews and fruit and vegetable processors could be exposed less directly. Yet, this is the only study found in the literature that evaluates occupational exposure of women to pesticides. This cross-sectional study, conducted in the Soviet Union, involved a clinical evaluation of over 600 female greenhouse workers and 300 women who cultivate vegetable gardens outdoors. The investigators point out that greenhouse conditions would be expected to enhance absorption of pesticides. Enhanced absorption would be due to the enclosed space (poor ventilation), high application rate, and high temperature and humidity, which increase dermal absorption. Planting and harvesting continuously throughout the year, as opposed to seasonal exposure of the control group, also would contribute to greater absorption of pesticides. The findings indicated that central nervous system problems were most prevalent. An increased prevalence of cardiovascular, respiratory, and liver dysfunction were noted. Dermatitis and allergic dermatitis were noted in 14 percent and 7.3 percent, respectively, of all the women in the study. No apparent differences were found between groups for sterility, menstrual dysfunction, "genital diseases of the inflammatory type" (p. 88), premature delivery, [infant] mortality, or spontaneous abortions. This was an ambitious clinical study that would have been enhanced by the inclusion of statistical analyses. Due to the absence of statistical results, the findings, both positive and negative, must be interpreted cautiously.

Pearn, J. H. (1985). Herbicides and congenital malformations: A review for the paediatrician. *Australian Paediatric Journal, 21,* 237–242.

Pearn provides a concise overview of human and animal studies of the structural teratogenic effects of 2,4-D, 2,4,5-T, and dioxin, which represent a small fraction of the herbicides that have ever been used. Some of the human studies reviewed were of environmental exposure, which is generally of a lesser magnitude than occupational exposure. The author points out that there is no evidence of a teratogenic effect of these herbicides in humans. However, the cited studies are generally methodologically weak (e.g., outbreak investigations, poorly defined exposure, or small sample size), are of a select subset of herbicides, and are limited to a single reproductive outcome. These limitations need to be taken into consideration by the reader.

Taylor, P. R., Stelma, J. M., & Lawrence, C. E. (1989). The relation of polychlorinated biphenyls to birth weight and gestational age in the offspring of occupationally exposed mothers. *American Journal of Epidemiology, 129,* 395–406.

This is a generally well-conducted study of women (*n* = 2,691) occupationally exposed to PCBs in the manufacture of capacitors between 1946 and 1977. It is one of the few reproductive cohort studies found in the literature. The study findings are important as PCBs are widely found, not only in various occupational settings, but also as a widespread environmental contaminant. A subsample of women under age 55 who had direct exposure to PCBs (*n* = 200) and indirect exposure to PCBs (*n* = 205; the comparison group) were interviewed to determine two reproductive endpoints (birth weight and gestational age) that indicate fetotoxicity. Linear regression was used to estimate highly chlorinated (and persistent) PCB body burdens at the time of each pregnancy for the primary exposure model. Other exposures that occurred during the manufacturing of capacitors (trichloroethylene, methyl isobutyl ketone, lead, zinc, tin, aluminum, iron, and epoxides) were not considered in the analysis. There was an inverse, but statistically non-significant, relationship between birth weight and the estimated PCB level when gestational age and confounders were controlled for in the analysis. The investigators suggest that the magnitude of the effect of PCBs on these reproductive outcomes "would have a negligible effect on perinatal and infant mortality and morbidity" (p. 405). This is a generally well-conducted study and confidence can

be placed in the validity of the findings. The advantage of using birth weight and gestational age in reproductive studies, as these investigators did, is that these outcomes can be verified from birth certificates. It would be desirable to replicate these findings using a similar cohort and follow them prospectively. In addition to the outcomes used in this study, it would be possible to include other reproductive outcomes of importance such as infertility, spontaneous abortions, and birth defects.

Organic Solvents

Lindbohm, M.-L., Taskinen, H., & Hemminki, K. (1985). Reproductive health of working women: Spontaneous abortions and congenital malformations. *Public Health Reviews, 13,* 55–87.

Lindbohm, M.-L., Taskinen, H., Kyyronen, P., Sallmen, M., Anttila, A., & Hemminki, K. (1992). Effects of parental occupational exposure to solvents and lead on spontaneous abortion. *Scandinavian Journal of Work and Environmental Health, 18*(Suppl. 2), 37–39.

Lindbohm and colleagues (1985) present a thorough overview of methodological issues related to occupational studies of spontaneous abortions and congenital malformations not limited to any particular class of chemical agents. They addressed many specific workplace hazards for women. Although this review article is somewhat dated, it is a very succinct summary of most relevant issues. The authors chose not to review anesthetic gases, but refer the reader to other sources. Adverse reproductive effects of antineoplastic drugs are not presented as this review was written prior to published reports of occupational reproductive effects of antineoplastic drugs. This article helps the reader to identify differences between occupational reproductive studies and studies of other occupational outcomes. This review article would provide a very good summary of most known reproductive hazards and methodological issues relevant for occupational health practitioners and researchers alike. The other article by Lindbohm et al. (1992) provides an excellent review of six case-control Finnish studies, which evaluated risk of spontaneous abortions among women exposed during the first trimester to solvents (three studies) or lead (one study). They also evaluated the risk of spontaneous abortion in wives of men exposed during spermatogenesis (80 days prior to conception) to solvents (one study) or lead (one study). For maternal exposure to solvents in general or specific solvents such as methylene chloride or tetrachloroethylene, the risk of spontaneous abortion was increased 50 percent to nearly 400 percent. At relatively low concentrations of blood lead in exposed women (most below 1.0 micromols/liter), no increased risk was observed. Men's exposure to solvents was associated with approximately a two-fold increased risk of spontaneous abortion. At the lowest concentration of lead exposure in men, no risk was detected, whereas at higher concentrations a modest increased risk was found (30 percent at 1.5–1.8 micromols/liter; 60 percent at ≥1.9 micromols/liter). It is interesting to note that, in general, the number of exposed cases was greater for each group or subgroup in the studies of wives of exposed men than in the studies of exposed women. As an excellent summary of risks associated with solvent and lead exposures in women and men, it also provides a fine example of the value of simultaneously examining occupational reproductive risks of women and men.

Huel, G., Mergler, D., & Bowler, R. (1990). Evidence for adverse reproductive outcomes among women microelectronic assembly workers. *British Journal of Industrial Medicine, 47,* 400–404.

A matched case-control study was conducted to examine risk of spontaneous abortion among women employed as microelectronic assemblers. Ninety pairs were matched on the following preemployment characteristics: ethnicity (white, Hispanic, other), age (±3 years for cases <45 years old; ±6 years for cases ≥45 years old), and number of pregnancies (0–5; 6+). Friends and relatives who had never worked in the microelectronics industry served as referents (controls). To avoid the lack of statistical independence associated with pregnancy outcomes in the same woman, the woman was used

as the unit of analysis. Women with pregnancies prior to employment as assemblers were not at increased risk of spontaneous abortion (OR = 0.9). However, women employed as microelectronic assemblers who had pregnancies subsequent to their employment were at increased risk compared to referents (OR = 5.6, $p < .01$; OR = 4.0, $p < .05$ when restricted to women who had no more than one spontaneous abortion). When analysis was restricted to women with pregnancies that occurred during their employment as assemblers, the risk increased to 15 ($p < .01$). The presumed agent(s) associated with these increased risks was solvents. However, the absence of industrial hygiene data precluded examination of specific solvents associated with the observed increased risks. Women were exposed to various combinations of chlorofluorocarbons, chlorinated cydrocarbons, glycol ethers, isopropanol, acetone, alcohol, toluene, and xylene. As a well-conducted study, the findings suggest that women employed in microelectronic manufacturing where solvent exposure occurs are at significantly increased risk for spontaneous abortion.

Bosco, M. G., Figa-Talamanca, I., & Salerno, S. (1987). Health and reproductive status of female workers in dry cleaning shops. *International Archives of Occupational and Environmental Health, 59,* 295–301.

This was a cross-sectional study of reproductive outcomes of women who work in dry cleaning establishments. The study of the health of women employed in the dry cleaning industry including reproductive outcomes is of considerable importance due to the toxicity of these solvents and the prevalence of women in this occupation. Currently, the primary exposure is to the organic solvent tetrachloroethylene. In the past, trichlorethylene was used, which has been associated with neurological and gastrointestinal problems. All pregnancies ($n = 102$) were used in the analysis, and confounders such as maternal age were not controlled for in the analysis. Spontaneous abortions were four times more frequent in women who worked "prior to and during pregnancy" (p. 300), which was not statistically significant.

Several methodological problems exist in this study. Exposure was poorly defined and the timing of exposure was not linked to specific reproductive outcomes. Other problems included the use of a small sample, limiting the sample to those currently employed, the use of multiple pregnancy outcomes in the same woman, and the lack of control for confounders. As such, these study findings were of borderline significance. It would be helpful to correct methodological weaknesses here in future studies so that reproductive risks of tetrachloroethylene, if any exist, can be determined.

Kilburn, K., Warshaw, R., & Thornton, J. C. (1989). Pulmonary function in histology technicians compared with women from Michigan: Effects of chronic low dose formaldehyde on a national sample of women. *British Journal of Industrial Medicine, 46,* 468–472.

Formaldehyde is used as a disinfectant and preservative for biological specimens, as a binder in plywoods, in the production of plastics and resins, and in urea-formaldehyde insulation. This is an important area of research as formaldehyde is a respiratory irritant and causes nasal cancer in animals. Formaldehyde is released from building materials and furnishings (e.g., carpet), so it may play a role in sick building syndrome, which is reviewed in the section on *Other Hazards.* Kilburn and colleagues used a repeated cross sectional study design to assess pulmonary function among nonsmoking female histology technicians (n = 240). Histology technicians are exposed to formaldehyde through the preparation and preservation of biological specimens in laboratories. The pulmonary function of these technicians was compared to a large population-based normative group of Michigan women. Compared to Michigan women, histology technicians had better pulmonary function for the first measurement period, but exhibited a greater decrement in pulmonary function five years later. The methodology used here could be repeated for groups of women exposed to formaldehyde and

other pulmonary irritants, including those associated with less clearly defined agents as in the case of sick building syndrome.

Lemasters, G. K., Samuels, S. J., Morrison, J. A., & Brooks, S. M. (1989). Reproductive outcomes of pregnant workers employed at 36 reinforced plastics companies. II. Lowered birth weight. *Journal of Occupational Medicine, 31,* 115–120.

This is a report of a case-control study of the association of styrene exposure on birth weight. Styrene is of interest because of its structural similarity to vinyl chloride, which is a mutagen and carcinogen. The findings of this study are important to women's occupational health as the reinforced plastics industries are often staffed with women and many are small operations that may be exempt from OSHA regulations. There were 229 styrene exposed and 819 unexposed live, singleton births available for analysis. Other solvent exposures in the reinforced plastics industry include acetone, methylethyl ketone, methylene chloride, toluene, and xylene; these solvents were not considered in the analyses. Several exposure models for styrene were used in the analyses including an estimated exposure dose for each pregnancy based on process, exposure intensity, and the product manufactured. There was no significant dose response detected. The investigators reported a power of 94 percent for detecting a 2 percent decrease in birth weight. This is an example of a well-conducted study in which there was no association found, as well as being one of few studies found in the literature in which a power analysis was reported. The power analysis allows the reader to determine the confidence one can place in a negative finding.

LaMarte, F. P., Merchant, J. A., & Casale, T. B. (1988). Acute systemic reactions to carbonless copy paper associated with histamine release. *Journal of the American Medical Association, 260,* 242–243.

Two indepth case studies of systemic reactions including laryngeal edema associated with exposure to an ingredient in carbonless copy paper are reported. The sensitizing ingredient is assumed by these reviewers to be an organic solvent or similar chemical. (The ingredient was not identified by LeMarte et al. through an agreement with the manufacturer.) The evidence is strong enough in these case reports to support a causal relationship. Carbonless copy paper is ubiquitous in a number of work settings including offices, health care settings, and general businesses. These findings are significant in light of the potentially life-threatening nature of the systemic reactions that are possible.

Pharmaceuticals

Vainio, H. (1982). Inhalation anesthetics, anticancer drugs and sterilants as chemical hazards in hospitals. *Scandinavian Journal of Work and Environmental Health, 8,* 94–107.

This is an excellent overview of several chemical hazards in hospitals (and other health care settings). Many anesthetic gases are abortifacents, carcinogens, and possibly teratogens. Ethylene oxide, which is used for cold sterilization of instruments and equipment in industry and health care settings, is suspected of being leukemogenic. Formaldehyde, also used for cold sterilization and as a laboratory solution (formalin), is associated with acute respiratory and mucous membrane irritation and dermatitis. Hexachlorophene, which was formerly used as a skin cleansing agent, is suspected of being a teratogen. At the time this review article was published, relatively little was known about the health effects of occupational exposure to anticancer drugs. In this regard, the article by Selevan et al. (1985) in which fetal loss is associated with occupational exposure to anticancer drugs is critiqued next.

Selevan, S. G., Lindbohm M.-L., Hornung, R. W., & Hemminki, K. (1985). A study of occupational exposure to antineoplastic drugs and fetal loss in nurses. *New England Journal of Medicine, 313,* 1173–1178.

Many antineoplastic drugs (cancer chemotherapy) are known to cause cancer in patients and birth defects in their offspring. Many nurses, pharmacists, and physicians prepare or administer these drugs for treating cancer and other nonmalignant disorders. Their widespread use has raised concern about reproductive and cancer risks in occupationally exposed workers. This is a case-control study in which nurses who experienced a fetal loss (based on last menstrual periods between October 1972 and March 1980) were compared to other nurses who had one or more live births (including congenital malformations or stillbirths), but no fetal losses, during the same period. Whenever more than one pregnancy outcome occurred during the study period, a pregnancy was randomly selected. Three controls were drawn from each hospital where the case mother was hospitalized, and these controls were matched to cases on age. Data were collected by self-administered questionnaires on the following: (a) health status, (b) alcohol and smoking habits, and (c) lifetime work and reproductive histories. In addition, respondents provided data regarding medication, illness, injury, alcohol and smoking habits, and exposure to antineoplastic drugs, X-rays, anesthetic gases, and ethylene oxide for a two-year period in relation to the case/control pregnancy. From the 650 study subjects selected, 89.2 percent of the case mothers and 98.1 percent of the control mothers responded. Using matched analysis, pregnancies ending in fetal loss were 2.30 times more likely to have first trimester exposure to antineoplastic drugs than control pregnancies. Fetal loss was not associated with cumulative exposure measures. This was a well-conducted occupational reproductive study in which Finnish registry data were used to identify cases and controls and to identify hospitals where antineoplastic drugs were used in large quantities. The results are consistent with those using animal models and patients. Since this classic report, a cross-sectional study has indicated that adverse pregnancy outcomes (spontaneous abortions and congenital malformations) were significantly associated with exposure to antineoplastic drugs during pregnancy (Rogers & Emmett, 1987). These findings indicate that adverse pregnancy outcomes are associated with occupational antineoplastic drug exposures, but further studies are needed. Cohort studies would be desirable and feasible.

Gardner, M. J., Coggon, D., Pannett, B., & Harris, E. C. (1989). Workers exposed to ethylene oxide: A follow up study. *British Journal of Industrial Medicine, 46,* 860–865.

Ethylene oxide is used in both industry and hospitals for cold sterilization of equipment and instruments. Ethylene oxide, a highly mutagenic agent, was previously found to be associated with an increased risk of spontaneous abortions among hospital nurses (Hemminki et al., 1982). As done in this study, it is particularly valuable to follow such an occupationally exposed cohort to determine if there is increased risk for other adverse health outcomes such as cancer. This standard mortality ratio (SMR) study investigated a population of workers in England and Wales who were thought to be exposed to ethylene oxide. The cohort consisted of 1,864 men, mostly chemical workers, and 1,012 women, almost entirely hospital workers. Exposure to ethylene oxide for chemical workers began before 1961, but only after 1961 for hospital workers. Three chemical workers, all men, died from leukemia. This was more than twice the expected number of deaths, but does not reach statistical significance. There were two cases of stomach cancer among hospital workers, compared to 0.86 expected, which also was not statistically significant. The relatively short follow-up period, especially for hospital workers, would likely yield low power for any cancer outcomes at this time. It is probable that this cohort will be followed for many years, yielding increasing power, to determine if ethylene oxide is a human carcinogen.

Rodriguez, W. J., Dang Bui, R. H., Connor, J. D., Kim, H. W., Brandt, C. D., Parrot, R. H., Burch, B., & Mace, J. (1987). Environmental exposure of primary care personnel to Ribavirin aerosol when supervising treatment of infants with respiratory syncytial virus infections. *Antimicrobial Agents and Chemotherapy, 31,* 1143–1146.

Decker, J. A., Seitz, T. A., Shults, R. A., Dietchman, S., Tucker, S. P., Belinky, R. R., & Clark, N. J. (1992). Occupational exposures to aerosolized pharmaceuticals and control strategies. *Scandinavian Journal of Work and Environmental Health, 18*(Suppl. 2), 100–102.

Acute symptoms as reported by Rodriguez and colleagues (1987) are an important area of research. Acute symptoms in health care workers exposed to Ribavirin, an antiviral agent, have been reported to the National Institute of Occupational Safety and Health. Ribavirin is an animal teratogen. This cross-sectional study was conducted to evaluate exposure and acute symptoms with 19 nonpregnant nurses as exposed subjects. The drug was delivered to pediatric patients by aerosolization through ventilators, oxygen tents, and oxygen hoods. Four non-pregnant nurses who did not work with patients receiving Ribavirin, but who worked in the same area, served as controls. No drug was detected in any of the participants, nor did the participants report any adverse reactions. Rodriguez et al. reported that the power to detect the outcomes measured was 84 percent. Because information regarding laboratory procedures and outcome measures is not fully developed in this article, its findings must be interpreted cautiously. In future studies, it would be desirable to use blood and urine samples from the pediatric patients at the same time to demonstrate that the laboratory method is adequate. In addition, it would be desirable to use an unexposed group from a unit where Ribavirin is not administered (e.g., newborn nursery).

The study by Decker and colleagues (1992) contributes substantially to the understanding of conditions in which Ribavirin and Pentamidine (another antiviral agent) become aerosolized into the environment and absorbed systemically by health care workers. Personal air samples of breathing zones were measured for seven nurses and six respiratory therapists (RTs). Personal air samples were reported as 8-hour time weighted averages (TWA) for five of seven nurses and two RTs, while short term (post-treatment) samples were analyzed for the remaining two nurses and five RTs. Urinary excretion levels were measured post-shift for nine nurses (22 samples) and eight RTs (17 samples). Nurses' personal air samples of Ribavirin ranged from below the level of detection to a high of 94 micrograms/cubic meter. Nurses' urinary excretion levels of the drug ranged from below the level of detection to 0.136 micromols per gram of creatinine. For RTs, personal air samples ranged from below the level of detection to a maximum of 83.3 micrograms/cubic meter. The mean urinary excretion level of Ribavirin was significantly greater for nurses compared to RTs. Consistent with the findings for Ribavirin, the personal air samples of Pentamidine indicated that contamination of breathing zones occurred, but varied considerably based on the method used for administering this treatment to patients. These two studies illustrate that the methods used in a study are critical to evaluate in relation to the reported findings. In contrast to the study by Rodriguez et al. (1987), the results from the study by Decker and colleagues (1992) clearly show that air contamination and biological absorption of pharmaceuticals occur in the workplace.

BIOLOGICAL HAZARDS

Owens, D. K. & Nease, R. F. (1992) Occupational exposure to human immunodeficiency virus and hepatitis B virus: A comparative analysis of risk. *American Journal of Medicine, 92,* 503–512.

The incidence of human immunodeficiency virus (HIV) infection among women is increasing. The health care industry is a major employer of women and much fear has been expressed over health care workers' potential occupational HIV exposure. Previous research has shown that occupational transmission of HIV is rare. Sadly, the fear of acquired immunodeficiency syndrome (AIDS) has overshadowed the fact that at least 200 health care workers in the United States die each year from occupational exposure to hepatitis B (HBV). The authors use a decision analytic model to estimate the occupational risk of HIV and HBV

infection in relation to expected loss of life. Loss of life expectancy was defined as the chance that a health care worker will seroconvert when exposed to the infection multiplied by the decrease in length of life associated with that infection. Using this approach allows for the comparison of a fatal disease with rare occupational transmission (e.g., HIV) to one which is less fatal but more readily transmitted (e.g., HBV). The following risks were estimated by the authors for a 30-year old female health care worker who is not immune to HBV. From a single needlestick, the health care worker would lose 39 days of life from a patient with advanced HIV infection, 17 days from a patient who is hepatitis B-surface antigen positive (HBsAg), and 38 days from a patient who is hepatitis B-e antigen positive (HBeAg). If vaccinated for HBV, the risk of HBeAG and HBsAg is reduced 10-fold. The authors also compared the loss of quality adjusted life expectancy by factoring in morbidity. Using the same 30-year old female health care worker, the number of quality adjusted days' loss from a single needlestick increases to: 45 with a HIV positive patient, 48 days with a HBsAg positive patient, and 109 days loss with a HBeAg positive patient. This article provides a reasonable approach for estimating health care workers' occupational risk of HIV versus HBV infection. In addition, the authors emphasize the importance of prevention. Wearing gloves reduces the amount of blood transmitted with a needlestick by 50 percent. In addition, over 90 percent of those vaccinated with the HBV vaccine are protected against HBV infection. Unfortunately, not all health care workers have received the vaccine and not all wear gloves when they should. Given the morbidity and the mortality associated with these infections, it is imperative that methods to protect health care workers be implemented, encouraged, and enforced.

Adler, S. P. (1989). Cytomegalovirus and child day care: Evidence for an increased infection rate among day care workers. *New England Journal of Medicine, 321,* 1290–1296.

Cytomegalovirus (CMV) is a known teratogen. Of infants born with congenital CMV, 25 percent die or suffer cognitive and neural damage.

Previous research indicated that day care workers do not carry a higher rate of CMV than other women who have frequent contact with children. This well-designed study contradicts those findings. Adler found a 5-fold increase in occupational risk for CMV infection among female day care workers than compared to a similar group of female hospital workers. Significant risk factors identified in the study were caring for children under 2 years of age and being a black female. Results of this study raise two concerns for working families. First, licensed day care facilities may fail to properly train their employees in infection control practices. Second, the majority of working families with young children use unlicensed day care providers, in which no training in infection control is required. Educational programs need to be provided for all day care workers to decrease this risk for women during child bearing years.

PSYCHOLOGICAL HAZARDS

Stress

Richardsen, A. M., & Burke, R. J. (1991). Occupational stress and job satisfaction among physicians: Sex differences. *Social Science and Medicine*, 33, 1179–1187.

This Canadian study surveyed 2,584 physicians about sources of job stress and satisfaction. Females comprised only 10 percent of the sample. Although both males and females reported similar job stressors, only the total number of hours worked and the threat of malpractice were predictive of overall stress for women. Interestingly, family or personal demands were not included by the authors as a potential stressor. The lack of including an important source of stress for working women may account for the low amount (6%) of overall stress explained. In addition, the small number of women in this sample, as compared to men, could also account for the poor prediction of overall stress for women. Family and personal demands, however, were included as an indicator of job satisfaction. For

women but not for men, sufficient time for family or for a personal life was predictive of job satisfaction. This study highlights the importance of including appropriate sources of stress for both men and women if analysis by gender is planned.

Baruch, G. K., Biener, L., & Barnett, R. C. (1987). Women and gender in research on work and family stress. *American Psychologist*, 42, 130–136.

In this review of 56 references, Baruch and colleagues identified several problems in the stress research of concern to women: lack of analysis of race, ethnic background, and social class interaction with stress; inappropriate measurement techniques; inappropriate generalization of findings of male studies to females; and lack of salient women's issues. Using current research, assumptions of workplace and family role stress are reexamined. Contrary to earlier predictions, the home does not serve as a buffer to stress for women. The authors argue that women's family and homemaker roles are more stressful due to a combination of high psychological demands and low control. Similarly, low level, low paying jobs are associated with stressors that negatively affect health. For many, the workplace provides more of a balance between control and demands. The overall effect of employment for women has been positive and may serve as a buffer to family role stress. What is critical is the perceived quality of women's role experiences, not just the role. This well-organized review successfully challenges the view that women become more susceptible to stress-related illness when the role of paid worker is added to family roles.

Repetti, R. L., Matthews, K. S., & Waldron, I. (1989). Employment and women's health: Effects of paid employment on women's mental and physical health. *American Psychologist*, 44, 1394–1401.

Using mainly longitudinal studies as data sources (67 references in all), this review article discusses several issues of interest related to women's employment and mental health. Mental health was measured in the various studies using self-report scales of anxiety and depression, and general psychological symptom scales. Employment does seem to have an effect on women's personal and work-related characteristics. Work impacts on women's mental health depending upon the marital status, maternal status (for black or unmarried women), employment attitudes, job demands, degree of job control, and the amount of job related social support. Findings are inconsistent from retrospective and cross sectional studies as to the overall effect of employment. Recommendations for future longitudinal research on employment's effect on women's mental health included the use of social support and overload as mediators. This article provides a succinct review of what is currently known about occupationally related stress in women workers.

Martocchio, J. J., & O'Leary, A. M. (1989). Sex differences in occupational stress: A meta-analytic review. *Journal of Applied Psychology, 74*, 495–501.

This meta analysis was limited to 15 studies that investigated the effects of workplace stress on both sexes. Contrary to qualitative reviews (e.g., Baruch et al. and Repetti et al.), no differences in gender were found in both physiological and psychological stress. This would be expected as the studies reviewed by Martocchio and O'Leary did not include any measures of family/home stress. The authors do provide, however, a good discussion of issues that should be addressed in future research: need for consistent definition of stress, lack of reported reliability and validity assessments, sparsity of psychometrically sound stress measures, deviations from equal numbers of male and female subjects, and lack of information regarding relationship between stress and moderating factors. The authors point out the need for longitudinal studies.

Klitzman, S., & Stellman, J. M. (1989). The impact of the physical environment on the psychological

well-being of office workers. *Social Science Medicine, 29,* 733–742.

Previous research on workplace stress focused on the psychosocial working environment, ignoring the possible effects of the physical working conditions on stress. Of the 1,830 nonmanagerial office workers from four different establishments who returned questionnaires in this study, 73 percent were females. Using factor analysis, the following variables were identified: physical environment (air quality, physical layout, traffic, privacy, and lighting); psychosocial work environment (relations with superiors, coworkers support, work load demand, job decision latitude, and job future); and psychological well-being (job satisfaction, office satisfaction, anxiety, irritation, and fatigue). Air quality, noise, ergonomic stressors, and privacy were physical environmental variables that significantly predicted worker psychological well-being. Although this well-designed study did not report gender as a variable, the findings are relevant as many women are employed in offices. Significant variables identified should be used in future research on occupational stress.

Ivancevich, J. M., & Matteson, M. T. (1982). Occupational stress, satisfaction, physical well-being, and coping: A study of homemakers. *Psychological Reports, 50,* 995–1005.

It is unusual within the occupational literature to study homemaker stress, but this study does so. Using a self-report questionnaire, the authors explored the stress and physical well-being of 307 middle and upper income full- and part-time homemakers. Ivancevich and Matteson concluded that the stress of homemaking varies. Full-time homemakers were most stressed with role issues related to the lack of being held in esteem by others. Part-time homemakers perceived more stress with spouse's unwillingness to share household responsibilities. Because most women who work outside the home are homemakers, further study in this area is important to better understand women's stress.

OTHER HAZARDS

Dusts

Zuskin, E., Kanceljak, B., Pokrajac, D., Schachter, E. N., & Witek, T. J. (1990). Respiratory symptoms and lung function in hemp workers. *British Journal of Industrial Medicine, 47*, 627–632.

This study analyzed respiratory symptoms and ventilatory capacity in hemp workers employed in 2 different mills. The women (n = 84) on average were exposed to 15.5 years of hemp dust, where the men (n = 27) had an average exposure of 20 years. Workers frequently rotated job responsibilities which means all workers were probably exposed to similar levels of dust. A control group consisted of 49 female and 30 male workers from a dust free industry. Controls were similar to the workers in age, smoking history, and length of employment. It is not surprising that the study found that the workers experienced increases in respiratory symptoms and decreases in ventilatory capacity at the end of the work shift as compared to the controls. What is surprising is that these mostly non-smoking female hemp workers, when compared with controls, had a higher prevalence of chronic respiratory symptoms than did the predominately smoking males. This is an important finding as smoking is usually associated with greater respiratory symptoms. However, this study does not mention the use of any protective equipment to prevent dust inhalation. It is not clear whether gender differences would persist if protective equipment were used. Unfortunately, women often have difficulty with protective equipment fitting properly since few are manufactured according to female body proportions.

Acheson, E. D., Gardner, M. J., Pippard, E. C., & Grime, L. P. (1982). Mortality of two groups of women who manufactured gas masks from chrysotile and crocidolite asbestos: A 40-year follow-up. *British Journal of Industrial Medicine, 39*, 344–348.

In reviewing National Health Service records of 757 English women, a higher rate of lung and ovarian cancer was found for those who had worked with crocidolite asbestos. In reviewing this and previous research on the possible association between asbestos exposure and ovarian cancer, the authors raised the concern that these women were possibly misdiagnosed. The authors believe that these women were more likely to have had peritoneal cancer (mesothelioma). The early signs of peritoneal cancer are very similar to those of ovarian cancer that have spread to the peritoneum. As more women hold "non-traditional" jobs as these women did during World War II, it is crucial that health professionals inquire about women's work histories, so that proper diagnosis and treatment are provided.

Sick Building Syndrome

Boxer, P. A., (1990). Indoor air quality: A psychological perspective. *Journal of Occupational Medicine, 32*, 425–428.

Hall, E. M., & Johnson, J. V. (1989). A case study of stress and mass psychogenic illness in industrial workers. *Journal of Occupational Medicine, 31*, 243–250.

In the past, unless unacceptable levels of chemical or other agents were detected, workers complaining about air quality were often labeled as mass psychogenic illness (MPI). Many labeled with MPI were women. Currently, it is recognized that very low levels of multiple chemicals occurring together can cause irritation. However, workers may still be diagnosed with MPI if no definitive cause can be found. Boxer asserts that reports of odors are often a triggering event in MPI. According to Boxer, the incidence of MPI differs from complaints of poor air quality or sick building syndrome. MPI occurs predominantly in industrial buildings with unskilled labor, where sick building syndrome is associated with office buildings and professional workers. The present study by Hall and Johnson used a sample (n = 179) of mostly female garment workers from three industrial facilities who had previously reported smelling "gas" at the worksite. This group was compared to a total of 34 men from the three facilities. The authors stated that work intensity, mental strain, work/home problems, education, and gender were predictive of overall severity of illness. Hall and Johnson suggested that these symptoms are consistent with MPI. However, given the small male sample size and the level of significance for gender considered acceptable ($p < .11$) by the authors, these conclusions are questionable. Further research in this area is needed.

Kreiss, K. (1989). The epidemiology of building-related complaints and illness. *Occupational Medicine: State of the Art Reviews, 4,* 575–591.

Twenty-four percent of office workers perceive that there are air quality problems at their worksites. This article is an excellent review (57 references in all) of building complaints with both known and unknown etiology. Recognized health effects include hypersensitivity pneumonitis, humidifier fever, building related asthma, and legionellosis. No abnormal levels of air quality contaminants are usually found. In the 1970s, workers whose air quality complaints were investigated by the government were often diagnosed with mass hysteria or psychogenic illnesses. These workers were mostly females. The author summarizes the classic European epidemiological and human panel studies. These studies clearly indicated that the symptoms experienced (lethargy, mucous membrane irritation, and headache) were remarkably uniform between a variety of different buildings and ventilation systems. These symptoms were not consistent with mass hysteria. Gender is not a factor when job categories are controlled.

Skov, P., Valjorn, O., & Pedersen, B. V. (1989). Influence of personal characteristics, job-related factors and psychosocial factors on the sick building syndrome. *Scandinavian Journal of Work and Environmental Health, 15,* 286–295.

In this follow-up to studies of Danish town halls, the authors found that the prevalence of work-related mucous membrane irritation and general symptoms were related to differences in building climate. Gender, job category, work functions, and psychosocial factors (dissatisfaction with co-workers and workload) were associated with both general and mucous membrane symptoms. Work functions that included handling carbonless paper, photocopying, and work at video display terminals, were highly predictive of symptoms. Women often perform these functions. Considering that the study is well-designed otherwise, it is curious that the authors did not report correlations between gender and work functions. It is very probable that work functions rather than gender are the issue here.

Work Patterns

Gold, D. R., Rogacz, S., Bock, N., Tosteson, T. D., Baum, T. M., Speizer, F. E., & Czeisler, C. A. (1992). Rotating shift work, sleep, and accidents related to sleepiness in hospital nurses. *American Journal of Public Health, 82,* 1011–1014.

Gordon, N. P., Cleary, P. D., Parker, C. E., & Czeisler, C. A. (1986). The prevalence and health impact of shiftwork. *American Journal of Public Health, 76,* 1225–1228.

Within the United States, over 50 percent of employees in major industries work either straight or rotating shifts. Previous studies have documented the physiological and psychological effects of shift work: sleep and eating disorders; disrupted family and social life; and increased cigarette, alcohol, and coffee consumption. Of those interviewed in the Gordon et al. study, 18 percent of the women and 26 percent of the men had rotating work schedules. Regardless of age, income, or education, females working rotating shifts used more sleeping pills or tranquilizers, were heavier drinkers, had lower social network scores, and perceived more severe job and more severe emotional problems than females working straight shifts. Results of previous studies indicating that shift workers consume more cigarettes and coffee were not substantiated. Although the Gordon et al. study did not measure the effects of different straight shifts (i.e., day versus night), rotating shift schedules are clearly more psychologically stressful than straight shifts. Increased on-the-job accidents and injuries have also been related to shift work and job stress. In the Gold et al. study of 635 nurses, nurses working either the night shift or rotated shifts had twice the number of errors or accidents as compared to nurses working day or evening shifts. Scheduling rotating shift workers to a forward rotation pattern (days to evenings, evenings to nights) has been shown to reduce some of the physical problems and to improve the quantity and quality of sleep.

Axelsson, G., Rylander, R., & Molin, I. (1989). Outcome of pregnancy in relation to irregular and inconvenient work schedules. *British Journal of Industrial Medicine, 46,* 393–398.

Although the authors investigated an interesting question, their study could be stronger methodologically. Thus, caution should be used in interpreting the results. The study sample consisted of women who were born after 1934 and who worked at a certain Swedish hospital between 1980 and 1984. The sample completed a questionnaire on pregnancy outcomes and working conditions during pregnancy. From the findings, the authors concluded that nonsmoking women who worked irregular hours ($n = 59$), evenings ($n = 6$), or rotated shifts ($n = 11$), delivered lower birth weight infants than nonsmokers who worked the day shift only ($n = 41$). These results occurred among women with at least one other child. Women working the night shift ($n = 70$), did not deliver significantly lower birth weight babies. This adds to the view that variable work schedules may be physiologically as well as psychologically stressful.

MORTALITY

Doebbert, G., Riedmiller, K. R., & Kizer, K. W. (1988). Occupational mortality of California women. *Western Journal of Medicine, 149,* 734–740.

This study contributes to the emerging body of knowledge on occupationally-related mortality for women. The results of the study demonstrated that women experience substantial differences in the risk of mortality by occupation. Dispelling the myth of "women's work is safe," these data suggest that health care providers must begin to consider occupational factors relating to many common diseases and injuries of women. This is an example of an informative standard mortality risk (SMR) study. The investigators found increased risk of mortality for a variety of female-dominated occupations including women in the health care, food service, laundry, communications, and cosmetology industries. To assess risks for specific categories of women workers, researchers need to conduct more SMR studies using large data bases. These studies would identify areas for further research on occupational mortality of women.

SOCIAL ISSUES

Clark, M. C. M. (1988). Working and non-working mothers' perceptions of their careers, their infants' needs and satisfaction with mothering. *Health Visitor, 61,* 103–106.

This study is an example of an investigation to determine the interrelationship of women's employment with their other societal roles. As increasing numbers of women with young children work outside the home, concerns have been raised about the effects of employment on mothers and their families. In this study, Clark compares attitudes of working and non-working mothers regarding their careers, their infants' needs, and satisfaction with mothering. Working mothers reported a significantly greater level of career orientation, as would be expected. Working women also reported being generally more satisfied with the mothering role than the non-working mothers and were less anxious about leaving their children while they worked. Since this report does not contain information about the reliability of the instruments used, caution must be used in the interpretation of the results. The article is of value for the issues raised by the author.

Ryan, A., & Martinez, G. (1989). Breast-feeding and the working mother. *Pediatrics*, 83, 524–531.

Key questions are raised by this comparison of the breastfeeding patterns of employed and unemployed mothers. Using data obtained through the Ross Laboratories Mother's Survey, responses were examined from a sample of 83,985 mothers with infants 6 months of age. Mothers' employment was associated with the duration of breastfeeding. Fifty-five percent of both employed and unemployed mothers in this sample breastfed in the hospital. More than twice as many unemployed mothers (24.3%) as employed mothers (10.0%) were still breastfeeding when these infants were 6 months of age. Also included in this article is an interesting comparison of ethnicity (black versus white) as a factor in breastfeeding for employed and unemployed mothers. This useful review of the literature addresses maternal employment policies as a possible factor in limiting breastfeeding duration for employed mothers. Unfortunately, this study does not address the reasons why this sample of employed mothers limited the duration of breastfeeding. The authors call for further examination of difficulties encountered by employed breastfeeding mothers. National health surveys could include additional data on possible difficulties for employed breastfeeding mothers.

Note: The authors wish to thank Faith Davis, PhD, for her critique of an earlier draft of the section of Methodological Issues. Dr. Davis is an Associate Professor, Division of Epidemiology and Biostatistics, School of Public Health, at the University of Illinois at Chicago.

Chapter 3

Women's Sexuality

Linda A. Bernhard

INTRODUCTION

This review covers the years 1988 through 1992. An extensive review of medical, nursing, psychology, sociology, social work, sexology, and women's studies journals, as well as a less-than-extensive review of book publications was conducted. Most of the citations are research studies; however, this fact could be a result of the search techniques used. Most articles that involved gender differences or comparisons only are not included. Such research has frequently been conducted with either explicit or implicit assumptions of male superiority, and is less useful for understanding *women's* sexuality.

During these years the most important explosion of literature concerns AIDS and AIDS prevention. There are several articles in this review about women's sexuality that were conducted directly or indirectly because of AIDS. Although the "sexual revolution" brought sexuality, and particularly women's sexuality, into the open, the AIDS epidemic has both pushed sexuality back into the bedroom, and made it front page news.

In the area of women's sexuality and AIDS, most of the research tries to describe women's sexual behaviors, with the primary purpose of educating women to prevent AIDS or AIDS transmission. Women who have been especially targeted are prostitutes, young heterosexually active women, and African-American women.

The most exciting additions to knowledge about women's sexuality published during these years include the number of articles concerning sexuality in diverse groups of women. Although the majority of articles in the chapter address white North American women, articles also address women from Africa, Asia, Australia, Europe, and South America. There are also articles on African-American women.

There are articles on adolescent, young adult, midlife, and old women. Further, there are articles concerning the sexuality of disabled women and inner-city women. Several articles concern lesbians and one article concerns transsexuals. Although the diversity is great, much more is needed.

Many articles in this chapter concern the sexuality of women experiencing various health or medical problems. Topics that were covered in volumes one and two of *Women's Health Perspectives: An Annual Review* included hysterectomy, cervical cancer, diabetes mellitus, pregnancy, and the menstrual cycle. New to this review of the literature are liver disease, multiple sclerosis, chemical dependency, and incest. As suggested by the number of medical articles in this review, the trend of medical and/or male control (including psychologists as well as physicians) of women and our sexuality continues.

Several of the studies emphasized concepts of importance to men rather than to women and clearly used traditional definitions of sexuality. For example, coital alignment and sexually explicit materials are topics of little interest to most women.

Studies about the Grafenberg spot and/or female ejaculation were included in each of the prior editions of this chapter. This time there were studies in which women were asked about their experience of the G-spot and female ejaculation, another study where researchers themselves tried to locate women's G-spots and produce ejaculations, and an essay about social construction.

These kinds of studies are consistent with the need to "help" women with their sexuality, but the particular "problem," as well as who defines the problem is often determined by men. This review includes work by physicians, psychologists, and nurses that aims to help women with their sexuality.

The focus of medical treatment is diagnosis and cure; consequently, medical personnel desire to help women with sexual problems related to various health problems. Unfortunately, many times the sexual "problems" result from the *treatment* of the health problem rather than from the problem itself. A desire to prevent sexual problems, rather than simply treat them, would be more helpful to women.

Women need to understand their sexuality, and medical descriptions can add to that understanding, but it would be most useful if women would define their sexuality. Women's health educators and researchers have encouraged a woman-oriented redefinition of sexuality. Women will define their own sexuality when given the space and time to do so. In her article, Simmonds specifically encourages black women to define their sexuality.

We still need a thorough understanding of "normal" women's sexuality, as we experience and describe it, rather than the medical view of women's sexuality as problematic. This means that there will not be one definition of women's sexuality, but rather, multiple definitions for diverse women.

To have women-oriented definitions of sexuality there must be more descriptions by women themselves about their sexuality. A few writers and/or researchers in this review did not pre-define sexuality. This perspective allowed women themselves to describe their sexuality or certain aspects of their sexuality, such as fantasy and preference for a circumcised partner.

When researchers pre-define sexuality and ask questions related to that definition, women most likely will respond to the researcher's definition. They may give completely different responses if asked open-ended questions. Greater use of qualitative methods seems to be what is needed to help women (re-)define their sexuality as they experience it.

Although it seems obvious that the context of women's lives affects sexuality, that fact has not often been included in research about women's sexuality, and is specifically missing in much of the newer physiological research on women's sexuality.

Another measure of who defines women's sexuality may be who conducts the research and writes the articles. The majority of articles in this chapter have at least one woman author. Moreover, the articles written by women only appear different from those by men in that women used more broad definitions of sexuality. In addition, when women head the research team, they may have final decision-making authority, and thus be more likely to take a women-oriented stance toward the research.

The articles concerning sexual dysfunction demonstrate this point. The research team headed by a woman (Osborn et al.) used a very different definition of sexual dysfunction than did the male writers of the other articles on dysfunction. Osborn et al. used a liberal definition of sexual dysfunction to define dysfunction in their population. They also asked the women in the study if the women thought they had experienced a sexual dysfunction; very few said they did, though they were not asked to describe what they meant or how they personally decided that they did or did not have a sexual dysfunction. Nonetheless, women's definitions may look quite different from traditional definitions.

In conclusion, trends observed in the literature over the past five years include: (1) emphasis on describing women's sexuality for AIDS prevention, (2) greater inclusion of a diversity of women, (3) women's sexuality continues to be defined by a masculine medical model, and (4) women-oriented definitions and descriptions of sexuality are becoming more prevalent.

BOOKS

Adamopoulos, D. A., Kampyli, S., Georgiacodis, F., Kapolia, N., & Abrahamian-Michalakis, A. (1988). Effects of antiandrogen-estrogen treatment on sexual and endocrine parameters in hirsute women. *Archives of Sexual Behavior, 17*(5), 421–429.

The purpose of this study was to investigate the effect of androgen on women's sexuality. Hirsute heterosexual women were treated with an antiandrogen and estradiol which resulted in reduced levels of free testosterone. There was no change in the amount of sexual activity (masturbation and intercourse), but after two months of treatment there was more frequent intercourse and less frequent masturbation. The authors conclude that this change may be due to improved feelings of self (since the hirsutism was reduced) that allowed the women to increase their sexual activity with partners. The overall conclusion was that androgen did not show any effects on the women's sexuality.

Alder, E., & Bancroft, J. (1988). The relationship between breast feeding persistence, sexuality and mood in postpartum women. *Psychological Medicine, 18,* 389–396.

This is a study conducted in Scotland of 91 primiparous women who were interviewed during and after pregnancy. Regardless of method of feeding the infant, there was a decline in sexuality postpartum. However, when compared to "artificial" feeders, at three months postpartum, breastfeeders waited longer to resume intercourse, experienced greater pain with intercourse, and reported decreased interest and enjoyment of sex. By six months postpartum the only difference between the groups was that breastfeeders still experienced dyspareunia. The authors acknowledge that sexuality postpartum is not simply related to breastfeeding but is multifactorial; however, the results should be useful for women who are concerned when they experience a decrease in sexual feelings postpartum. They can be counselled that they may expect their feelings to return before six months.

Andersen, B. L., Anderson, B., & deProsse, C. (1989). Controlled prospective longitudinal study of women with cancer: I. Sexual functioning outcomes. *Journal of Consulting and Clinical Psychology, 57*(6), 683–691.

The first author has conducted several studies concerning sexuality in women with cancer. This is another prospective study, comparing women with gynecologic cancers with women who have benign gynecologic disease and women who have no apparent gynecologic disease. The results showed no global sexual behavior disruption in women with gynecologic cancers, but 30 percent of the women experienced sexual dysfunctions, as diagnosed by DSM-III criteria. Of interest was that sexual excitement was diminished for women experiencing both cancer and benign gynecologic disease, but more so for the women with cancer. The most useful aspect of the article is that the authors propose directions for interventions to minimize sexual difficulties in women with cancer.

Arthritis Foundation. (1990). *Living and loving: Information about sex.* Atlanta: The Foundation.

This patient education pamphlet provides brief, but helpful guidelines for women who have arthritis to think of their sexuality in broad terms. It also provides line drawings and descriptions of positions for sexual intercourse for women with specific arthritic joints.

Bach, N., Schaffner, F., & Kapelman, B. (1989). Sexual behavior in women with nonalcoholic liver disease. *Hepatology, 9*(5), 698–703.

The authors believe their study to be the first that has investigated the relationship between sexual functioning and liver disease in women. Basically no differences were found between women in this study and the results of other large studies of sexuality in "normal" adult women; thus, the authors conclude that women with liver disease can experience normal sexual relations. One very positive component of the article is that the data gathering instrument is included. Other researchers interested in

studying this population of women might use the instrument and thus be able to compare results.

Bachmann, G. A. (1990). Psychosexual aspects of hysterectomy. *Women's Health Issues, 1*(1), 41–49.

This is a comprehensive review of research studies and general articles, between 1941 and 1989, concerning the emotional and sexual effects of hysterectomy on women. Although there is no consensus in the literature, Bachmann concludes that women with hysterectomies and *without* oophorectomies should not have sexual difficulties, unless they have personal characteristics or consequences that would put them at risk. She encourages physicians to identify preoperatively the characteristics of women at risk and to provide them with counselling and education before surgery. She does not address women with hysterectomies *and* oophorectomies, even though the literature review strongly suggests that these women may very well experience sexual difficulties following hysterectomy.

Bachmann, G. A., Leiblum, S. R., & Grill, J. (1989). Brief sexual inquiry in gynecologic practice. *Obstetrics and Gynecology, 73*(3, Part 1), 425–427.

The purpose of this research was to determine whether a brief sexual inquiry (two or three questions) would elicit sexual concerns from women in a private gynecology practice. The impetus was the recognition by gynecologists that they should assess sexual concerns, but the recognition that such assessment was frequently not performed. Over a 15-month period 887 women, ages 12–78 years, were questioned. Three percent of the women shared sexual concerns as the reason for their visit. An additional 16 percent shared sexual concerns when the brief sexual inquiry was used. The concern shared by almost half of the women was dyspareunia. Other studies have reported a much higher incidence of sexual problems among women, and the authors propose reasons why their numbers are smaller. However, it is unfortunate that physicians must limit their assessment of women's sexual concerns to two or three questions. A more thorough assessment probably would uncover other problems that may be even more serious for women's health.

Bahen-Auger, N., Wilson, M., & Assalian, P. (1988). Sexual response of the type I diabetic woman. *Medical Aspects of Human Sexuality, 22*(10), 94–100.

The manner in which the data are presented in this brief article makes it somewhat difficult to understand, but the topic of the research is important. Studies of sexuality in diabetic women should identify whether the women have Type I or Type II diabetes. In this study, sexual variables were compared by length of time Type I diabetic women had the disease. Illustrative case studies reinforce the findings.

Bailey, V. R. (1989). Sexuality—Before and after birth. *Midwives Chronicle and Nursing Notes, 102*(1212), 24–26.

This is a brief, but accurate discussion of the changes in sexuality experienced by many women during pregnancy, labor and delivery, and postpartum. Most of the changes discussed are those related to sexual intercourse. Suggestions are provided for women and their partners about how to manage the changes. The author acknowledges that there is very little empirical evidence that documents the changes she describes.

Bancroft, J., Sherwin, B. B., Alexander, G. M., Davidson, D. W., & Walker, A. (1991). Oral contraceptives, androgens, and the sexuality of young women: I. A comparison of sexual experience, sexual attitudes, and gender roles in oral contraceptive users and nonusers. *Archives of Sexual Behavior, 20*(2), 105–120.

Bancroft, J., Sherwin, B. B., Alexander, G. M., Davidson, D. W., & Walker, A. (1991). Oral contraceptives, androgens, and the sexuality of young women: II. The role of androgens. *Archives of Sexual Behavior, 20*(2), 121–135.

These two papers report the results of a study that compared 55 college student oral contraceptive users with 53 nonusers. The mean age of both groups was 21.6 years. Pill users reported more liberal sexual attitudes and interactions than nonusers, but there were no differences in masturbation and fantasy. Although the researchers expected to find an "activating effect" of free testosterone (blood levels) on sexual behavior in both groups, that was not the result. There was an association between testosterone levels and sex with a partner, but not masturbation in contraceptive users; and the results were opposite for the nonusers. The authors attempted to explain their "paradoxical" results by suggesting that activation effects were obscured by psychosocial factors. Although other research has suggested that testosterone is important in sexual functioning, this study did not show that. It may be the small sample or the young age of the participants, but researchers should acknowledge their findings and conduct further studies before accepting (or rejecting) developing theory.

Bergstrom-Walan, M., & Nielsen, H. H. (1990). Sexual expression among 60–80 year old men and women: A sample from Stockholm, Sweden. *Journal of Sex Research, 27*(2), 289–295.

The results of a random survey of old Swedes is presented, and comparisons by gender are made. Attitudes toward sexuality were liberal. Sexual activity and importance decreased with advancing age; however, 50 percent of the women reported that sexuality was important to them. Of those with a partner, 57 percent still engage in intercourse, and one-third of all the women masturbate. Twenty-nine percent reported no sexual satisfaction. These are interesting descriptive results from a population typically perceived as sexually liberated. However, since it is survey data, no explanations can be determined.

Bernhard, L. A. (1992). Consequences of hysterectomy in the lives of women. *Health Care for Women International, 13*(3), 281–291.

Sixty-three women who underwent hysterectomy were followed for about two years. Three months after surgery, the women's sexuality was significantly improved from the day before surgery. However, nearly two years after hysterectomy, the women were not as positive about their sexual or other outcomes of hysterectomy. This was a small study, but its longitudinal aspect is a strength. It may be that something changes over time that causes a negative, long-term sexual outcome for some women following hysterectomy, even though the short-term outcome appears positive. More research is needed.

Bishop, G. (1989). Sex and UTI in older women. *Medical Aspects of Human Sexuality*, 23(11), 65–69.

This article is primarily an admonition to primary physicians who care for older women that if the women present with dysuria, the cause may be urethral trauma resulting from sexual activity. Because many physicians do not think older women are sexual, and because many older women are embarrassed to discuss their sexuality, the cause of many urinary tract infections may be undiagnosed. Physicians are urged to conduct sexual histories to determine whether sexual activity may be the cause of infection. Prevention of continued infections may be possible if women can modify their sexual activities; for example, with less vigorous activity or the use of vaginal creams.

Brashear, D. B., & Munsick, R. A. (1991). Hymenal dyspareunia. *Journal of Sex Education and Therapy*, 17(1), 27–31.

The authors surveyed 31 women who had undergone hymenectomies for treatment of dyspareunia. Prior to surgery, all women had inadequate hymenal ruptures. All but three of the women reported improvement or relief of the pain, and 77 percent said the surgery significantly improved their sex lives. Many of these women had been to more than one physician seeking help for the dyspareunia, but did not receive it. This study demonstrates a physical source of dyspareunia that was apparently discounted by gynecologists as unimportant and/or psychological.

Bretschneider, J. G., & McCoy, N. L. (1988). Sexual interest and behavior in healthy 80- to 102-year-olds. *Archives of Sexual Behavior*, 17(2), 109–129.

This very interesting study was conducted with physically and mentally healthy elderly persons living in retirement facilities in California. They tended to be well-educated and of middle and upper socioeconomic status. Even though this is a select sample, it is a sample of both women and men that have barely been studied with regard to sexuality. The three most frequently experienced sexual activities (touching and caressing without sexual intercourse, masturbation, and sexual intercourse) were the same for women as they were for men, but more men engaged in the activities. However, 53 percent of the men reported having a sexual partner, while only 25 percent of the women did. Correlations between past and present frequency and enjoyment of sexual behaviors were strong for all activities except sexual intercourse.

Catania, J. A., Dolcini, M. M., Coates, T. J., Kegeles, S. M., Greenblatt, R. M., Puckett, S., Corman, M., & Miller, J. (1989). Predictors of condom use and multiple-partnered sex among sexually-active adolescent women: Implications for AIDS-related health interventions. *Journal of Sex Research*, 26(4), 514–524.

Considerable research is now being conducted concerning condom use as an AIDS prevention measure. This study was conducted with primarily white young women from blue collar families in a high AIDS-incidence area (California). The mean age was 17.9 years. All of the women were heterosexual and sexually active. The mean frequency of vaginal intercourse in the previous two months was 15.1 times, but the mean frequency of condom use in the previous two months was only 2.6. The only statistically significant predictors of condom use among these women were greater enjoyment of condoms and greater willingness to request partners to use condoms. Thus, the authors suggest that when intervening with adolescents for AIDS prevention, ways must be found for adolescents to enjoy condom use. Although there is concern that prediction of condom use is insufficient for AIDS prevention, it is a starting point for working with women whose sexual behaviors put themselves at risk for developing AIDS, now or in the future.

Charmoli, M. C., & Athelstan, G. T. (1988). Incest as related to sexual problems in women. *Journal of Psychology and Human Sexuality*, 1(1), 53–66.

In this survey, adult women who had experienced incest were compared with adult women who had not experienced incest. The results are consistent with other studies on this topic that show that women who experienced incest reported significantly more vaginal problems, negative emotional reactions to sex, and compulsive sex behaviors than did women who have not experienced incest. One difference between the findings of this and other studies was that these women did not report differences with regard to orgasm. Variables associated with the greater number of sexual problems were perpetrator at least six years older than the victim, victim less than eight years of age at onset, occurrences more often than once per month, and negative reactions of others when she told them about the experience. The authors are careful to not generalize the findings because many of the incest survivors were in therapy at the time of the study, but consistency of the results with other research suggests that much work needs to be done to aid survivors in terms of their sexuality, but even more importantly, to work for the prevention of childhood sexual abuse.

Cole, E., & Rothblum, E. D. (1991). Lesbian sex at menopause: As good as or better than ever. In B. Sang, J. Warshow, & A. J. Smith (Eds.), *Lesbians at midlife: The creative transition* (pp. 184–193). San Francisco: Spinsters Book Company.

According to the authors, this was the first systematic study of lesbian sexuality at menopause. The sample included 41 Caucasian lesbians whose mean age was 51.5 years. Most of these women reported sex as good as or better than before menopause, and they emphasized sexuality in relationships. Any "changes" in sexuality were described as "differences," rather than "problems." The authors acknowledge several methodological limitations of the study, but the study is still valuable as a beginning understanding of one unique aspect of lesbian sexuality.

Cole, E., & Rothblum, E. D. (Eds.). (1989). *Women and sex therapy.* Binghamton, NY: Haworth. (Published as *Women and Therapy*, Vol. 7, Nos. 2/3, 1988).

Although the editors indicate that this volume is addressed to mental health professionals who want to learn more about sex therapy issues for women and to sex therapists who are interested in women's perspectives, the volume is useful to anyone who is interested in broad perspectives about the role of sexuality in women's lives. The papers, written by a variety of professionals, include topics that are divided into the sections of historical and political perspectives, theoretical considerations, physiological conditions and issues, and clinical implications for particular populations. Attention was paid to inclusion of not only diverse topics, such as infertility, AIDS, and interstitial cystitis, as well as sexual abuse and dysfunction, but also to diverse groups of women, such as ethnic and minority women, lesbians and bisexuals, as well as divorced and disabled women. This volume is a valuable resource for a better understanding of women's sexuality as defined by women.

Conway-Turner, K. (1992). Sex, intimacy and self esteem: The case of the African-American older woman. *Journal of Women and Aging, 4*(1), 91–104.

This is a very interesting, beginning study of urban, old, noninstitutionalized, married African-American women (mean age, 75 years).

The women were interviewed and completed questionnaires about their intimate relationships and their self-esteem. Similar to studies of old white women, these women kissed and sexually touched their partners frequently, and these behaviors were positively associated with self-esteem. However, the frequency of sexual intercourse depended on the health of the partner.

Dackman, L. (1990). *Up front: Sex and the post-mastectomy woman.* New York: Viking.

A 34-year-old heterosexually experienced, single woman tells the story of her own mastectomy, reconstruction, and the re-establishing of her sexuality. The focus is on her mastectomy, not on cancer. Issues related to dating and telling men about her surgery are covered in detail, and she clearly reports a "no fairy tale" ending. The book would be very valuable for young, single women who face or have had mastectomies.

Darling, C. A., Davidson, J. K., Sr., & Conway-Welch, C. (1990). Female ejaculation: Perceived origins, the Grafenberg spot/area, and sexual responsiveness. *Archives of Sexual Behavior, 19*(1), 29–47.

Darling, C. A., Davidson, J. K., Sr., & Cox, R. P. (1991). Female sexual response and the timing of partner orgasm. *Journal of Sex and Marital Therapy, 17*(1), 3–21.

Darling, C. A., Davidson, J. K., Sr., & Jennings, D. A. (1991). The female sexual response revisited: Understanding the multiorgasmic experience in women. *Archives of Sexual Behavior, 20*(6), 527–540.

Davidson, J. K., Sr., & Darling, C. A. (1989). Self-perceived differences in the female orgasmic response. *Family Practice Research Journal, 8*(2), 75–84.

Davidson, J. K., Sr., & Darling, C. A. (1988). The sexually experienced woman: Multiple sex partners and sexual satisfaction. *Journal of Sex Research, 24,* 141–154.

Davidson, J. K., Sr., Darling, C. A., & Conway-Welch, C. (1989). The role of the Grafenberg spot and female ejaculation in the female orgasmic response: An empirical analysis. *Journal of Sex and Marital Therapy, 15*(2), 102–120.

These six articles all report findings of a large (n = 2,175) anonymous survey of professional nurses from 16 states. Each article focuses on a separate analysis of some subsample (typically about 800 heterosexual married women) who completed certain questions on the 122-item questionnaire. Titles of the articles include the specific variables described in each article, but most concern orgasm and ways women achieve or do not achieve orgasm and satisfaction in their sexual relationships. Literature reviews are carefully done for each article. Many significant differences are reported, but the authors do not acknowledge that these differences could be due primarily to the large sample, and the use of individual items for correlations. Nonetheless, this is an interesting research study which helps to describe the sexuality of a specific group of women.

DeHaan, C. B., & Wallander, J. L. (1988). Self-concept, sexual knowledge and attitudes, and parental support in the sexual adjustment of women with early- and late-onset physical disability. *Archives of Sexual Behavior, 17*(2), 145–161.

Since so few studies of sexuality in disabled women have been conducted, this is an important study of sexuality among women disabled by neuromuscular or orthopedic conditions. College students who were nondisabled were compared with students disabled after the age of 18 (late-onset) and those disabled from birth or before the age of three (early-onset). The early-onset disabled women were significantly different from the other two groups in frequency and satisfaction with sexual activities. Women with late-onset disabilities differed from nondisabled women only in the difference between their desired and actual enjoyment of sexual activities. However, self-concept, sexual knowledge, and parental support for sexual development did not differ among the groups. The results suggest a need for more research that could explain reasons why women with early-onset disabilities have more sexual problems, and could develop methods to assist women who have such disabilities with their sexuality.

Dow, M. G. T., & Gallagher, J. (1989). A controlled study of combined hormonal and psychological treatment for sexual unresponsiveness in women. *British Journal of Clinical Psychology*, 28, 201–212.

Thirty heterosexual couples, in whom the primary complaint was sexual unresponsiveness in the (premenopausal) woman were randomly assigned to one of three treatments: sexual counselling plus testosterone, sexual counselling plus placebo, or testosterone only. When compared to the testosterone only group, both counselling groups had significant improvements in several measures of sexuality. The authors conclude that testosterone therapy has no advantage over sexual counselling for treatment of a general population of couples experiencing sexual unresponsiveness in the woman. The study was conducted in Australia and shows that medication cannot simply be used to treat a presumed female sexual dysfunction.

Eichel, E. W., Eichel, J. D., & Kale, S. (1988). The technique of coital alignment and its relation to female orgasmic response and simultaneous orgasm. *Journal of Sex and Marital Therapy*, 14(2), 129–141.

The purpose of this article was primarily to describe the Alignment technique, a position for sexual intercourse said to enhance women's orgasm during intercourse, as well as to aid in simultaneous orgasm for the couple. A small sample of persons who had been taught the technique were compared with a sample of persons who had not been taught the technique. The women who had learned the technique reported significantly greater satisfaction concerning several aspects of orgasm that were studied. However, the technique requires considerable physical, emotional, and attitudinal behaviors on the part of both partners for it to be employed. It clearly places emphasis for the

sexual activity on orgasm, which is probably not most women's primary interest. Further, even though it may increase sexual satisfaction, it is not very practical, and one might wonder how many women and couples could actually use it for any of their sexual encounters.

Evans, B. A., Bond, R. A., & Macrae, K. D. (1988). Sexual behaviour in women attending a genitourinary medicine clinic. *Genitourinary Medicine*, 64, 43–48.

The purpose of this study was to determine the incidence of women's sexual behaviors that may place them at risk for sexually transmitted diseases, including AIDS. One thousand women, ages 14 to 75 who attended a genitourinary clinic in London were surveyed. Over half of the women had five or more sexual partners in their lifetime, but only 9 percent had had that number in the past year. One-fifth of the women practiced anal intercourse and 70 percent practiced fellatio. Black women had fewer numbers of partners, and participated less frequently than white women in both anal intercourse and fellatio. Although the motivation for these types of studies is disease, they do provide data that describes at least some of women's sexual activities.

Fisher, W. A., & Gray, J. (1988). Erotophobia-erotophilia and sexual behavior during pregnancy and postpartum. *Journal of Sex Research*, 25(3), 379-396.

Erotophobia-erotophilia is a learned personality characteristic, now determined through research to determine a person's general avoidance or approach of sexuality. The concept was studied in 50 married couples, where the woman was in the second trimester of pregnancy; 25 couples also responded two-to-three months postpartum. Results showed that erotophilic women were more interested in sex, engaged in sexual behavior more frequently, were more sexually satisfied, and were more willing to experiment with new sexual techniques during their pregnancies than were erotophobic women. Further, the erotophilic women resumed intercourse sooner postpartum and were more likely to breastfeed their infants than were erotophobic women. This was correlational research, and although the concept of erotophobia-erotophilia seems to be a predictor of women's sexual behavior during later pregnancy and postpartum, causation cannot be assumed. It seems unlikely that a single variable is the determining factor in prediction of something as complex[a] as sexual behavior during pregnancy and postpartum.

Freund, M., Leonard, T. L., & Lee, N. (1989). Sexual behavior of resident street prostitutes with their clients in Camden, New Jersey. *Journal of Sex Research*, 26(4), 460–478.

A concern about heterosexual transmission of AIDS between female prostitutes and their paying and non-paying partners prompted this descriptive study of the sexual behaviors performed by prostitutes in one urban area. Twenty female prostitutes, with a mean age of 30 years, most of whom were other than Caucasian, were interviewed during the daytime, while they were working, concerning their sexual activities of the previous 24 hours. Each prostitute was interviewed at least five times over a seven-month period. The most frequent type of contact was penile-oral, almost three times more common than penile-vaginal. Kissing and penile-anal contact were rare. The prostitutes reported having about four clients per day, and they worked four or five days each week. Repeat contacts with the same clients accounted for about half of the prostitutes' sexual contacts. Condoms were used in 74 percent of the sexual contacts described in the study, and most of the prostitutes reported working during their menstrual periods. The results of this study show that both these women and their sexual partners are at high risk for the development of AIDS. It is unfortunate that the motivation for this study was AIDS rather than women's health or sexuality. Prostitutes have had considerable blame placed on them for the spread of AIDS, but because AIDS is transmitted more easily from male to female, the prostitute herself (as well as her paying and non-paying partners) should be concerned about acquiring AIDS.

George, W. H., Gournic, S. J., & McAfee, M. P. (1988). Perceptions of postdrinking female sexuality: Effects of gender, beverage choice, and drink payment. *Journal of Applied Social Psychology*, 18(15), 1295–1317.

This research was conducted to study the ways in which persons view women's drinking of alcohol and its effects on their sexuality. College students responded to vignettes about a heterosexual couple on a date. Both male and female students reported the woman in the vignette to be more sexual (but less socially skillful and more aggressive) if she drank alcohol than if she drank cola. Further, if a man paid for the drinks, rather than the woman paying for her own, the subjects also rated the woman's sexuality as enhanced. These results validate popular beliefs held, especially by college age young people, that women's sexuality is enhanced by drinking alcohol. Unfortunately, these types of misconceptions may lead to unwanted sexual activity or rape for young women.

Glatt, A. E., Zinner, S. H., & McCormack, W. M. (1990). The prevalence of dyspareunia. *Obstetrics and Gynecology*, 75(3, Part 1), 433–436.

For this study dyspareunia was defined as "pain or discomfort in the labial, vaginal, or pelvic area during or after sexual intercourse." A survey of 314 women, in their 30s provided the data. Using content analysis 39 percent of the women had never had dyspareunia, 27.5 percent had experienced dyspareunia which had resolved, and 33.5 percent had dyspareunia at the time of the study. Most of the women had discussed it with their partners, but not with anyone else, including their physicians. Most did not know the cause of their problem. Although a broad definition of dyspareunia was used, the incidence is relatively high and of concern, since dyspareunia limits women's sexual expression.

Goldstein, M. K. (1991). Gynecologic factors in sexual dysfunction of the older woman. *Clinics in Geriatric Medicine*, 7(1), 41–61.

The authors reviewed literature on sexual dysfunction in older women, and although they define sexual dysfunction as problems with sexual desire, arousal, orgasm and coital pain; the literature they reviewed covers many other sexual problems. The authors also reviewed studies on prevalence of sexual concerns in old women, but conclude that the prevalence is unknown. The article is written for clinicians and encourages them to take seriously old women's sexuality.

Hagstad, A. (1988). Gynecology and sexuality in middle-aged women. *Women and Health, 13*(3/4), 57–80.

A random sample of women 37 to 46 years of age living in Goteborg, Sweden was used for this study. The participation rate was 77 percent, so the results should be very representative of urban Swedish women in midlife. Furthermore, a strength of the study is that a clinical population was *not* used. The first part of the article deals with gynecological health, and the latter part involves sexual health. Almost all of the women reported a stable sexual relationship and considered sexual activity important for a relationship. However, over half of the women reported a coital frequency that differed from their desired frequency. Almost all experienced orgasm with intercourse and, although the majority had masturbated, the frequency of masturbation was very low. These results are very interesting for they represent what can be assumed to be typical sexual behaviors for a specific group of women. More studies like this one would be helpful for understanding women's sexuality.

Hallstrom, T., & Samuelsson, S. (1990). Changes in women's sexual desire in middle life: The longitudinal study of women in Gothenburg. *Archives of Sexual Behavior, 19*(3), 259–268.

This study of 497 Swedish midlife women measured sexual desire at two times, six years apart. Two-thirds of the women reported no change in desire; most of those who changed reported less desire after six years. No women over 50 reported strong sexual desire. The study demonstrates general stability of libido

in midlife women. The strength of the study is self-report rather than lab measurement.

Hart, J., Cohen, E., Gingold, A., & Homburg, R. (1991). Sexual behavior in pregnancy: A study of 219 women. *Journal of Sex Education and Therapy, 17*(2), 86–90.

The purpose of this study was to describe married Israeli women's sexual behavior during pregnancy. Women were invited to participate two-to-four days postpartum; 26 percent of those approached refused participation on religious grounds. Results showed a gradual decline in libido and coital frequency during pregnancy, greatest in the third trimester and greater in women with high libido before pregnancy. Half the women reported dyspareunia at some time during the pregnancy. This study is consistent with other similar studies, but adds information about a unique population of women who have been less studied.

Heiman, J. R., Rowland, D. L., Hatch, J. P., & Gladue, B. A. (1991). Psychophysiological and endocrine responses to sexual arousal in women. *Archives of Sexual Behavior, 20*(2), 171–186.

This laboratory study was conducted to determine whether a biological (endocrine) mechanism facilitates sexual arousal. Thirteen volunteers submitted to biological and psychological measurement of their sexual arousal during and after viewing sexually explicit videotapes. Differences between the control and experimental group were identified, but could be explained in different ways. This study suffers from a small sample as well as its attempt to explain women's sexuality on the basis of women viewing films which they may or may not prefer for sexual arousal.

Herold, E. S., & Way, L. (1988). Sexual self-disclosure among university women. *Journal of Sex Research, 24*, 1–14.

Using a newly developed tool to measure sexual self-disclosure, based on Jourard's Self-Disclosure Questionnaire, the authors studied a convenience sample of 203 college women, ages 18 to 22. The women were asked about the level of their sexual self-disclosure to their mother, father, close female friend, and dating partner. The women were classified as virgin or nonvirgin on the basis of having participated in sexual intercourse. The amount of reported sexual self-disclosure was fairly low overall, and particularly low to parents. The only difference between virgins and nonvirgins with regard to amount of sexual self-disclosure was that nonvirgins were more disclosing to their dating partners. Because the tool is new and psychometrics have not been established, and because of the non-random and relatively small sample, few conclusions can be made, though the data seem to affirm an assumption that women rarely reveal themselves sexually.

Holland, J., Ramazanoglu, C., & Scott, S. (1990). Managing risk and experiencing danger: Tensions between government AIDS education policy and young women's sexuality. *Gender and Education*, 2(2), 125–146.

Holland, J., Ramazanoglu, C., Scott, S., Sharpe, S., & Thomson, R. (1990). Sex, gender and power: Young women's sexuality in the shadow of AIDS. *Sociology of Health and Illness*, 12(3), 336–350.

These two articles concern an AIDS project for 16–21 year-old-women in London and Manchester, England. The project involves discovering the processes these young women use to define their sexuality and sexual practices, as well as the implications these processes have for the sexual transmission of HIV. These young women most typically defined sex as penile-vaginal intercourse with male orgasm. A feminist analysis related to issues of power and control shows that these women perceive little control over their heterosexual relationships, even though some do resist male pressure.

House, W. C., Faulk, A., & Kubovchik, M. (1990). Sexual behavior of inner-city women. *Journal of Sex Education and Therapy*, 16(3), 172–184.

Poor urban young women attending a family planning clinic were interviewed about their sexuality. The only significant difference by race was that white women reported a higher desired frequency for sex than black women. The women were generally satisfied with their sexual relationships, though only 31 percent reported ever masturbating. The results were contrasted with other studies of middle class women and provide interesting data to begin to understand possible differences in women's sexuality by class.

Hurlbert, D. F. (1991). The role of assertiveness in female sexuality: A comparative study between sexually assertive and sexually nonassertive women. *Journal of Sex and Marital Therapy*, 17(3), 183–190.

Using a tool for sexual assertiveness that he developed (and is printed in the article), 100 healthy women, married to military men, were categorized using a median split, as sexually assertive or nonassertive. The women kept a diary of their sexual desire, activity, and orgasms for four weeks. Sexually assertive women had higher frequencies of sexual activity and orgasms, greater subjective sexual desire, and greater marital and sexual satisfaction. The author suggests that these results support sexual assertiveness training for women. The assumption is clearly that more is better; however, this is not what many women would say. Moreover, the unstated purpose of the study seems to be to get more women into sexual counselling/therapy.

Hurlbert, D. F., & Whittaker, K. E. (1991). The role of masturbation in marital and sexual satisfaction: A comparative study of female masturbators and nonmasturbators. *Journal of Sex Education and Therapy*, 17(4), 272–282.

Hurlbert again studied women married to military men to determine the relationship between masturbation to orgasm and nonmasturbation. Women who masturbated to orgasm ($n = 41$) were matched with women who had never masturbated to orgasm ($n = 41$). Using a variety of quantitative measures, women who masturbated had significantly more orgasms, greater sexual desire and satisfaction, higher self-esteem, and were aroused more quickly than women who did not masturbate. This study, although limited by its lack of qualitative information, shows some of the benefits of masturbation for women.

Jani, N. N., & Wise, T. N. (1988). Antidepressants and inhibited female orgasm: A literature review. *Journal of Sex and Marital Therapy, 14*(4), 279–284.

Segraves, R. T. (1988). Psychiatric drugs and inhibited female orgasm. *Journal of Sex and Marital Therapy, 14*(3), 202–207.

These two articles review literature that suggests that antidepressant and antipsychotic medications affect orgasm in women. The effect may be decreased strength of orgasm, increased time to reach orgasm, or inability to have orgasm. The physiologic mechanism is not understood, but several hypotheses are given. Since women are frequently prescribed these medications, study of their effects is important. The authors, all psychiatrists, encourage assessment of women's sexual function when taking these drugs.

Jindal, U. N., & Dhall, G. I. (1990). Psychosexual problems of infertile women in India. *International Journal of Infertility, 35*(4), 222–225.

Two hundred women (122 Hindus and 78 Sikhs) seen consecutively at a tertiary care infertility clinic in India were interviewed about the psychosexual aspects of their infertility. Half (n = 105, 52%) reported at least one psychosexual difficulty. The most frequently reported problem (n = 81) was anorgasmia; however, 52 of the women also indicated that they were not worried about this problem. Decreased frequency of intercourse was the next most frequently reported problem (n = 56). Women believed the lack of intercourse was related to their loss of libido, subsequent to their unfulfilled aim of pregnancy. The authors report that in India the cultural pressure

on males to have a child (i.e., son) is so great that their entire sexual relationship is oriented toward the goal of fertility. Moreover, women are *always* assumed at blame for an infertility problem; infertility in males is not believed possible. Consequently, infertile women are thought unimportant and worthless.

Kahn, A. P., & Holt, L. H. (1990). *The A—Z of women's sexuality.* New York: Facts on File.

This book, written for a general audience, is a dictionary of terms concerning sexuality and reproduction. Although the definitions are somewhat simplistic, it is useful, and there are many cross-referenced terms. The book also contains an extensive bibliography, divided into topical areas.

Kane, S. (1990). AIDS, addiction, and condom use: Sources of sexual risk for heterosexual women. *Journal of Sex Research, 27*(3), 427–444.

Two case studies of African-American women—one an IV drug user and the other, a partner of an IV drug user—are presented and analyzed. These cases come from an AIDS prevention project on the South Side of Chicago, which began with an attempt to understand women's sexual behavior. The author concludes that the cultural context and how that context is shaped and experienced by each individual woman affects greatly the kinds of risk-reducing behavior that she will use.

Kehoe, M. (1988). Lesbian relationships and homosexuality. *Journal of Homosexuality, 16*(3/4), 43–52.

Each article in this issue presents different results of a survey of 100 lesbians over 60 years of age. Topics include lifestyle, social life, services for older women, family, health, and demographics. This article concerns sexuality and relationships. The author concluded from the total survey that sexuality was not a major concern of these women. Over half of the women had not engaged in any sexual activity within the past year; friendship and intimacy seemed to be more important than sex. The author acknowledges the lack of representativeness of the sample; however, the importance of the study must also be acknowledged. To understand sexuality in all women, from their own perspectives, this type of study must be conducted. It is interesting and informative.

Kippax, S., Crawford, J., Waldby, C., & Benton, P. (1990). Women negotiating heterosex: Implications for AIDS prevention. *Women's Studies International Forum, 13*(6), 533–542.

This is a very interesting report of results of a study of midlife Australian women's sexuality using the method of memory work (which is described). The purpose was to examine women's sexual negotiations prior to AIDS, under the assumption that women's sexual negotiations have probably changed since AIDS. The authors conclude that a permissive, rather than a restrictive, discourse about sexuality is necessary for educating women about AIDS prevention.

Kockett, G., & Fahrner, E. M. (1988). Male-to-female and female-to-male transsexuals: A comparison. *Archives of Sexual Behavior, 17*(6), 539–546.

This is a follow-up study of 58 transsexuals, 37 male-to-female and 21 female-to-male. Personal interviews regarding partnership and sexual behavior, relationships with family, friends, sex role, occupation, and somatic conditions were conducted with the subjects. The results were consistent with other such studies: female-to-male transsexuals were significantly more likely to be in lasting partnerships and to experience greater sexual satisfaction than were male-to-female transsexuals. The authors' explanation is that female-to-male transsexuals are more likely to have lived the masculine gender role and established a satisfactory relationship before the gender reassignment surgery was performed. Although this may be true in Germany where the study was conducted, that may not be true elsewhere. What was not studied and could be more explanatory is the major gender change

of giving up the social power and status of being male, to become a female with its lack of social power and status.

Kost, K., & Forrest, J. D. (1992). American women's sexual behavior and exposure to risk of sexually transmitted diseases. *Family Planning Perspectives, 24*(6), 244–254.

This analysis of epidemiological data on young women in 1988 and 1989 shows that 70 percent of the women had at least one heterosexual nonmarital sexual partner. The analysis was performed by the Alan Guttmacher Institute, and bias toward marital sexual monogamy is clear. The study was performed to describe women's risk of STDs, including AIDS, simply on the basis of one risk factor—multiple heterosexual partners. Women's having multiple partners was clearly demonstrated, but that avoids consideration of many other risk factors, and does not help us understand women's sexuality.

Lawrence, K., & Herold, E. S. (1988). Women's attitudes toward and experience with sexually explicit materials. *Journal of Sex Research, 24,* 161–169.

This survey was conducted to determine whether women's presumed sexual freedom extended to their attitudes and experience with sexually explicit materials (SEM), which were defined as erotic novels, *Playboy*-type magazines, *Playgirl*-type magazines, and X-rated films. The sample included 198 women who were members of a fitness center in Canada. Attitudes were equally divided between positive and negative. Slightly more than one-third of the women had not used erotic novels in the past year, and over half had not used the other types of materials. For those who had used SEM, the most frequent reason for novels was entertainment. For the other types of SEM the most frequent reason for use was chance occurrence. Consistent with a strong feminist opposition to pornography, a strong feminist orientation was associated with unfavorable attitudes toward SEM and infrequent use. However, for some women SEM is an acceptable part of their sexual experiences. To have a complete understanding of women's sexuality, these perspectives must be studied.

Leiblum, S. R. (1990). Sexuality and the midlife woman. *Psychology of Women Quarterly, 14*(4), 495–508.

This is a literature review of aging, hormonal changes, menopause, and hysterectomy as negative influences on the sexuality of midlife women. The article concludes with brief suggestions about how practitioners might manage the problems discussed. Although the author is to be commended for the review she did, the review only makes clearer the lack of information available about midlife women's sexuality, and that there is a great need for study of the positive, as well as negative, aspects of midlife women's sexuality.

Leigh, B. C. (1989). Reasons for having and avoiding sex: Gender, sexual orientation, and relationship to sexual behavior. *Journal of Sex Research, 26*(2), 199–209.

This study was conducted to identify differences between heterosexual and homosexual women and men with regard to reasons for having and avoiding sex. A large random sample of persons living in San Francisco completed a questionnaire with closed-ended questions. Differences were found between men and women, regardless of sexual orientation, and between heterosexuals and homosexuals regardless of gender. The strongest differences, however, were between men and women, and support previously published information that suggests that women are more likely to engage in sexual behavior for emotional closeness, while men engage in sexual behavior for conquest and sexual pleasure. In all cases the differences were small and the authors suggest that attention be paid to the similarities rather than the differences. Although this is a comparative study the results of heterosexual and lesbian women are of interest in understanding women's sexuality.

Lightfoot-Klein, H. (1989). Rites of purification and their effects: Some psychological aspects of female genital circumcision and infibulation (Pharaonic circumcision) in an Afro-Arab Islamic society (Sudan). *Journal of Psychology and Human Sexuality, 2*(2), 79–91.

Lightfoot-Klein, H. (1989). The sexual experience and marital adjustment of genitally circumcised and infibulated females in the Sudan. *Journal of Sex Research, 26*(3), 375–392.

Even though Pharaonic circumcision was declared illegal under Sudanese law in 1956, the law has never been implemented. The practice is still almost universally performed on young girls in the Sudan, and the day of circumcision is considered to be the most important day of a woman's life. Circumcision is considered the only way of protecting a woman's status and her sexual purity. In these two articles the author presents the findings of her qualitative, anthropological research in the Sudan, during which she interviewed more than 400 persons representing all walks of life. Pharaonic circumcision consists of the excision of the clitoris, labia minora, and the inner parts of the labia majora; and the suturing of the remaining labia majora together so that the only opening is no more than pinhole-sized. At marriage it may take anywhere from days to months for the male to penetrate the female, and with extreme pain to her. After delivery of a baby, the women's infibulation is often resewn. Despite this extreme genital mutilation, and despite the cultural prohibitions of a woman showing any interest in sexual intercourse, most Sudanese women do experience sexual desire, pleasure, and orgasm. Very few of the women interviewed knew that there are other options in the world for what they experience as "normal." The first article focuses more on psychological aspects and the second article on sexual aspects of Pharaonic circumcision, but read together, the articles provide a great deal of information about this extreme form of female mutilation. A more thorough treatment of the subject can be found in the author's book, *Prisoners of Ritual*, Haworth Press, Binghamton, New York, 1989.

Lunde, I., Larsen, G. K., Fog, E., & Garde, K. (1991). Sexual desire, orgasm, and sexual fantasies: A study of 625 Danish women born in 1910, 1936, and 1958. *Journal of Sex Education and Therapy, 17*(2), 111–115.

A random sample of Danish women who were 70, 40, and 22 years of age at the time of the study was obtained to describe their sexual fantasies and the relationship of their fantasies to their orgasms. Roughly half of the women had experienced a great variety of fantasies, most often during masturbation, but the women had difficulty sharing their fantasies with the (female physician) interviewer. This is an important study that demonstrates a difficulty in sex research, even with a population (Danes) generally viewed as sexually liberal.

Malatesta, V. J., Chambless, D. L., Pollack, M., & Cantor, A. (1988). Widowhood, sexuality and aging: A life span analysis. *Journal of Sex and Marital Therapy, 14*(1), 49–62.

This study was undertaken to identify (1) which changes in physical and emotional states and environmental context that interfere with widows' ability to meet their sexual and affectional needs; (2) the level of unhappiness widows experience because they no longer have various sexual and heterosocial activities; and (3) the degree to which certain activities satisfy widows' sexual and affectional needs. A select group of 100 widows, ages 40 to 89 years, living in the community, and who were generally educated, financially stable, socially active, and in good health was surveyed. Younger widows experienced more barriers and unhappiness with regard to their sexual and affectional needs; advancing age was associated with fewer sexual needs. Among all the widows, children and grandchildren, wearing attractive clothing, and spirituality were the most helpful vicarious activities that helped meet their needs. That their clothing and hair were important expressions of their sexuality is important; too often these variables are not included in sexuality. Although this was a very unique group of widows, it is a beginning study that helps to understand some

sexual needs of older widows—an understudied group with regard to their sexual needs. However, the results do not generalize to all older widows or older women, and much more research is needed to understand the sexuality of this group.

Metz, M. E., & Seifert, M. H. (1988). Women's expectations of physicians in sexual health concerns. *Family Practice Research Journal, 7*(3), 141–152.

This study shows that women want their physicians to discuss sexual health with them, even though it may be a stressful topic. However, when given a choice, the women in the study said they would be most likely to talk with their spouse and good friends before talking with a physician about sexual health concerns. The women did choose a physician (before mental health professional, nurse, or clergyperson) as the first professional with whom they would discuss their concern. The results suggest that many women do not have good information about their sexual concerns, and that primary care physicians, in particular, must be more careful about addressing the sexual health of their female clients.

Meuwissen, I., & Over, R. (1992). Sexual arousal across phases of the human menstrual cycle. *Archives of Sexual Behavior, 21*(2), 101–119.

These researchers conducted three experiments to test whether sexual arousal in women varies across the menstrual cycle. Australian women were the participants. Results were consistent with other research, and provide insufficient evidence to suggest that sexual arousal changes systematically across the menstrual cycle in women, either subjectively or physiologically. However, many women frequently report such changes.

Morokoff, P. J. (1988). Sexuality in perimenopausal and postmenopausal women. *Psychology of Women Quarterly, 12*, 489–511.

This article is a review of research and related literature from the past 20 years, concerning the relationship of both natural and surgical menopause to sexual functioning in women. The major conclusions are that most women continue sexual activity, are not sexually dysfunctional, and do not experience a decline in their sexual functioning during and after the climacteric. With regard to hormonal function, testosterone is clearly important in women's sexuality, but the role of estrogen is unclear. The author suggests numerous questions for future research so that a better understanding of the relationship of menopause to women's sexuality will be achieved.

Osborn, M., Hawton, K., & Gath, D. (1988). Sexual dysfunction among middle aged women in the community. *British Medical Journal, 296*, 959–962.

This was a study of the prevalence of sexual dysfunction among a random sample, stratified by age, of 35- to 59-year-old heterosexual partnered women in England. Although the definitions of sexual dysfunction are not consistent with many clinical definitions of dysfunction, they are operationally defined in the article. Although the definitions used are less stringent than many sex therapists would use, the incidence of sexual dysfunction (33% overall) can be considered low. However, the investigators also asked the women if they themselves thought they had a "problem with sex," and only 10 percent said they did. The only gynecological problem associated with sexual dysfunction was urinary incontinence. This is an interesting descriptive study that supports the presence of sexual health in many women, even when researchers expect to find otherwise.

Palace, E. M., & Gorzalka, B. B. (1992). Differential patterns of arousal in sexually functional and dysfunctional women: Physiological and subjective components of sexual response. *Archives of Sexual Behavior, 21*(2), 135–159.

This might be considered a "state of the art" physiological study of women's sexual arousal: the newest and most refined equipment was used. Further, sexually dysfunctional women were compared with functional women; and dysfunctional women had subjectively and physiologically less arousal than functional women. The authors conclude that subjective experience and genital vasocongestion are two primary components of sexual arousal. Since these two components are correlated, it seems that practitioners ought to simply respect women's subjective reports about sexual functioning and avoid invasive procedures.

Pelletier, L. A., & Herold, E. S. (1988). The relationship of age, sex guilt, and sexual experience with female sexual fantasies. *Journal of Sex Research, 24*, 250–256.

Little research has been conducted about fantasy as an aspect of female sexuality. In this study of 136 single college women, 97 percent reported that they had experienced sexual fantasies. More women experienced fantasies in nonsexual than in sexual situations. The most frequently reported fantasy was sexual intercourse with a boyfriend or future husband. Frequency of fantasies, number of different fantasies, and erotic content of the fantasies were all strongly negatively associated with sex guilt and sex anxiety. The importance of this study is that nearly all of the women reported having fantasies. Women were asked to describe their favorite fantasy, as well as to indicate the frequency with which they experienced each of 25 fantasies, during masturbation, sexual intercourse, and nonsexual situations. Some women indicated that they had experienced every one of the 25. Interestingly, when asked to describe their favorite fantasy, 33 percent described a fantasy that did not include any sexual behavior. In terms of women's sexuality this may suggest that women experience even more fantasies than it has been thought, since most measurement of sexual fantasies has included a given list from which women simply choose. Further research should include options for women to describe, rather than simply choose from a list the fantasies they experience.

Purifoy, F. E., Grodsky, A., & Giambra, L. M. (1992). The relationship of sexual daydreaming to sexual activity, sexual drive, and sexual attitudes for women across the life-span. *Archives of Sexual Behavior, 21*(4), 369–385.

Sexual daydreaming, spontaneous sexual thoughts unrelated to the task at hand (the scale used to measure sexual daydreaming is reproduced in the article), was assessed in 117 women, ages 26–78, and associated with other sexual behaviors. Daydreaming was associated with sexual interest and activity, positively under 35 years, and negatively in older women. The authors conclude that sexual daydreaming reflects a positive orientation toward sexuality and reflects the current concerns of women. This is a new and interesting approach to understanding other than traditionally defined sexual behaviors of women.

Rice, S. (1989). Sexuality and intimacy for aging women: A changing perspective. *Journal of Women and Aging, 1*(1/2/3), 245–264.

Rice's "changing perspective" is a woman-oriented definition of female sexuality. By considering broadly both sexuality and intimacy, she suggests new ways of viewing older women and their sexuality. She discusses the issues of ageism, changing societal attitudes toward sexuality, widowhood, physical diseases, institutionalization, and elder abuse; and the effects of these on older women's sexuality. This is a very interesting article that should be read by anyone who cares for older women, and also by anyone interested in women-oriented definitions of sexuality.

Richardson, L. (1988). Sexual freedom and sexual constraint: The paradox for single women in liaisons with married men. *Gender and Society, 2*(3), 368–384.

In this interesting research, indepth interviews were conducted with 65 women who were at the time, or had been in sexual liaisons with married men. From the women's perspective, it is women who are in control of their sexuality by relating to a married man and who use the liaison to become less sexually repressed, to receive sexual affection without intercourse, to avoid sexually transmitted diseases, and to explore their sexual orientation. However, the author recognizes, though the women seemed not to, that if the woman "fell in love" with the man, the dynamics of the relationship changed, so that the woman was no longer in control, but was, in fact, disadvantaged. Hence, her recognition of sexual freedom and constraint, as the title of the article suggests. The author's feminist beliefs allowed her to hear what these liaisons meant to the women from their own perspectives. Her research is valuable as an addition to understanding the ways in which women define and live their own sexuality.

Rosenzweig, J. M., & Dailey, D. M. (1989). Dyadic adjustment/sexual satisfaction in women and men as a function of psychological sex role self-perception. *Journal of Sex and Marital Therapy, 15*(1), 42–56.

The Bem Sex Role Inventory (BSRI), Hudson Index of Sexual Satisfaction, and the Dyadic Adjustment Scale were administered to women and men. Results were as expected, and similar for both women and men: those who were classified as androgynous were significantly more sexually satisfied and maritally adjusted than those classified as sex typed. The participants also completed the BSRI for themselves concerning a sexual situation. Interestingly, about half of both females and males reported feminine sex typing in that situation. The authors discuss the results and suggest a need for qualitative research that may explain the results better than the use of the quantitative methods of the study.

Rosenzweig, J. M., & Lebow, W. C. (1992). Femme on the streets, butch in the sheets? Lesbian sex-roles, dyadic adjustment, and sexual satisfaction. *Journal of Homosexuality, 23*(3), 1–20.

The BSRI was used to classify lesbians' (*n* = 111) "global" behavior and their behavior in a sexual situation. Only the women who were globally typed as feminine (*n* = 16) did not change significantly during a sexual situation; others increased in femininity. Consequently, the title of the article is misleading, and is used only to attract readers. These lesbians reported high levels of dyadic adjustment and sexual satisfaction. Interesting suggestions for future research are provided.

Savitz, L., & Rosen, L. (1988). The sexuality of prostitutes: Sexual enjoyment reported by "streetwalkers." *Journal of Sex Research, 24,* 200–208.

Sexual response in 46 prostitutes was studied through structured interviews. The authors' purposes were to address the stereotypes of prostitutes as sexually nonresponsive and as lesbian. The women were selected from women in Philadelphia convicted of prostitution or a prostitution-related crime. However, the women were quite heterogeneous with regard to personal characteristics. Results showed that most of the prostitutes experienced sexual pleasure with both their clients and private partners, but the sexual enjoyment was higher with private partners. Over 60 percent were usually or always orgasmic with clients, and all reported being orgasmic with their private partners. Receiving oral sex was the most pleasurable sexual activity with both clients and private lovers. None of the prostitutes identified themselves as lesbian, and only five women identified themselves as bisexual. The authors (both male) state that they believe the costs of prostitution outweigh any erotic benefit, but they also believe they have contradicted widely held beliefs about prostitutes.

Schover, L. R. (1988). *Sexuality and cancer: For the woman who has cancer, and her partner.* New York: American Cancer Society.

The breadth of topics related to sexuality in women who have cancer addressed in this 40-page educational booklet is remarkable. Although the major emphasis is on reproductive cancers, topics such as the effects of cancer treatments on women's sexual response and desire are of use to women with many types of cancers. What the booklet gains in breadth,

however, it loses in depth. In some cases non-empirically based generalizations are made; in other cases, topics are treated very simplistically. Numerous other resources, including reading materials, films, and organizations are listed at the end. Women who have cancer and their partners should find this booklet a very useful resource.

Schover, L. R., Fife, M., & Gershenson, D. M. (1989). Sexual dysfunction and treatment for early stage cervical cancer. *Cancer, 63*(1), 204–212.

This is a prospective study of sexuality in 61 women treated for cervical cancer. The results compare women treated with radical hysterectomy only versus women treated with radiation with or without surgery. The researchers used a broad definition of sexuality and provided brief sexual counselling to all women in the study. The most important findings were that although there were basically no differences between the groups at six months post-treatment, at one year post-treatment there were significant differences. The women treated with radiation experienced more dyspareunia and decreased sexual desire than the women treated with hysterectomy only. Further, the women treated with radiation experienced other lifestyle changes that suggest a decreased quality of life. The authors note that generally the total group of women had few sexual changes, and attribute that to the counselling which they provided. Consequently they appropriately urge sexual education and counselling for women experiencing cervical cancer, and particularly urge sexual follow-up at one year post-treatment.

Schumacher, D. (1990). Hidden death: The sexual effects of hysterectomy. *Journal of Women and Aging, 2*(2), 49–66.

This article reflects the personal experience and bias of the author that hysterectomy results in significant loss to women's sexual functioning. She argues that this loss (the hidden death) is not acknowledged, and suggests 18 factors that contribute to the ongoing use of hysterectomy. The author's anger and pain are clear, but she, as others have, equates hysterectomy and hysterectomy with oophorectomy, which are not equivalent. Some women *do* have sexual difficulties following hysterectomy, but many do not; the author would have readers believe that all women do.

Simmonds, F. N. (1988). *She's Gotta Have It:* The representation of black female sexuality on film. *Feminist Review, 29,* 10–22.

She's Gotta Have It is a film, written and produced by Spike Lee, a young black filmmaker, who also plays a role in the film. The entire cast is black. This article is a critical review of the film with regard to sexuality—black *female* sexuality, but sexuality as defined by men for men. The author, a black woman herself, discusses how the title of the film, as well as the images, all present a negative definition of black female sexuality, both heterosexual and lesbian. She challenges black women to define their own sexuality.

Slob, A. K., Koster, J., Radder, J. K., & Van Der Werff Ten Bosch, J. J. (1990). Sexuality and psychophysiological functioning in women with diabetes mellitus. *Journal of Sex and Marital Therapy, 16*(2), 59–69.

Dutch women with Type I diabetes (*n* = 24) and healthy women (*n* = 10) were shown a sexually explicit film to determine sexual arousal by measuring temperature of the labia minora. Labial temperatures were higher in the diabetic women, but when women were matched for their initial labial temperatures, there were no differences in subjective arousal or labial temperature increases. The researchers suggest that the results are because the diabetic women did not have serious neuropathy; however, results could also be because the women did not find the films sexually arousing.

Stanislaw, H., & Rice, F. J. (1988). Correlation between sexual desire and menstrual cycle characteristics. *Archives of Sexual Behavior, 17*(6), 499–508.

The purpose of this article was to describe research results testing the hypothesis that women's sexual desire is hormonally based. The research was a large, prospective study of women from five countries (Canada, Colombia, France, Mauritius, United States) who were using the sympto-thermal method of natural family planning. The authors are careful to indicate that the women did not know that this was, in any way, a study of sexuality, but they did mark on the daily calendars that they kept, when they experienced sexual desire. It is not clear from the article, however, whether the women marked *every* day that they experienced desire, or only the day of *onset* of sexual desire. Presumably the latter is correct, since the authors wanted to show that desire is hormonally based and not the result of sociocultural or other factors; but, if it is, the operational definition of "onset of sexual desire" requires clarification. The conclusion reached from the study is that sexual desire is associated with the basal body temperature shift. The authors do admit that hormones are not the only factor in sexual desire and that the specific hormones have not been identified.

Teets, J. M. (1990). What women talk about: Sexuality issues of chemically dependent women. *Journal of Psychosocial Nursing and Mental Health Services, 28*(12), 4–7.

The author reports about three years of unstructured discussions about sexuality with women recovering from chemical dependency. The most frequent areas of discussion were having sex when sober, values regarding sex, incest, rape, and battering, and other reproductive and sexual health concerns. The study confirms the importance of sexuality in the lives of recovering women, as it is for all women.

Thompson, S. (1990). Putting a big thing into a little hole: Teenage girls' accounts of sexual initiation. *Journal of Sex Research, 27*(3), 341–361.

The title of this article provides only half of the picture. The author conducted in-depth interviews with 400 teenage young women who described their first experiences with intercourse. This article presents findings of a representative sample of 100 of these young women. There were lesbian as well as heterosexual women; some were teen mothers. About 30 percent were African-American or Hispanic. These young women reported their first experience of sexual intercourse in one of two "stories." The first story was the one about putting a big thing into a little hole. These young women had essentially no preparation of masturbation, petting, foreplay, desire, or contraception. They had difficulty remembering the experience. The other story was told by young women who felt positively about their sexuality. They had prior experiences of desire, masturbation, childhood sex play, and heavy petting, and they had talked with their mothers about sex. These young women remembered the experience in great detail, partially, at least, because they made the decision to participate. This is a very interesting article, with many implications concerning sex education for young women.

Thornton, N. G., & Dewis, M. (1989). Multiple sclerosis and female sexuality. *Canadian Nurse*, 85(4), 16–18.

Written for nurses, this article provides a brief overview of some of the sexual changes and concerns in women who have multiple sclerosis. Sexual difficulties, such as lack of orgasms, decreased libido, and decreased vaginal lubrication occur in women with multiple sclerosis. General muscular weakness and spasticity may also affect sexual activity. Many of the sexual changes result directly from the demyelination that occurs with the disease. Since demyelination is not predictable, neither general nor sexual symptoms can be accurately predicted, and women may experience times of improvement and times of deterioration. Sexual difficulties may also represent a psychological reaction to the disease. Helpful and specific suggestions are provided for nurses to use when assisting women who have sexual difficulties as a result of multiple sclerosis.

Tolman, D. L. (1991). Adolescent girls, women and sexuality: Discerning dilemmas of desire. *Women and Therapy, 11*(3/4), 55–69.

This is a theoretical article, written for therapists, about the dilemmas for adolescent women, of experiencing sexual desire. Tolman suggests that girls may deny sexual desire or discuss it only in code, rather than talk explicitly about their desire. She believes that this is because society does not want to accept that females are sexual. Brief suggestions are provided for how to assist young and adult women to talk about their sexual desires, as well as the socially created negative feelings that talking openly about sexuality engenders.

Van de Wiel, H. B. M., Schultz, W. C. M. W., Hallensleben, A., Thurkow, F. G., & Bouma, J. (1988). Sexual functioning following treatment of cervical carcinoma. *European Journal of Gynaecologic Oncology, 9*(4), 275–281.

This study was conducted in the Netherlands where usual treatment for cervical cancer is radical hysterectomy. Eleven women (10 heterosexual and one lesbian) were followed for six months post-treatment. The authors' interpretations of their results may go beyond the data presented. They suggest that these women, six months after treatment, even though there were no changes in overt sexual behaviors, valued sexuality less than before treatment, and adapted to their partners' sexual needs because of their own lowered self-esteem. The tool used to measure sexuality was a broad quantitative measure, but the interpretation is based on a very traditional "love ethos," that women have a duty to give their partners love and attention and sacrifice for them. That is, the researchers seem to interpret negatively, positive findings.

Wakefield, J. (1988). Female primary orgasmic dysfunction: Masters and Johnson versus DSM-III-R on diagnosis and incidence. *Journal of Sex Research, 24*, 363–377.

One wonders what the real purpose of this article is. The stated purpose is to demonstrate that the diagnosis of Primary Orgasmic Disorder (POD) cannot be justified for most of the women who have it. To make the point, the author suggests that Masters' and Johnson's criterion for POD allows women to be diagnosed with POD who do not have it. They may never have had sexual experience or they may not have had sufficient sexual stimulation (specifically masturbation according to the author) to warrant a diagnosis of POD. The well-known masturbation therapy of Lonnie Barbach is used to demonstrate that sufficient stimulation (i.e., masturbation) results in orgasm, and thus the women so treated really did not have a disorder. Wakefield finally makes it clear that he wants the DSM-III-R criteria to be even more specific than they are for diagnosing POD, and that he supports a psychiatric diagnosis for POD, rather than the non-psychiatric label used by Masters and Johnson and many others. Although the reader could believe that Wakefield is concerned about women's sexual health, it appears that what he really wants is a psychiatric label, for which therapy should be given.

Walling, M., Andersen, B. L., & Johnson, S. R. (1990). Hormonal replacement therapy for postmenopausal women: A review of sexual outcomes and related gynecologic effects. *Archives of Sexual Behavior, 19*(2), 119–137.

This is an excellent review of the effects of hormone replacement therapy (HRT) on women's sexuality. Studies were carefully analyzed for their methods, as well as results. The authors conclude that (1) estrogen has a positive effect on sexual functioning in postmenopausal women; (2) progestin does not alter that effect; and (3) androgens have a positive effect if estrogen does not. However, the authors also suggest specific kinds of research studies that should be conducted to illuminate understanding of the effects of hormones on postmenopausal women's sexuality.

Weinberg, M. S., & Williams, C. J. (1988). Black sexuality: A test of two theories. *Journal of Sex Research, 25*(2), 197–218.

This study is not specifically about female sexuality; it is a comparison of sexuality between black and white women and men. Data from three earlier studies were used to test two hypotheses: (1) black men and women are more sexually permissive than are white men and women, but the differences are more a function of class than race; and (2) differences in sexual permissiveness between white men and women are greater than they are between black men and women because black women have more power in the family. Neither hypothesis was supported. The motivation for this type of study seems unclear, yet, the authors' concluding statement that new theories are needed to deal with the complexities of race, class, and gender concerning sexuality is certainly true.

Whipple, B., Ogden, G., & Komisaruk, B. R. (1992). Physiological correlates of imagery-induced orgasm in women. *Archives of Sexual Behavior, 21*(2), 121–133.

The purpose of this study was to determine whether women's self-reported "imagery-induced" (without physical stimulation) orgasms produced physiological changes similar to masturbation induced orgasms. Ten paid volunteers participated in a lab setting. Physiological measures were comparable across the two kinds of orgasms, and the authors conclude that results warrant a reassessment of the nature of orgasm.

Whitam, F. L., & Mathy, R. M. (1991). Childhood cross-gender behavior of homosexual females in Brazil, Peru, the Phillipines, and the United States. *Archives of Sexual Behavior, 20*(2), 151–170.

Heterosexual and lesbian adult women from the four countries were questioned about their "cross-gender" behaviors and interests during childhood. The questions were very stereotypically gender identified (e.g., boys played with cars and soldiers while girls played with dolls). Multiple chi square analyses demonstrated that lesbians, across the cultures, had more cross-gender behaviors and interests in their childhood than heterosexual women. The researchers' underlying hypothesis appears to be essentialism: they imply that the cross-cultural findings suggest that cross-gender behaviors in childhood are precursors of adult sexual orientation.

Williamson, M. L., & Williamson, P. S. (1988). Women's preferences for penile circumcision in sexual partners. *Journal of Sex Education and Therapy, 14*(2), 8–12.

The hypothesis of this study was that most American women prefer a circumcised penis in their sexual relations. The participants were 145 Midwestern adult women who had given birth to a son within the previous month. Nearly all (89%) of the sons had been circumcised. The majority of women preferred a circumcised male for the four sexual activities studied: sexual intercourse (71%), viewing a nude penis for sexual arousal (76%), giving manual stimulation (76%), and giving fellatio (83%). The two most common reasons for preference of a circumcised penis were cleanliness and sexier appearance. The authors conclude that women prefer circumcision for sexual reasons, and that fact may account for the continued high rate of circumcision, at a time when pediatricians and others are attempting to convince the public to abandon routine circumcision. The authors recommend replication of the study in a location where most males are not circumcised. This is a fascinating study, but the results could simply mean that women prefer what they have experienced. No statistical analyses were computed comparing the preferences of the women (only 16% of the total) who had sexual experience with both circumcised and noncircumcised males.

Winter, E. J. S., Ashton, D. J., & Moore, D. L. (1991). Dispelling myths: A study of PMS and relationship satisfaction. *Nurse Practitioner, 16*(5), 34–45.

Women with PMS were compared to women who did not report PMS on marital, sexual, and family satisfaction. Women with PMS had significantly less marital and sexual satisfaction, but not significantly different family satisfaction. There is very little literature or research concerning the sexuality of women with PMS, though work on PMS frequently suggests sexual problems in these women. This study systematically compared a small group of women on one variable (satisfaction), which is positive, but much more research must be conducted to understand the sexuality and possible alterations in sexuality of women with PMS.

Winton, M. A. (1989). Editorial: The social construction of the G-spot and female ejaculation. *Journal of Sex Education and Therapy, 15*(3), 151–162.

The author believes that research supports the facts that all women have G-spots, orgasm and ejaculation are separate processes for women, few women do ejaculate, and the fluid ejaculated is not urine. Nonetheless, he also believes that the G-spot and female ejaculation have *not* been socially constructed and therefore are not socially accepted. He presents a model based on power and sexual scripts for defining sexuality. Interestingly, he includes feminists and sexologists as those who have power to define sexuality. This is an extremely interesting essay.

Wood, P. J., & Giddings, L. S. (1991). The symbolic experience of hysterectomy. *Nursing Praxis of New Zealand, 6*(3), 3–7.

The letters women wrote in response to a questionnaire on hysterectomy in a New Zealand women's newspaper were analyzed. Four themes, one of which was sexuality—redefining sexual experience, were identified. The majority of redefinition concerned sexual intercourse, and although a third reported improvement in their sexual relationship following hysterectomy, many women were displeased by the cavalier and negative attitudes of their physicians toward their sexuality and how it could be influenced by hysterectomy. This study also demonstrates positive sexuality outcomes for women following hysterectomy, and is in contrast to Shumacher's (1990) report, on page 87.

Wyatt, G. E. (1989). Reexamining factors predicting Afro-American and white American women's age at first coitus. *Archives of Sexual Behavior, 18*(4), 271–298.

Wyatt, G. E., & Dunn, K. M. (1991). Examining predictors of sex guilt in multiethnic samples of women. *Archives of Sexual Behavior, 20*(5), 471–485.

Wyatt, G., & Lyons-Rowe, S. (1990). African-American women's sexual satisfaction as a dimension of their sex roles. *Sex Roles, 22*(7/8), 509–524.

Each of these three articles reports results of a very carefully executed study, using probability sampling techniques, of 126 African-Americans and 122 Caucasian women, 18–36 years of age, and living in Los Angeles. The 478 item Wyatt Sex History Questionnaire was used. The first two articles compare African-American and white women, and the third describes findings in only the African-American sample. Much was learned from this research, including a similar mean age (16.6 years) of onset of coitus for both groups; but the research is especially valuable in providing new and useful information about the sexuality of African-American women.

Wyatt, G. E., Peters, S. D., & Guthrie, D. (1988). Kinsey revisited, Part I: Comparisons of the sexual socialization and sexual behavior of white women over 33 years. *Archives of Sexual Behavior, 17*(3), 201–239.

Wyatt, G. E., Peters, S. D., & Guthrie, D. (1988). Kinsey revisited, Part II: Comparisons of the sexual socialization and sexual behavior of black women over 33 years. *Archives of Sexual Behavior, 17*(4), 289–332.

These two articles compare data from the Kinsey studies with data from a study conducted by the first author in 1986; thus, 33 years is the time difference between the Kinsey and Wyatt studies, not the ages of the women. In fact, the women were 18–36 years and college-educated. Part I concerns white, non-Hispanic women, and Part II concerns a diverse group of African-American women who were raised in the United States. The purpose of the research was to compare the sexual behaviors of women from two

different eras; white women were *not* compared with black women. Numerous differences were found in the areas of sexual socialization and education, as well as in particular sexual behaviors between the time periods for both groups of women. The results reflect relaxed societal norms in sexual behaviors for women. Additionally, more women in the current studies reported child sexual abuse.

Young, E. W., Koch, P. B., & Bailey, D. (1989). Research comparing the dyadic adjustment and sexual functioning concerns of diabetic and nondiabetic women. *Health Care for Women International, 10,* 377–394.

Thirty diabetic women were compared with a sample of 30 nondiabetic women, matched for age, race, and marital status. There were no differences in dyadic adjustment between the groups. However, the diabetic women reported significantly more problems with sexual repulsion, vaginal lubrication, ability to reach orgasm, dyspareunia, and performance anxiety than did nondiabetic women. Research on sexuality of diabetic women is very limited, and this study adds to the available information; however, methodological problems limit the results. Thus, one must be very careful about concluding that diabetic women are more limited in their sexuality than are nondiabetic women.

Zaviacic, M., Zaviacicova, A., Holoman, I. K., & Molcan, J. (1988). Female urethral expulsions evoked by local digital stimulation of the G-spot: Differences in the response patterns. *Journal of Sex Research, 24,* 311–318.

This study, conducted in Czechoslovakia, was conducted to further understand the phenomena of the G-spot and "female ejaculation." Twenty-seven women who were undergoing work-ups for their infertility were the subjects. The "stimulatory technique" is described for how the G-spot was found and ejaculation sought by the investigators (three males and one female). A G-spot was identified in all of the women; however, only ten could be stimulated to ejaculation. These women were further categorized with regard to their ejaculations as relatively hard-to-induce, easily induced, and intermediate; and descriptions of the groups were delineated. Interestingly, the authors report that women in the easily induced and intermediate groups were generally not sexually aroused by the stimulation or ejaculation. This could suggest many things including that the women believed themselves being treated for infertility, and thus they simply were "putting up" with the treatment, in the hopes of a cure; that the position was uncomfortable; or that they simply were not sexually aroused by having two physicians stimulating their vaginas.

Zhou, X. (1989). Virginity and premarital sex in contemporary China. *Feminist Studies, 15*(2), 279–288.

In this article about sexuality and power in young women in modern China, the author interviewed rural and urban women, mostly in their twenties, to explore their beliefs about sexuality. Traditional beliefs about female virginity prior to marriage still exist; however, most urban women (87%) in her sample engaged in premarital sexual intercourse. Fewer rural women (11%) did, though she suggests an increase there as well. Women have power in their relationships with men by maintaining their virginity, and that power is lost when they lose their virginity. Thus, there are many reasons why men and men's families (especially their mothers) try to have women give up their virginity. Using a feminist perspective, the author discusses this "difficult and painful dilemma" for young women in China today.

Chapter 4

Contraception

Theresa Lawlor McDonald
Susan R. Johnson

INTRODUCTION

During the 1990s, we finally saw progress in availability of contraceptive methods over the previous decade. During the 1980s, the United States struggled with a conservative political climate, cuts in funding, and lawsuits brought against contraceptive products. As a result, drug companies faced high premiums or no insurance for contraceptive products. Investment in research and development to produce new contraceptive products for worldwide testing was cut drastically as well. In 1970, 13 drug companies conducted contraceptive research and development (R & D) whereas by 1987 there were only four such companies. Ortho, the only large U.S. drug company still doing significant contraceptive R & D, points out just how extremely dependent upon other countries for new contraceptive products we have become. Far more important than the situation in our country, however, is the major impact of R & D losses for future generations throughout the world (Diczfalusy, 1991).

Increased contraceptive use is essential for a more peaceful world. History is quite clear on this point: The result of overpopulation is disease, war, and famine. Currently, we appear to be reaching critical mass when comparing earth resources to our population. Only rapid advancements in and worldwide distribution of contraceptive technology can alter these inevitable consequences. Today the world population is 5.3 billion. The United Nations, for one, has low, medium, and high population projections depending upon how long it will take to reach replacement level of fertility worldwide (approximately 2.1 children per couple).

Year Level Reached:	*World Population Stabilized At:*
2010 (Low Projection)	8 billion by end of 21st century
2035 (Medium Projection)	10 billion by end of 21st century
2065 (High Projection)	14 billion by end of 21st century

Within the next 40 years there may be twice as many people on earth. Restricting final world population to 10 billion calls for increasing contraceptive use by married women of reproductive age from 51 percent to 58 percent before the year 2000 and to 71 percent by 2020. Unfortunately due to the cultural, social, and political status of women in the world this will be difficult to achieve. The World Health Organization (WHO) indicates that although one third of the households in the world are headed by women and women make up one third of the world's work force, they perform two thirds of the total hours worked, receive 10 percent of the world's income, and own less than 1 percent of its property. As a result, many women cannot afford contraception, especially young unmarried women who are often denied contraception (Diczfalusy, 1991).

In the United States, young unmarried women are our greatest concern. By age 14, approximately 15 percent of boys and over 7 percent of girls have had sexual intercourse. By age 17, almost half of all teens have had intercourse, with only half of these teens using any method of birth control (including withdrawal) at first intercourse. Even worse, the average delay between first intercourse and a clinic visit to obtain contraception is one year—and then the visit is usually prompted by a pregnancy scare. Some of the most common reasons teens give for delaying the visit are: they believe that there are barriers to health care for them, they fear certain contraceptives or the pelvic exam, and they don't want to acknowledge they are sexually active or even talk about it. In addition, they have the sense of invulnerability characteristic of the teen years (Committee on Adolescence, 1990).

In Europe and Canada, on the other hand, these factors do not prevent many more teens at the same ages from obtaining and using contraception. In fact, unintended pregnancy rates in European countries are 50 percent to 85 percent lower than in the United States (Woods, 1991).

Why is this? Problems specific to the United States include teens having limited access to health care and limited resources to pay for services. In addition, many health care providers fail to offer contraceptive services as part of routine adolescent care, often due to unwarranted fear of promoting sexual promiscuity (Committee on Adolescence, 1990).

Changes must be made in the way health care is provided, especially to teenagers. Health practitioners need to keep in mind the special concerns of teens when providing contraception advice and technology. Teens need a supportive, nonthreatening, confidential relationship. They need enough time for counseling, education, and problem solving. And they need periodic reassessment due to sometimes rapid changes in their sexual relationships (Committee on Adolescence, 1990). They need both verbal and written information; they may be too anxious to hear verbal information and may throw written information away immediately to avoid having it found at home (Hillard, 1989). When possible, practitioners may try to facilitate communication between teenagers and family members to gain much needed support for the teen. Adolescents also need education on effective methods and usually assistance in obtaining a method. Withdrawal is commonly used by teens as a method of birth control since many believe it is the only "method" available to them. Even though withdrawal has a high failure rate and does not protect against infection, teens deserve praise for their concern about pregnancy prevention. Although it is helpful for teens to be informed of periodic abstinence and fertility awareness, these methods are unreliable, too complicated, and require too much abstinence for most teens (Committee on Adolescence, 1990).

Oral contraceptives are the choice of the majority of teenage women but, again, providers must be aware of the special concerns of teens, including: weight gain, nausea, breakthrough bleeding, and amenorrhea. Appropriate counseling on these side effects will decrease discontinuation of oral contraceptives (Woods et al., 1992).

As advances are made in providing oral contraceptives with lower doses of hormone, women at either end of the age spectrum—teenagers and premenopausal women—are receiving more attention from oral contraceptive providers. However, young and poor women continue to have difficulty obtaining oral contraceptives because they must have an examination (which many young women greatly fear) before receiving a prescription. In this regard, many health practitioners also are sensitive to educating women, and sometimes couples, on use of barriers and spermicides for contraception. Hopefully, more and more practitioners are also spreading the word on use of barriers and spermicides for sexually transmitted disease (STD) protection. An area practitioners must not neglect here is education on the importance of using barriers and spermicides *in addition to other contraceptive methods* which offer no STD protection, such as oral contraceptives (OCs), intrauterine devices (IUDs), and natural methods.

Practitioners must understand the seriousness of their responsibility to educate so that clients can protect themselves and others against disease. In the process, practitioners also must be aware of how easily they may remove a client's right to choose a specific contraceptive method, for example, by using undo influence. Physicians and nurse practitioners, males and females alike, influence in different ways, but they do influence. With this in mind, articles on health care providers were chosen to remind both providers and users of the influence providers have over users' birth control method choices.

The growing need for health education and preventive care calls for health professionals, other than physicians, who have prescriptive privileges to provide services in a more cost-effective way. For this reason, among the reviews selected here is an article on prescriptive privileges for health professionals. Limiting prescription of contraceptive devices to physicians, especially in regard to female barriers, is often expensive and inconvenient for users, particularly those in rural or inner city areas where physicians are in short supply.

In an effort to counteract many unreasonable fears about birth control pills, the reviewed articles also include client misconceptions and reactions to side effects, such as break-through bleeding, controversies about pills, and health benefits of pills. Continuing concerns about cancer, heart, and vascular disease prompted the inclusion of articles on the effects pills have on lipid and carbohydrate metabolism and the relationship of OCs to cancer of the breast and reproductive organs. Articles of great interest to clinicians were reviewed on the topics of the effect of tetracycline and missing pills on OC effectiveness, decreased incidence of chlamydial pelvic inflammatory disease (PID) despite the increased incidence of chlamydial cervical infections, OC interchangeability (or not!), and 7-week OC cycles. In addition, there are several review articles that describe methods still being re-searched. The transdermal patch, a delivery system providing estrogen and progestin, is one of the experimental methods.

Other interesting topics not reviewed but included in the reference sec-tion are mortality and contraceptive delay after OC use, the pharmacology of contraceptives, OCs and Down syndrome (of interest due to delayed child-bearing), physiologic reactions to incorrect pill taking, and OC effect on bone density. The article on pharmacology discusses the fact that the ethinyl estradiol and norethindrone combination in Ortho Novum 7/7/7/ and Tri-norinyl pills are partially deactivated in the liver (the "first pass" effect) while levonorgestrel in Triphasal and TriLevlen is 100 percent available. This may explain the decreased breakthrough bleeding claimed by producers of levonorgestrel products. However, the apparently increased potency of monophasic levonorgestrel pills may increase risk of progestational side ef-fects, including increases in serum low density lipoproteins (LDL) which may increase risk of coronary heart disease.

An article on the three new progestins is reviewed. Two of the pro-gestins, desogestrel and norgestimate, have been approved for use in the United States. All three progestins are similar to levonorgestrel in control of breakthrough bleeding but do not have significant effects on low density lipoproteins (LDL) as does monophasic levonorgestrel. This means they are not as likely to cause thrombophlebitis as levnorgestrel. Two of the pro-gestins, norgestimate and gestogen, are 100 percent available like levon-orgestrel. The other progestin, desogestrel, undergoes two chemical changes before it is active in the body.

For women who have children, are breastfeeding, and want a hormonal contraceptive which will not affect their baby or their milk supply, there is a reviewed article on the currently available progestin-only pill.

Several more articles reviewed cover the long-acting progestins, Nor-plant and Depo-Provera, since they were recently approved by the Food and Drug Administration (FDA), and more articles are listed in the references section. Articles on Depo-Provera indicate it causes no major changes in lipoproteins, does not significantly effect children born to mothers using Depo-Provera during pregnancy, has a protective effect against endometrial cancer up to 8 years after use is discontinued, and does not alter the risk of ovarian cancer. This finding is surprising considering OCs decrease ovarian cancer risk by preventing ovulation. In addition, Depo-Provera causes no in-creased risk of liver cancer in areas where hepatitis B is endemic. Since the risk of liver cancer caused by OCs is lower where hepatitis B is endemic, studies are needed in areas where hepatitis B is *not* endemic. In addition, a study on injectable contraceptives and cervical cancer is included in the re-view section.

Contraceptive vaccines are still in the research phase. Although no arti-cles on contraceptive vaccines were reviewed, there is an article on vaccines listed in the reference section.

As for the intrauterine device (IUD), reviewed articles cover the protective effect of the new Progestacert IUD against pelvic inflammatory disease (PID) with its complications of ectopic pregnancy and infertility, and the relationship between the IUD and human papilloma virus (HPV).

Several articles on the diaphragm were chosen for review because of its importance in decreasing both the incidence of STDs, and the risk of cervical intraepithelial neoplasia (CIN) which may be a precursor to cancer of the cervix. We also included an article on the association between bacterial vaginosis and acute cystitis among diaphragm users and reviewed an article on non-menstrual toxic shock with barrier contraceptives.

Vaginal rings, as they have been proposed, are simply a new delivery system for contraceptive hormones. Currently being researched are rings with progestin only and rings with both estrogen and progestin. Although the concept is attractive, unacceptable bleeding has been a problem in development thus far.

Ever since the FDA approved the Prentif Cervical Cap with the requirement that there be Pap smears after 3 months of use to look for abnormality in the smears, there have been questions as to the necessity of this requirement. Gollub and Sivin (1989) reviewed Bernstein's study upon which the FDA judgment was based and concluded that Bernstein misinterpreted his data—that, in fact, there were not more abnormal Pap smears among cap than diaphram users. Bernstein wrote a response to their critique and they responded to his response. The critique and both replies are listed in the references section. The review also includes a large clinical study on cervical cap effectiveness which found use effectiveness to be somewhat higher than several other studies.

Currently being researched in this regard is a new cervical cap: the silicone rubber Femcap with a new "sailor cap" design. An article on the Femcap is included in the review section.

Noted in the reference section is an article on why women initiate and discontinue sponge use. Dissatisfaction with birth control methods currently available, ease of purchase, and selective marketing by drug companies strongly influence women in their contraceptive choices. The contraceptive sponge is an example of widespread marketing of a method which is considerably less effective for women who have had vaginal deliveries. Like the condom, it may be easily purchased at drug or grocery stores without a prescription. Ease of purchase could make this an acceptable method for some teenage women, many of whom have intercourse on the spur of the moment.

The AIDS epidemic has increased both interest in and use of condoms, female barrier methods, and spermicides. Condoms for males are now packaged to attract women and a female condom (called *Reality*) is expected on the market soon. It will probably be approved for both contraception and STD protection although the initial market is expected to be for STD protection alone. Because it is important to be knowledgeable on issues related to protection against STDs, several of the articles reviewed cover testing male and female condoms, as well as research on the increasing incidence of allergy to latex condoms. In fact, this allergy may be related to increased use of latex gloves. Also reviewed is an article describing how vaginal lubrication produced by foreplay may reduce condom breakage. Since condom breakage is found in increased numbers with specific couples, education in condom usage is very important.

The reference section also contains articles on the new tactylon male condom, promoting condom use through educating clients, and the inadequacy of both tensil strength and air testing of condoms in predicting condom breakage. An article on current and experimental male contraception and another on the polymer sling is important here. The researcher of the polymer sling reports that it works two ways. It decreases sperm counts with body heat by holding the testicles up against the body and by electromagnetic charges from the polymer which interfere with sperm production. In this small study of 14 men wearing the sling for 12 months, all subjects became azospermic (no sperm present) in 140 days, plus or minus 21 days. Sperm production resumed after subjects stopped wearing the sling. Although this study is quite small, it does indicate a more serious consideration of experimental male contraception methods. However, more research on *effectiveness*, not just low sperm counts, is required.

Breastfeeding is considered the oldest method of birth control. Because of society's current negative attitude about breastfeeding, women attempting to use this as their contraceptive method need a great deal of support and education. Several articles cover breastfeeding alone and in combination with the progestin-only pill.

There has long been an interest in devices to detect ovulation. Thus, articles are presented on two types of ovulation monitors in the reference section. They may be used with natural family planning methods of birth control or alone, though reasons for why one would *not* want to use them alone are made clear in the articles. Several articles reviewed point out the difficulties encountered in evaluating effectiveness of natural family planning methods and the difficulty of comparing natural family planning methods with other contraceptive methods.

Female sterilization is the most popular method of birth control in the United States. Many women maintained that they had longer, heavier menstrual periods after tubal ligation sterilization. Several studies found little change. One study found no significant changes in menstrual blood loss after four different sterilization techniques. A description of a new sterilization technique, currently being researched, which can be done in a physician's office has been included among the referenced articles. Also included is an article on characteristics of women who seek and then have a tubal reanastamosis (rejoining).

One of the reviewed articles covers the effectiveness of a variety of postcoital or emergency contraceptives (also called "the morning after pill") which was calculated from 21 studies. The four contraceptive methods reviewed were (1) high doses of estrogen-only hormones, (2) combined estrogen-progestin hormones, (3) danazol, and (4) insertion of an IUD. Effectiveness rates of the four methods ranged from 98.2 percent to 99.9 percent.

Two reviewed articles of great importance research contraceptive effectiveness. One article points out how short-term failure rates multiply enormously over time and the other article discusses how methodological problems might have a major effect on reports of contraceptive effectiveness.

Although the area of contraception is moving according to Kaeser (1990) "at a snail's pace," it is at least finally moving forward and not backward.

REFERENCES

Bain, J. (1989). Male Contraception. *Advances in Contraception, 5,* 263–269.

Beckman, L., Murray, J., & Harvey, S. (1989). The contraceptive sponge: Factors in initiation and discontinuation of use. *Contraception, 40*(4), 481–496.

Bernstein, G., Freziers, R., & Clark, V. (1990). Letter to the editor. *Contraception, 42*(2), 241–246.

Bracken, M., Hellenbrand, K., & Holford, T. (1990). Conception delay after oral contraceptive use: The effect of estrogen dose. *Fertility and Sterility, 53.*(1), 21–26.

Chilvers, C., McPherson, K., Peto, J., Pike, M., & Vessey, M. (1989). Oral contraceptive use and breast cancer risk in young women. *The Lancet,* May 6, 973–982.

Committee On Adolescence. (1990). Contraception and adolescents. *Pediatrics, 86*(1), 134–137.

Diczfalusy, E. (1991). Contraceptive prevalence, reproductive health and our common future. *Contraception, 43*(3), 201–225.

Garza-Flores, J., De la Cruz, D., Valles de Bourges, V., Sanchez-Nuncio, R., Martinez, M., Fuziwara, J., & Perez-Palacios, G. (1991). Long-term effects of depot-medroxyprogesterone acetate on lipoprotein metabolism. *Contraception, 44*(1), 61–69.

Goldzieher, J. (1989). Pharmacology of contraceptive steroids: A brief review. *American Journal of Obstetrics & Gynecology, 160*(5), Part 2, 1260–1264.

Gollub, E., & Sivin, I. (1990). Letter to the editor. *Contraception, 42*(2), 247–251.

Gollub, E., & Sivin, I. (1989). The prentif cervical cap and pap smear results: A critical appraisal. *Contraception, 40*(3), 343–349.

Guillebaud, J. (1990). Oral contraceptives in risk groups: Exclusion or monitoring? *American Journal of Obstetrics & Gynecology, 163*(1), Part 2, 443–446.

Hamilton, C., & Hoogland, H. (1989). Longitudinal ultrasonographic study of the ovarian suppressive activity of a low-dose triphasic oral contraceptive during correct and incorrect pill intake. *American Journal of Obstetrics & Gynecology, 161*(5), 1159–1162.

Harvey, S., Beckman, L., & Murray, J. (1989). Factors associated with use of the contraceptive sponge. *Family Planning Perspectives, 21*(4), 179–183.

Holt, V., Daling, J., McKnight, B., Moore, D., Stergachis, A., & Weiss, N. (1992). Functional ovarian cysts in relation to the use of monophasic and triphasic oral contraceptives. *American Journal of Obstetrics & Gynecology, 79*(4), 529–533.

Kallen, B. (1989). Maternal use of oral contraceptives and Down Syndrome. *Contraception, 39*(5), 503–506.

Kessel, E. (1989). Pelvic inflammatory disease with intrauterine device use: A reassessment. *Fertility & Sterility, 51*(1), 1–9.

Koetsawang, S., Ji, G., Krishna, U., Cuadros, A., Dhall, G., Wyss, R., Rodriquez la Puenta, J., Andrade, A., Khan, T., & Kononova, E. (1990). Microdos intravaginal levonorgestrel contraception: A multicentre clinical trial: I. Contraceptive efficacy and side effects; II. Expulsions and removals; III. The relationship between pregnancy rate and body weight; IV. Bleeding patterns. *Contraception, 41*(2), 105–167.

Levine, S., Fagan, S., Pessin, M., Silbergleit, R., Floberg, J., Selwa, J., Vogel, C., & Welch, K. (1991). Accelerated intracranial occlusive disease, oral contraceptives, and cigarette use. *Neurology,* December, 1893–1901.

Lloyd, T., Buchanan, J., Ursino, G., Myers, C., Woodward, G., & Halbert, D. (1989). Long-term oral contraceptive use does not affect trabecular bone density. *American Journal of Obstetrics & Gynecology, 160*(2), 402–404.

Murray, P., Stadel, B., & Schlesselman, J. (1989). Oral contraceptive use in women with a family history of breast cancer. *Obstetrics & Gynecology, 73*(6), 977–983.

Notelovitz, M., Levenson, I., McKenzie, L., & Khan, F. (1991). The effect of low-dose oral contraceptives on lipids and lipoproteins in two at-risk populations: Young female smokers and older premenopausal women. *Contraception,* 44(5), 505–513.

Panser, L., & Phipps, W. (1991). Type of oral contraceptive in relation to acute, initial episodes of pelvic inflammatory disease. *Contraception, 43*(1), 91–97.

Russell-Brown, P., Piedrahita, C., Foldesy, R., Steiner, M., & Townsend, J. (1992). Comparison of condom breakage during human use with performance in laboratory testing. *Contraception, 45,* 429–437.

Schlesselman, J. (1989). Cancer of the breast and reproductive tract in relation to use of oral contraceptives. *Contraception, 40*(1), 1–27.

Shafik, A. (1992). Contraceptive efficacy of polyester-induced azoospermia in normal men. *Contraception, 45,* 439–451.

Steinberg, W. (1989). Oral contraception: Risk and benefits. *Advances in Contraception, 5,* 219–228.

Talwar, G., Hingorani, V., Kumar, S., Roy, S., Shahani, S., Krishna, U., Dhall, K., Sawhney, H., Sharma, N., Singh, O., Gaur, A., Rao, L., & Arunan, K. (1990). Phase I clinical trials with three formulations of anti-human chorionic gonadotropin vaccine. *Contraception, 41*(3), 301–316.

Trussell, J., Warner, D., & Hatcher, R. (1992). Condom performance during vaginal intercourse: Comparison of Trojan-Enz and Tactylon condoms. *Contraception, 45*(1), 11–19.

Turjanmaa, K., & Reunala, T. (1989). Condoms as a source of latex allergen and cause of contact urticaria. *Contact Dermatitis, 20,* 360–364.

Vessey, M., & Grice, D. (1989). Carcinoma of the cervix and oral contraceptives: Epidemiological studies. *Biomedicine & Pharmacotherapy, 43,* 157–160.

Vessey, M., Villard-Mackintosh, L., McPherson, K., & Yeates, D. (1989). Mortality among oral contraceptive users: 20-year follow-up of women in a cohort study. *British Medical Journal, 299,* December 16, 1487–1491.

Wilcox, L., Chu, S., & Peterson, H. (1990). Characteristics of women who considered or obtained tubal reanastomosis: Results from a prospective study of tubal sterilization. *Obstetrics & Gynecology, 75*(4), 661–665.

Wolner-Hanssen, P., Eschenbach, D., Paavonen, J., Kiviat, N., Stevens, C., Critchlow, C., DeRouen, T., & Holmes, K. (1990). Decreased risk of symptomatic chlamydial pelvic inflammatory disease associated with oral contraceptive use. *Journal of the American Medical Association, 263*(1), 54–59.

Woods, E. (1991). Contraceptive choices for adolescents. *Pediatric Annals, 20*(6), 313–321.

Woods, E., Grace, E., Havens, K., Merola, J., & Emans, S. (1992). Contraceptive compliance with a levonorgestrel triphasic and a norethindrone monophasic oral contraptivea in adolescent patients. *American Journal of Obstetrics & Gynecology, 166*(3), 901–907.

World Health Organization Collaborative Study of Neoplasia & Steroid Contraceptives. (1991). Depot-medroxyprogesterone acetate (DMPA) and risk of epithelial ovarian cancer. *International Journal of Cancer, 49*, 191–195.

World Health Organization Collaborative Study of Neoplasia & Steroid Contraceptives. (1991). Depot-medroxyprogesterone acetate (DMPA) and risk of liver cancer. *International Journal of Cancer, 49*, 182–185.

World Health Organization Collaborative Study Of Neoplasia & Steroid Contraceptives. (1991). Depot-medroxyprogesterone acetate (DMPA) and risk of endometrial cancer. *International Journal of Cancer, 49*, 186–190.

Wu, D. (1989). An overview of the clinical pharmacology and therapuetic potential of gossypol as a male contraceptive agent and in gynaecological disease. *Drugs, 38*(3), 333–341.

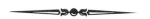

BOOKS AND ARTICLES

Albert, A., Hatcher, R., & Graves, W. (1991). Condom use and breakage among women in a municipal hospital family planning clinic. *Contraception, 43*(2), 167–176.

This study reports on male condom use from a woman's point of view. Information was collected through questionnaires given to women at a Family Planning Clinic. Thirty-six percent of 106 women reported condom breakage in 1 out of 100 acts of intercourse. One pregnancy occurred for every 19 times a condom broke.

In the past year, one in four women reported condom slipping, in effect, one slippage for every 30 acts of intercourse. Fourteen percent of the women used two condoms at once, no doubt because 80 percent of them had experienced previous condom breakage. One must remember that the information collected from the women depended upon their memory of the past year and may have considerable recall bias.

Twelve of the 106 women experienced 35 percent of condom breaks, implying that behavior during intercourse may be an important factor in breakage. Most of the condoms which broke were prelubricated. However, decreased lubrication of the woman may be a factor here. Teens had less breakage than women aged 25 or older. In 65 percent of the breakages, foreplay lasted 0 to 5 minutes and in 22 percent of the breakages, foreplay lasted 6 to 15 minutes. In an effort to decrease breakage, the authors recommend spending more time in foreplay, using additional non-oil based lubrication if necessary, using the condom once, and (easier said than done) checking the condom for tears just prior to ejaculation.

Ansbacher, R. (1991). Interchangeability of low-dose oral contraceptives: Are current bioequivalent testing measures adequate to ensure therapeutic equivalency? *Contraception, 43*(2), 139–147.

It is this author's opinion that current FDA guidelines for assessing differences in bioavailability between generic oral contraceptives (OCs) and brand-name products are inadequate to insure therapeutic equivalence. He proposes placing oral contraceptives in the critical drug category so that generic substitution for brand names would not be allowed.

Ansbacher states that the FDA considers two products pharmaceutically equivalent if they contain the same active ingredients and are identical in strength, route of administration, and dosage form (a capsule cannot be substituted for a tablet). Notwithstanding such identities, the two products may differ in inert substances. Under present guidelines, the maximum concentration of a generic product must fall between 80 percent and 120 percent of the values for the brand-name product based on plasma concentration of the hormones on a single day of testing, not on every day of a 28-day cycle. In addition, the FDA allows a $-/+5$ percent lot-to-lot variation. If the hormones in OCs were 20 percent lower than the brand-name product, in some individuals blood levels of the hormones would be below this 20 percent minimally acceptable value. These women could experience pregnancy or breakthrough bleeding. In addition, an imbalance in the estrogen-to-progestogen ratio might increase side effects.

Ansbacher gives the cost in 1985 of an uncomplicated vaginal delivery as $2,923, a Cesarean delivery as $4,862, and the cost of raising a child to age 18 as $53,000. He makes the point that the risks of an unwanted pregnancy do not justify the perceived savings of generic substitution.

Brache, V., Alvarez-Sanchez, F., Faundes, A., Tejada, A., & Cochon, L. (1990). Ovarian endocrine function through five years of continuous treatment with Norplant subdermal contraceptive implants. *Contraception, 41*(2), 169–177.

This long-term study reveals that women using Norplant implants have a variable degree of ovarian activity compared with more complete depression of ovarian function seen with oral and injectable contraceptives. Although luteal activity increases with time, Norplant cycles are not necessarily anovulatory—the implants are at least as effective as oral contraceptives or injectables. The fluctuating estrogen levels combined with continuous progestin may protect against bone loss and explain rapid resumption of ovulation and return to fertility after discontinuation of Norplant.

Brinton, L. (1991). Oral contraceptive and cervical neoplasia. *Contraception, 43*(6), 581–591.

Recent studies show some evidence of a relationship between cervical neoplasia and long-term OC use. Results of studies are difficult to interpret because of bias and confounding variables. There may be increased risk of cervical neoplasia with multiple sexual partners, a history of genital infections, and among women who have never used barrier contraception, all of which suggests OCs may act as co-carcinogens with transmissible agents such as the human papilloma virus (HPV). The increased risk with smoking usually is not enough to account for the increased risk in OC users.

There appears to be a higher risk associated with recent use of OCs and possibly with higher estrogen doses. There is also a suggestion of a stronger effect for adenocarcinomas than for squamous cell tumors. It is known that OCs cause a marked increase in glandular-to-squamous ratio of cervical epithelium, and microglandular hyperplasia is recognized as an OC related lesion. Oral contraceptives may cause endocervical adenocarcinomas by long-term stimulation of the proliferating glandular epithelium. A relationship is biologically possible, given that there are hormone receptors in cervical tissue and that OCs have been found to induce cervical hyperplasia. However, pathologic studies do cast some doubt on this hypothesis since microglandular hyperplasia has not been established as a precursor of adenocarcinoma.

In addition, OCs may cause growth of human papillomavirus (HPV) infections, the leading suspect in cervical cancer. After adjustment, detection bias among OC users from having more regular Pap smears does not seem to be a factor in increased risk.

Controls in this study were women not using contraceptives and women who used the IUD for contraception. Use of the IUD in relation to cervical cancer risk has not been well investigated and women not using contraception may be at decreased risk of cervical cancer for reasons unknown to these researchers. If that were true, this comparison would result in an apparent increased risk of cervical cancer among OC users when in fact there is only a decreased risk among controls. Further studies are needed to clarify the relationship between OCs and cervical neoplasia. Meanwhile, women on OCs should have annual Pap smears.

Broome, M., & Fotherby, K. (1990). Clinical experience with the progestogen-only pill. *Contraception, 42*(5), 489–496.

Three pregnancies occurred in 358 women using the progestin-only pill (POP) for 18,125 women months of use. The Pearl Index of effectiveness was 0.2 per 100 woman years. For women who discontinued the POP, the main reason was menstrual irregularity (47.5%) although almost 40 percent had mostly regular menstraul patterns. The high effectiveness in this study is credited to taking the POP at the same time each day. The authors claim that the effect of POP in rendering cervical mucus impenetrable by spermatozoa is maximal about 4 hours after pill intake and begins to decline after about 22 hours. Ideally, the POP should be taken at least 4 hours and not more than 20 hours before intercourse. The data in this study suggest that the POP is more effective and better tolerated than is commonly believed.

Coker, A., Hulka, B., McCann, M., & Walton, L. (1992). Barrier methods of contraception and cervical intraepithelial neoplasia. *Contraception, 45*(1), 1–9.

This study examined risk factors for cervical intraepithelial neoplasia (CIN). There were 103 cases and 258 controls. Compared with controls, cases were half as likely to have used barrier contraception (diaphragms and condoms) indicating the protective effect of barriers. Use of spermicide alone was not associated with reduced risk of CIN. Recent use, latency, and age at first barrier method use were all associated with a reduced risk of CIN.

Czegledy, J., Gergely, L., & Batar, I. (1989). Human Papillomavirus in cervical smears taken from women wearing an intrauterine contraceptive device. *Archives of Gynecology & Obstetrics, 244,* 87–89.

This is an interesting study on incidence of various types of the human papillomavirus (HPV) in IUD wearers. Cervical cells were screened for human papillomavirus (HPV) infections in 108 women wearing intrauterine devices (IUDs). The

cells were tested for HPV types 6, 11, 16, and 18. The researchers found 20 percent (22 women) were positive for HPV. Types 6 and 11 were found in 17 women (3 women had both), 4 women had type 16, and 1 woman had type 18. All five of the women with types 16, and 18 had normal Pap smears and no abnormalities were seen on colposcopy. These rates of HPV detection are similar to those found in other sexually active populations.

Dicker, D., Wachsman, Y., Feldberg, D., Ashkenazi, J., Yeshaya, A., & Goldman, J. (1989). The vaginal contraceptive diaphragm and the condom—A reevaluation and comparison of two barrier methods with the rhythm method. *Contraception, 40*(4), 497–504.

Good news for those who want relatively harmless and complication-free contraception! This 2-year study found the effectiveness of diaphragms to be 97.5 percent, condoms 96.8 percent, and rhythm 94.8 percent. The study size was reasonable with 85 diaphragm users, 98 condom users, and 64 rhythm users. All subjects chose the method they wanted to use and were highly motivated, the key to effectiveness with any method. However, both accidental pregnancy rates and discontinuation rates increased with duration of use. This is in contrast to many other studies which have found accidental pregnancy rates for users often dropping with increase in duration and experience of method use. The authors conclude that these methods are reasonably effective, acceptable, safe, with no medical contraindications to their use. Clinicians should not discourage satisfied users, and should encourage motivated couples to consider these methods. In this time of concern about sexually transmitted diseases, this study is good news for contraceptive users and educators. However, this study does indicate that the effort to increase compliance may lead to laxity and discontinuation of the methods with time.

Drew, W., Blair, M., Miner, R., & Conant, M. (1990). Evaluation of the virus permeability of a new condom for women. *Sexually Transmitted Diseases, 17*(2), 110–112.

A new barrier contraceptive device for internal use by women should soon be approved for general use by the FDA. The brand name is *Reality*. It is a disposable device consisting of a soft, loose-fitting polyurethane sheath with two diaphragm-like flexible polyurethane rings. One ring lies inside the sheath and serves as an insertion mechanism fitting up around the cervix like a diaphragm. The other ring remains outside the vagina, protecting the labia and base of the penis. The condoms tested were unlubricated, unpowdered, and without spermicide. The study was designed to test for permeability of the condom to the human immunodeficiency virus (HIV) that can cause AIDS and the cytomegalovirus (CMV). Viral leakage was not observed in three trials for each virus. The attraction of the female condom is that it allows women to protect themselves against STDs rather than depending upon male partners to provide protection.

This study was supported by the drug company that is producing the condom.

Droegemueller, W., Katta, L., Bright, T., & Bowes, W. (1989). Triphasic randomized clinical trial: Comparative frequency of intermenstrual bleeding. *American Journal of Obstetics & Gynecology, 161*(5), 1407–1411.

Hillard, P. (1989). The patient's reaction to side effects of oral contraceptives. *American Journal of Obstetrics & Gynecology, 161*(5), 1412–1415.

Schilling, L., Bolding, O., Cheault, C., Chong, A., Fleury, F., Forrest, K., Glick, H., Hasson, H., Heil, C., & London, R. (1989). Evaluation of the clinical performance of three triphasic oral contraceptives: A multicenter, randomized comparative trial. *American Journal of Obstetrics & Gynecology*, Part 2, *160*(5), 1264–1268.

The above three articles are grouped together because they are concerned with intermenstrual bleeding that commonly accompanies oral contraceptive pill use. Two of the studies specifically address the lower dose triphasic pills. The lower doses have led to increased incidence of breakthrough bleeding (BTB) and amenorrhea (absent periods) which are frequently reasons for discontinuing birth control pills. On the positive side, there is often a decreased incidence of other nuisance side effects, which are also common reasons for discontinuing pills.

Droegemueller et al. found that Tri-Norinyl had the highest incidence of intermenstrual bleeding (63%), Ortho-Norvum 777 was next (44%), and Tri-Levlen had the least (33%). Only the difference between Tri-Levlen and Tri-Norinyl was statistically significant.

Schilling et al. studied Triphasal, Ortho-Novum 777, and Tri-Norinyl. Different starting days were used but no significant differences were seen in BTB from using different starting days. Compared with Triphasil, the rate of spotting and bleeding with Tri-Norinyl was 3 times greater. When comparing Tri-Norinyl to Ortho-Novum 777, bleeding was 2 to $2^1/_2$ times greater.

Both studies found that while products with levonorgestrel (Triphasil and Tri-Levlen) had less spotting and breakthrough bleeding, the product with norethindrone, Tri-Norinyl, had the most. Availability for use in the body of these two progestins varies. According to Droegemueller et al., Tri-Levlen and Triphasal have 100 percent availability of the progestin, Ortho Novum 777 has 73 percent availability, and Tri-Norinyl 47 percent availability. Differences in BTB between the three contraceptives might be explained both by availability of the progestins and by the phasing of both estrogen and progestin in Tri-Levelen and Triphasal. Variable absorbtion of the progestin component, norethindrone, in Tri-Norinyl and Ortho-Novum 777 may also contribute to increased BTB with these products.

Hillard's article points out that although BTB is often considered a minor side effect, it is a major reason for discontinuing pills. It is the unpredictability of the bleeding, rather than the amount of bleeding, that prompts women to stop taking pills. Not taking pills as directed increases BTB and one study found that only 28 percent of women took pills correctly. When amenorrhea is present, women become very concerned about pregnancy and need a pregnancy test for reassurance. When women have bleeding or amenorrhea, they frequently call their practitioner for reassurance which adds to the cost of health care. Even with reassurance, they may lose confidence in the method. Studies have concluded that women's independent judgements were more important in the decision to stop or continue pills than medical advice. Practitioners should emphasize that if a woman has side effects, she should call then rather than discontinuing her pills.

Fasoli, M., Parazzini, F., Cecchetti, G., & La Vecchia, C. (1989). Post-coital contraception: An overview of published studies. *Contraception, 39*(4), 459–467.

Women frequently request contraception after unprotected intercourse. There are two main types of post-coital contraception, hormones and intrauterine devices (IUDs). This article reviews studies for the effectiveness of various methods. The pooled failure rates for various methods are:

0.6%	High doses of ethinylestradiol (4 studies)
1.1%	High-doses of other estrogens (2 studies)
1.8%	Combined estrogen/progestin (11 studies)
2.0%	Danazol (3 studies)
0.1%	IUD (9 studies)

The authors report that although their review is limited by an over-representation of optimistic results and an absence of direct comparison between treatments in several studies, it suggests that the IUD and high-dose ethinylestradiol are more effective than danazol or combined contraceptives. However, the side effects of high-dose estrogen—nausea, vomiting, and cycle disturbance—are not acceptable as a routine method and IUDs are not for everyone. These results should be reconsidered when antiprogestins allowing medical abortion in the 4th through 6th weeks of pregnancy become more widely available.

Flynn, A., Pulcrano, J., Royston, P., & Spieler, J. (1991). An evaluation of the Bioself 110 electronic fertility indicator as a contraceptive aid. *Contraception, 44*(2), 125–139.

The Bioself 110 is a hand-held electronic device that combines the basal body temperature (BBT) and calendar methods of fertility regulation for planning or preventing pregnancy. The device signals fertility status by colored lights.

This research reports on a pilot study of 1,238 cycles of 131 women with 5 planned and 24 unplanned pregnancies. Of the unplanned pregnancies, 2 were related to the device, 9 were related to condom failures, 2 to withdrawal failures, and 11 to unprotected intercourse during "unsafe" times. One of the 2 device failures occurred when the woman incorrectly read the device and the other was believed to have occurred due to device failure. The authors conclude that the Bioself is a reliabale and acceptable contraceptive aid for couples not wishing to use hormonal or invasive means of contraception and they call for larger clinical studies, possibly randomized with the symptothermal method as a control, to verify the usefulness of this device.

Franklin, M. (1990). Recently approved and experimental methods of contraception. *Journal of Nurse-Midwifery, 35*(6), 365–374.

For those who have little time to find and read articles on the newer methods of birth control, this article has thorough but brief reviews of the Paragard Copper T 380A intrauterine device, the Prentif Cervical Cap, Norplant progestin implants, the Reality vaginal pouch, Depo-Provera and norethindrone injectable progestins, the hormonal vaginal ring, transdermal patches, experimental male methods (testosterone, Sulfasalazine, gossypol, and reversible vasectomy), a gonodal hormone that controls the follicle stimulating hormone called inhibin, and contraceptive vaccines.

In discussing effectiveness, the author points out that a study by the Alan Guttmacher Institute suggests contraceptive failure rates may be up to 30 percent higher because abortions are underreported. The author mentions the two primary ways to compute contraceptive effectiveness: the Pearl index and life table analysis. However, the author does not point out the differences between them and how they can skew effectiveness rates of contraceptives although she does discuss at length the differences between method (theoretical) and user failure rates.

Grimes, D. (1992). The safety of oral contraceptives: Epidemiologic insights from the first 30 years. *American Journal of Obstetrics & Gynecology, 166*(6), Part 2, 1950–1954.

Established health benefits and potential risks of oral contraceptive (OC) use are delineated in this article. The newer low dose OCs do not appear to be associated with an increased risk of myocardial infarction or stroke. After evaluating the information from various studies, the author concludes that although breast cancer is the most important safety concern, the bulk of recent data suggests that oral contraceptives (OCs) have no overall impact on a woman's risk of developing this disease. The effect of OCs on development of cervical cancer is less clear. In recent years, several studies have reported an increased risk of cervical cancer after five or more years of OC use. Confounding factors that are sources of confusion in research studies when examining associations between cervical cancer and OCs are sexual activity, regular Pap smear screening of OC users, and smoking.

Harkless, G. (1989). Prescriptive authority: Debunking common assumptions. *Nurse Practitioner, 14*(8), 57–61.

Prescriptive privilege is essential in providing primary care to healthy as well as ill people. Women are especially affected by limiting prescriptive privileges because the most effective contraceptives are restricted to prescription only. The author reviews the historical background for the physician monopoly on prescriptive privilege.

He also covers many other issues connected to prescriptive authority. This article will help practitioners, politicians, and patients understand the history of prescriptive privilege in the United States. It also presents the logic for making necessary changes that will help bring our health care system into the 21st century so that quality care will be available to larger numbers of people.

Harvey, S., Beckman, L., & Murray, J. (1989). Healthcare provider and contraceptive care setting: The relationship to contraceptive behavior. *Contraception, 40*(6), 715–729.

This study examined three factors in provision and use of contraceptives: (1) the role of the health care provider in the selection and consistent use of contraceptive methods, (2) provider-client relationships including information given and client satisfaction, and (3) characteristics of the environment. Approximately 90 percent of subjects were seen by a gynecologist or other physician specialist of whom 77 percent were male. Approximately two thirds of all providers, physician and non-physician, were male. Forty-eight percent of clients were seen in private offices, 30 percent in private group practices, and 22 percent in family planning or other public clinics. Forty-five percent of clients reported that the provider recommended a specific contraceptive method to them, with the birth control pill, vaginal sponge, and diaphragm most frequently recommended. Methods least frequently recommended were rhythm and male sterilization. Females were more likely than males to recommend the diaphragm. Methods most frequently discouraged were the pill, IUD, and sponge. Non-MDs were more likely to discourage the sponge. Males and females were equally likely to encourage or discourage any method. Non-MDs generally provided more information, especially on how the method works.

No significant differences were found between care given in the private and clinic settings. However, clients were somewhat more likely to receive information in the clinic setting. The majority of women (83%) were satisfied that their birth control needs were met. Women were more satisfied with female providers, regardless of whether they were MDs or non-MDs. The setting, private or clinic, was not a significant issue in satisfaction.

The most frequent negative comments were that the practitioner was not friendly enough and that he or she did not spend enough time with the client. The authors point out that the literature indicates greater compliance in contraceptive users is associated with giving more information. In this study, only two-thirds of the practitioners provided information on three of the items examined, and only three-fourths discussed the effectiveness of contraceptive methods. Nurses gave more information, asked more open-ended questions, and provided more overall communication. Although physicians spent an average of 16 minutes with each patient, only 1 minute was spent giving information.

Hatcher, R., Stewart, F., Trussell, J., Kowal, D., Guest, F., Stewart, G., & Cates, W. (1990). *Contraceptive Technology*, 15th Edition. New York: Irvington Publishers.

For many health practitioners, *Contraceptive Technology* has been "the bible" for contraceptive health care. A glance at the table of contents shows why. It starts with principles of family planning and the patients' "Bill of Rights" and goes on to sexuality (normal and dysfunctional), that great mystery the menstrual cycle, menstrual and gynecologic problems, sexually transmitted diseases, all kinds of contraceptive methods, abortion, pregnancy including adolescent pregnancy, infertility, counseling and education, and global population information. It contains many client education samples. This book is an excellent resource for clients, clinicians, and educators.

Herrero, R., Brinton, L., Reeves, W., Brenes, M., de Britton, R., Tenorio, F., & Gaitan, E. (1990). Injectable contraceptives and risk of invasive cervical cancer: Evidence of an association. *International Journal of Cancer, 46*, 5–7.

This study examines the relationship between invasive cervical cancer and two injectable contraceptives (IC), depot-medroxyprogesterone acetate (DMPA or Depo-Provera) and norethisterone enanthate (NE). A total of 759 cases and 1,467 controls were interviewed to find 32 cases and 82 controls who had ever used injectable contraceptives. Other risk factors for invasive cervical cancer were controlled including sexual behavior of women and their partners and infection with the human papillomaviruses (HPV).

Women who had used IC for less than 5 years had a relative risk (RR) of 0.5 but users for 5 or more years had a RR of 2.4. The effect of prolonged IC use was stronger for women reporting first use 10 or more years before the interview (RR 3.4) and if it was more than 5 years since the IC was last used (RR 5.3). Cervical cancer risk was particularly high among women who had never had a Pap smear and where the last Pap smear was 2 or more years before the interview (RR 6.3). The reduced cervical cancer risk associated with short-term IC use may reflect more frequent Pap smear screening as the method is initiated. Although the numbers in this study are small, they suggest an increased risk of cervical cancer with long-term IC use. Monitoring long-term IC users for cervical disease with annual Pap smears is indicated until more conclusive results are available.

Hooton, T., Fihn, S., Johnson, C., Roberts, P., & Stamm, W. (1989). Association between bacterial vaginosis and acute cystitis in women using diaphragms. *Archives of Internal Medicine, 149*, September, 1932–1936.

For many years, the assumption had been made that pressure of the diaphragm rim on the urinary bladder caused urinary tract infections (UTI). Research by these authors indicates that this may not be the only reason for UTIs. Their data indicates that there is an alteration of vaginal flora in women who use diaphragms. The reason for this is not known. This change in flora results in an increased vaginal pH, an abnormal vaginal fluid pattern (indicated by gas-liquid chromatography), a decrease in the normal lactobacilli bacteria, and an increase in Escheria coli around the vaginal opening. The authors speculate that the changes could result from diaphragm use or from associated events, such as sexual activity or spermicide use. A major problem with this study is that its authors studied only women with symptoms similar to those seen with cystitis and did not study asymptomatic women for comparison. Until healthy women are studied, this information is only of academic interest.

Kaeser, L. (1990). Contraceptive development: Why the snail's pace? *Family Planning Perspectives*, 22(3), 131–133.

This study summarizes "Developing New Contraceptives: Obstacles and Opportunities," a report on a 2-year study of contraception in the United States by the Committee on Contraceptive Development. The committee was composed of practitioners, public health personnel, legal experts, drug company executives, researchers, economists, and demographers. They found that many population subgroups are not comfortable with the contraceptives currently available. Subgroups of concern include teenagers, women who are breastfeeding, and older couples who do not want sterilization. Many of the "new" contraceptives are not new, in fact, but simply involve new delivery systems for hormones.

The most serious obstacles to contraceptive development in the United States are attitudes of the American public, the organization of and resources available for research, federal regulations, and product liability. Although American society seems permissive and sexually liberated, attitudes toward reproduction and contraceptive use have been remarkably conservative. Perhaps this conservatism is a result of the country's religious roots. In addition, there is little demand for new contraceptive methods. Even groups where support would be expected, such as feminist and consumer groups, are among the most critical of newer contraceptive methods as being potentially dangerous or unhealthy. In general, the net impact of the nation's values has been to slow contraceptive development and reduce support for research. Only one large drug company in the United States (Ortho Pharmaceutical Corp.) is still involved in contraceptive research. Activity by small single-purpose firms, universities, and nonprofit organizations has increased but only large companies can underwrite full-scale development and marketing. Federal funding for research appears to have increased modestly since the mid-1970s but federal contributions to applied contraceptive development have declined. Private foundation support for basic research in reproductive sciences has declined dramatically.

The time involved, the amount of data required, and the enormous costs for Food and Drug Administration (FDA) approval has reduced incentives to do research by shortening the product's patent life on the open market, thus reducing its profitability. Although patents grant 17 years of exclusive rights, the patent generally must be acquired long before FDA approval to market the product is obtained. The average time it takes to go through the FDA process has shortened the time from FDA approval to patent expiration from 14.4 years in 1967 to 7.9 years in 1984. FDA approval of contraceptives is more demanding because users are healthy. The FDA does not see a need here to balance benefits against serious illness or death as it does for drugs used to treat illness. Apparently, the FDA does not take into consideration the serious consequences of pregnancy and delivery for many women when effective birth control methods are not available. The committee that performed the present study concluded with several recommendations, among them that the FDA assign more importance to effectiveness and convenience of new birth control methods, that the FDA follow approved methods by long-term studies, that there be federal statutes giving some liability protection to manufacturers, and that the National Institutes of Health give more funding to encourage research in contraception which will attract young scientist to this field of research.

Kennedy, K., Rivera, R., & McNeilly, A. (1989). Consensus statement on the use of breastfeeding as a family planning method. *Contraception*, 39(5), 477–487.

An interdisciplinary international group of researchers in lactational infertility met to arrive at consensus about conditions under which breastfeeding can be used as a safe and effective method of family planning. Data from 13 prospective studies in 8 countries were reviewed. The consensus of the group was that the maximum birth spacing effect of breastfeeding is achieved when a mother fully or nearly fully breastfeeds and remains amenorrheic. When these two conditions are fulfilled, breastfeeding provides more than 98 percent protection from pregnancy in the first 6 months after delivery. High suckling frequency and avoidance of long intervals between feeds day and night prolongs the period of infertility. Pacifiers and feeding bottles should not be used.

Klavon, S., & Grubb, G. (1990). Insertion site complications during the first year of Norplant use. *Contraception, 41*(1), 27–37.

This study examines 2,674 Norplant users from 7 countries who were followed for 1 year. One-year incidence rates of infection (0.8%), expulsion (0.4%), and local reaction (4.7%) varied widely among countries and at clinics within a country. In contrast to reports that insertion site complications occur during the first few weeks of use, these data show that 34.6 percent of insertion site infections and 64.3 percent of implant expulsions were reported after the first 2 months of use and that 35.7 percent of local reactions were reported after 4.5 months of use. It is possible that low-grade infections begin soon after insertion but remain subclinical for several weeks, although probably not for several months. Of the 16 women with infections who did not have the implants removed immediately, half of them required or requested removal indicating that immediate removal in case of infection may be appropriate. This study contains much valuable data on insertion site complications.

Kornaat, H., Geerdink, M., & Klitsie, J. (1992). The acceptance of a 7-week cycle with a modern low-dose oral contraceptive (Minulet). *Contraception, 45*(2), 119–127.

For various reasons, women taking oral contraceptives (OC) want to postpone withdrawal bleeding. Despite wide use of this practice, few articles have been published on the topic. This study examines menstrual patterns when OC hormone pills were taken continuously for 6 weeks rather than the usual 3 weeks.

The OC chosen for this study is Minulet, a low-dose oral contraceptive (OC) containing gestodene 75 micrograms and ethinylestradiol 30 micrograms. A group of 55 women took the

OC for 42 consecutive days. During this time, 96 percent experienced no breakthrough bleeding (BTB), and 81 percent experienced no BTB or spotting. Eight women reported side effects of breast tenderness, nausea, abdominal bloating, headache, and dysmenorrhea. When compared with an earlier study of a 7-week cycle with another OC, Minulet offered excellent cycle control.

Landgren, B-M., & Csemiczky, G. (1991). The effect on follicular growth and luteal function of "missing the pill": A comparison between a monophasic and a triphasic combined oral contraceptive. *Contraception, 43*(2), 149–158.

This study examines the effects on follicular growth and hormonal levels of prolonging the pill-free interval from 7 to 10 days. In earlier studies, these authors determined that monophasic levonorgestrel OCs remained an effective contraceptive when pills were missed for 2 consecutive days at various phases of the cycle. The women in this study missed the first three pills in a cycle of monophasic combined desorgestrel oral contraceptives (OC) and in a cycle of triphasic combined levonorgestrel OCs. There were two groups of 10 women each. Ovulation occurred in one woman in each group. Four women in each group had follicular activity only. Five women in the monophasic group and three women in the triphasic group had complete ovarian suppression. Two women taking the triphasic preparation showed follicular growth followed by insufficient luteal function. There seemed to be a considerable gap between the appearance of ovarian activity and ovulation, with wide interindividual variation within the two treatment groups. Still there was less suppression of follicular development during the prolonged pill-free interval in the triphasic group. The authors state that these findings indicate there is a minor risk of escape ovulation when the pill-free interval is prolonged to 10 days. This is in agreement with Killick et al. who concluded that even increasing the pill-free interval to 11 days would not result in pill failure. However, it is in contrast with the well-established fact that a restoration of endogenous ovarian activity occurs during the pill-free interval of 7 days in women taking low-dose combined OCs. More discussion is needed on whether shortening the pill-free interval to 5 days would reduce the risk of escape ovulation, making the method more effective. The gain seems negligible. However, the regimen might reduce breakthrough bleeding.

Leeper, M., & Conrardy, M. (1989). Preliminary evaluation of Reality, a condom for women to wear. *Advances in Contraception, 5,* 229-235.

The polyurethane *Reality* female condom has several advantages over use of male condoms. It is less disruptive during sexual activity as there is no need to wait until the man's penis is erect to place the condom, the man should have less decreased sensitivity, the female condom is stronger (therefore less likely to break), more resistant to oils, and it provides better protection against sexually transmitted diseases (STD) since it covers the labia.

Three studies were conducted to evaluate the risk of barrier failure allowing semen into the vagina. The combined risk of barrier failure for *Reality* used 1,000 times in the three studies was 3 percent. The combined risk of failure for male condoms used 700 times was 11.6 percent. Although most women will use the female condom for STD protection, it may prove to be a more effective contraceptive than the male condom.

Letterie, G., & Chow, G. (1992). Effect of "missed" pills on oral contraceptive effectiveness. *Obstetrics & Gynecology, 79*(6), 979-982.

This study was done to determine whether missing pills at varying times in an oral contraceptive (OC) cycle resulted in follicular growth and ovulation. Fifteen women (who desired tubal reanastamosis) were randomized into three groups and issued packs of Ortho Novum 777 with four consecutive pills missing in specific sequences: group I, days 1-4; group II, days 3-6; and group III, days 6-9. Serum was examined for levels of lutinizing hormone (LH), follicle stimulating hormone (FSH), estradiol (E2), and progesterone, and serial ovarian

ultrasound examinations were done to determine follicular development throughout the cycle at 4-day intervals. No subject ovulated as suggested by serum progesterone levels and ultrasound assessment of follicular development. It appeared that OC exerted a similar degree of pituitary and ovarian suppression even when the subjects missed four pills at varying times in the cycle. The anovulatory effect persisted for the rest of the cycle after the pills were restarted and taken correctly.

Louv, W., Austin, H., Perlman, J., & Alexander, W. (1989). Oral contraceptive use and the risk of chlamydial and gonococcal infections. *American Journal of Obstetrics & Gynecology, 160*(2), 396-402.

This study examined rates of cervical infection with gonorrhea and chlamydia in 617 oral contraceptive (OC) users compared with 158 sterilized women and 43 intrauterine device (IUD) users who acted as controls. Compared with non-users, rates of infection with both gonorrhea and chlamydia were found to be increased in OC users by approximately 70 percent. Cervical columnar epithelium (vascular, mucus producing glandular tissue) may be responsible for the increased rate of chlamydial infections but not gonorrheal infections. Rates of infection with gonorrhea were higher in women using pills that were more androgenic (male hormone).

As in determining risk of cervical cancer, the confounding variables make determining cause and effect extremely difficult. This article makes a valuable contribution toward understanding at least some of the issues involved.

Mishell, D., Connell, E., Haney, A., Hodgen, G., & Speroff, L. (1989). Oral contraception for women in their 40s. *The Journal of Reproductive Medicine,* (Supplement), *35*(4), 447-479.

This is a report on a panel discussion at the 37th Annual Meeting of the American College of Obstetricians and Gynecologists in 1989. The discussion centers around the fact that women over age 35 have limited contraceptive choices. These include sterilization, barriers, intrauterine devices (IUD), and natural family planning. What follows is an interesting in-depth discussion of studies, risk factors, benefits, drug potency, drug interactions, metabolic effects and side effects, drug labeling, and prescribing practices for oral contraceptives use in women over 40. An excellent article!

Murphy, A., Zacur, H., Charache, P., & Burkman, R. (1991). The effect of tetracycline on levels of oral contraceptives. *American Journal of Obstetrics & Gynecology, 164*(1) Part 1, 28–32.

The controversy about possible decreased effectiveness of oral contraceptives (OCs) while taking antibiotics started in 1971 when Reimers and Jeyeck noted increased abnormal vaginal bleeding in OC users on rifampin and other anti-tuberculosis drugs. Other case reports followed. The postulated mechanism was that the antibiotics altered the normal flora of the gut so that less estrogen was absorbed. The relationship has not previously been studied despite widespread use of antibiotics, particularly tetracycline for acne and sexually transmitted disease treatment in teenagers. In this study, seven normal women on a common monophasic 1/35 OC took tetracycline 500 mg q 6 hours for the first 10 days of the cycle. Blood levels of tetracycline and the two hormones in the pill were measured before starting the medications, then eight times on day 1 and levels of the drugs were measured again between days 5 and 10. No significant decrease of either the hormones or tetracycline was seen at any time. However, the sample size was quite small.

Negrini, B., Schiffman, M., Kurman, R., Barnes, W., Lannom, L., Malley, K., Brinton, L., Delgado, G., Jones, S., Tchabo, J-G., & Lancaster, W. (1990). Oral contraceptive use, human papillomavirus infection, and risk of early cytological abnormalities of the cervix. *Cancer Research, 50*, 4670–4675.

The Pap smears from 1,964 women were examined to determine if oral contraceptive (OC) use was a risk factor for cytological abnormalities of the cervix. Pap smears were divided into three groups: atypia, low grade squamous

intraepithelial lesion (SIL/LG), and high grade squamous intraepithelial lesion (SIL/HG). A subset, which included most of the women with SIL low or high grade, was also tested for human papilllomavirus (HPV). It is widely believed that HPV infection may produce high grade cervical neoplasia only in the presence of cofactors. OC use was not related to atypia and SIL/LG but was associated with an elevated risk of SIL/HG that increased with longer duration of OC use (RR 4.6). HPV infection was associated with both low and high grade SIL but not with atypia. Taking the HPV results into consideration did not alter the OC findings. There was no evidence that OC use synergistically increased the risk of cervical neoplasia among HPV-infected women, although small numbers prevented a reliable evaluation for high grade SIL. OC use did appear to increase the detection of HPV types 16 and 18 but the etiological importance of this finding is unclear.

The authors state that they considered and controlled for the fact that contraceptive methods (such as barriers) used by controls might actually decrease the risk for cervical neoplasia. This was not believed to be a factor because many subjects in the control group had not used any contraceptive method.

Parazzini, F., Negri, E., La Vecchia, C., & Fedele, L. (1989). Barrier methods of contraception and the risk of cervical neoplasia. *Contraception, 40*(5), 519–530.

The authors state that several studies have shown barrier contraceptives protect against cervical cancer. They wish to provide more quantitative data on the relationship between barrier contraceptives and invasive and non-invasive cervical cancer. The researchers looked at two sets of data: (1) 367 subjects with invasive cervical cancer and 323 controls, and (2) 316 subjects with non-invasive cervical cancer and 258 controls.

Subjects reported on personal characteristics and habits, related medical history, gynecologic and obstetric information (including frequency of Pap smears), sexual habits, and lifetime use of contraceptives. Use of a barrier was reported by 6 percent of subjects with invasive cervical cancer and 12 percent of their controls while use of a barrier was reported by 16 percent of subjects with non-invasive cervical cancer and 22 percent of their controls. Regardless of whether cancer only involved the cervix or had invaded other tissues, use of a barrier method appeared to reduce risk of cancer. Greater risk reduction (50%) was seen with invasive cancer compared with a 27 percent reduction for women with non-invasive cancer. This may mean that earlier detection through routine gynecological exams is a contributing factor.

Pardthaisong, T., Yenchit, C., & Gray, R. (1992). The long-term growth and development of children exposed to Depo-Provera during pregnancy or lactation. *Contraception, 45,* 313–324.

Most investigations of children exposed to synthetic progestins during pregnancy have been done on children exposed because of threatened abortion, not for contraceptive use. None of these studies examined the long-term effects of exposure to systemic contraceptive drugs such as depot-medroxyprogesterone acetate (DMPA) which have a prolonged action and are known to cross the placenta. There has been concern over the use of hormonal contraceptives during lactation as well as during pregnancy. Although the progestin-only contraceptives such as DMPA do not affect milk volume, they are transferred through breast milk and could potentially affect health and development of nursing infants. Studies have found that women using DMPA had smaller children. These investigators noted in a previous study that women using DMPA were of a lower socioeconomic status than mothers in the control group which would explain the smaller infants. No impairment in growth during childhood or at puberty was found except for reported (though not observed) delayed appearance of pubic hair in DMPA-exposed girls.

Rebar, R., & Zeserson, K. (1991). Characteristics of the new progestogens in combination oral contraceptives. *Contraception, 44*(1), 1–9.

This is a good review of studies done on the three new low-dose oral contraceptives (OCs),

two of which have been approved for use in the United States. The new OCs—desogestrel, norgestimate, and gestodene—have three chemically different progestogens which are potent but have few androgenic (male hormone) side effects. They have few, if any, estrogenic effects and weak antiestrogenic effects. These OCs are the results of an ongoing effort to reduce the total amount of steroids in OCs. However, it is important to remember it is the *biological activity* of the steroid (a combination of both the *dose and potency* acting together) and *not number of milligrams* that is important when comparing and contrasting different OCs. This article contains chemical structures of the four old, as well as the three new, progestogens to assist in understanding the differences between the pills. Desogestrel must be transformed in two steps to its active form. Norgestimate and gestodene are active in their original form although a small proportion of norgestimate is metabolized to levonorgestrel. Because of the different metabolism, the three new progestogens may have different metabolic effects.

Gestodene appears to have the most potent progestogenic activity. All progestogens bind to other steroid receptors. Because of the tendency of gestogene to bind to mineralcorticoid receptors, it may be helpful for women who have elevated blood pressure, although clinical use is needed to bear out this hypothesis. In general, these new progestogens appear to have few or no effects on carbohydrate or lipid metabolism, or on clotting factors. The authors report a small increase has been seen in high density lipoprotein (HDL) with desogestrel and a small but significant decrease in clotting time with gestodene as is seen with levonorgestrel. Clinical trials have not shown any increased risk of blood clots with gestodene compared with older OC formulas. When considered together, the authors conclude, there appears to be little difference between the new progestogens and low-dose OCs currently in use.

Richwald, G., Greenland, S., Gerber, M., Potik, R., Kersey, L., & Comas, M. (1989). Effectiveness of the cavity-rim cervical cap: Results of a large clinical study. *Obstetrics & Gynecology, 74*(2), 143–148.

This is one of the largest studies of the cervical cap done in the United States. Information was gathered from 3,433 women at 15 sites from 1981 to 1988. The number of women-years of use was not given. Method effectiveness rate for the cap was 96.2 percent and user effectiveness rate was 88.7 percent. The mean age of the subjects was 29, 91 percent were white and had completed high school, 80 percent were unmarried, and 60 percent were college graduates.

Factors associated with increased risk of pregnancy were age under 30 years, no college degree, plans to have more children, sexual intercourse more than three times a week, lower income, previous pregnancies including abortions, no previous experience with the cap, wearing the cap for longer time periods, and cap dislodgement. Twenty percent of users reported problems with cap dislodgement, cap odor, or partner discomfort. This study indicates that when cap size is selected by experienced fitters, women are highly motivated and well instructed in correct use, and they use the cap as instructed. In this regard, the cap can be approximately as effective as birth control pills for a select group of educated women age 30 or older.

Ross, J. (1989). Contraception: Short-term vs. long-term failure rates. *Family Planning Perspectives, 21*(6), 275–277.

Small risks taken repeatedly accumulate to very large risks over a long period of time. This author states that a young couple of average fertility not using any birth control method has a 15 percent to 20 percent chance of pregnancy each month. If they use a contraceptive that is 95 percent effective, the risk of pregnancy is lowered to about 1 percent each month. A 1 percent risk per month over 10 years accumulates to a 70 percent chance of pregnancy occurring in that 10-year time period. Approximately one-fifth of pregnancies end in spontaneous abortions or miscarriages which results in a 62 percent chance of a pregnancy that leaves the woman with the choice of having an abortion or a child. Considering that

most women need contraception for at least 20 years, this indicates there have been, and will be, many unwanted children. Fortunately, fertility declines with aging. But these numbers indicate the importance of using the most effective birth control methods available. This is an excellent article and should be mandatory reading for anyone counseling contraceptive users.

Sahwi, S., Toppozada, M., Kamel, M., Anwar, M., & Ismail, A. (1989). Changes in menstrual blood loss after four methods of female tubal sterilization. *Contraception, 40*(4), 387–398.

Although many women have claimed that their periods were longer or heavier after sterilization procedures, recent studies have not substantiated these subjective evaluations. The results of this study are in agreement with several larger prospective studies which have failed to find effects of sterilization on menstrual patterns.

Schwartz, B., Gaventa, S., Broome, C., Reingold, A., Hightower, A., Perlman, J., & Wolf, P., Toxic Shock Syndrome Study Group (1989). Nonmenstrual toxic shock syndrome associated with barrier contraceptives. *Reviews of Infectious Diseases*, II, Supplement 1, January–February, S43–S48.

Toxic shock has been a concern with female barrier contraceptive use. This group of authors examined potential risk factors for non-menstrual toxic shock syndrome (TSS) in 28 subjects and 100 controls. Both sponges and diaphragms were associated with a significant, though low, increased risk of toxic shock. Although there were not enough cap users for a meaningful evaluation of the association with TSS, the information collected indicates an increased risk similar to the sponge and diaphragm. Based on this study, the authors estimate that approximately 40 sponge users and 54 diaphragm users have TSS in the United States per year. With deaths at 8 percent of total cases, approximately eight deaths occur per year from TSS.

The authors point out that the risk of TSS is low when compared to the risk of pregnancy or the risk of complications related to other contraceptive methods. Although this study is quite small to use in projecting the number of cases of and deaths from TSS per year, still this information should be considered when making birth control choices.

Shihata, A., & Trussel, J. (1991). New female intravaginal barrier contraceptive device: Preliminary clinical trial. *Contraception, 44*(1), 11–19.

This is a report on a study of the effectiveness and acceptability of a new silicone rubber cervical cap called the Fem Cap. The Fem Cap, which is shaped like a sailor's hat, has a dome that covers the cervix, a rim that fits snugly into the vaginal fornices, and a brim that adheres and conforms to the vaginal wall. It is reusable for 2 to 3 years and has an applicator to facilitate insertion, if needed.

Of 106 study participants with a total of 1,300 cycles of exposure, 5 became pregnant. Two reported dislodgement of the cap during intercourse and the other three did not use the cap consistently. Six more women reported dislodgement of the Fem Cap during intercourse but did not become pregnant. All women were instructed to use spermicide with the cap.

The Pap smears of two participants converted from Class I to Class II. Both had human papillomavirus (HPV). Four converted from Class II to Class I. None had Class III Pap smears. None of the women or their partners reported any discomfort.

The Fem Cap may be another acceptable choice for some women but the number of dislodgements in 7 of 106 women indicates it is less than an ideal method.

Shoupe, D., Mishell, D., Bopp, B., & Fielding, M. (1989). Norplant: Subdermal implant system for long-term contraception. *American Journal of Obstetrics & Gynecology, 160*(5), Part 2, 1286–1292.

This is an excellent review of studies on the levonorgestrel delivery system, Norplant. Insertion, removal, and patient management of problems are covered along with effectiveness, drug metabolism, mechanism of action, metabolic changes, contraindications to use, side effects, complications, and user acceptance.

Shoupe, D., & Mishell, D. (1991). The significance of bleeding patterns in Norplant implant users. *Obstetrics & Gynecology, 77*(2), 256–260.

This study was done to examine bleeding patterns of 234 Norplant users during 5 years of use and to identify the bleeding patterns of users who conceived. It is important to note that all but 60 women in this study had implants with a denser type of silastic tubing which released less hormone than the tubing currently used. In the first year of use, 26.65 percent of users had regular cycles, 66.3 percent had irregular cycles, and 7.1 percent had no menstrual periods. By the 5th year of use all had menstrual periods; 62.5 percent had regular cycles and 37.5 percent had irregular cycles. Of the 10 users who became pregnant, 8 had regular menstrual cycles in the 6 months before the diagnosis of pregnancy, 1 had irregular cycles and 1 did not keep a record of bleeding. All but one of the method failures occurred in women who had the more dense silastic tubing which results in lower rates of diffusion, therefore lower blood levels of levonorgestrel. Three of the pregnancies in this study were ectopic which is similar to the 20 percent rate of ectopic pregnancies reported by others. Weight of the women was not a factor in these method failures.

The conclusions to be drawn from this study are: (1) to suspect pregnancy in Norplant users who miss a period after several months of regular cycles, (2) to establish the location of the pregnancy early since 20 percent are ectopic, and (3) reassure women who are amenorrhic that their method is effective and that they do not need periodic pregnancy tests.

Shuber, J. (1989). Transcervical sterilization with use of methyl 2-cyanoacrylate and a newer delivery system (the Femcept Device), *American Journal of Obstetrics & Gynecology, 160*(4), 887–889.

This procedure for sterilization avoids the risk of injuries and death associated with procedures requiring anesthesia and surgery. Liquid Methyl 2-Cyanoacrylate was introduced into the woman's tube where it joins the uterus. The substance was placed in the tubes by blowing up a balloon in the uterus which forced the liquid into the tubes. No pain medication or tranquilizers were used on the 34 women having the procedure. The procedure took less than 5 minutes and was performed in a same-day surgery facility. All women were able to leave the operating table within 2 minutes after the procedure was completed. The stay in the recovery room averaged $1^3/_4$ hours with 86 percent leaving in less than $2^1/_2$ hours. Approximately half of the women asked for pain medication in the recovery room. The authors report no significant differences in menstrual function before and after the procedure, but give no information on how this was determined.

On follow-up, 88 percent of the women had complete bilateral obstruction of the tubes, as desired. All except one of the women, including those for whom the procedure failed, said they would have the procedure again if necessary and would recommend it to others.

Additional contraception is needed for 4 months until a hysterosalpingography (x-ray exam of uterus and tubes using dye) is done to check for blockage of the uterine tubes.

Since this method could be done in a physician's office or clinic with no special equipment, it might make sterilization available to more women provided they had access to X-ray equipment for the 4-month follow-up.

Soper, D., Brockwell, N., & Dalton, H. (1991). Evaluation of the effects of a female condom on the female lower genital tract. *Contraception, 44*(1), 21–29.

This study was done to determine if use of the polyurethrane Reality female condom was traumatic to the vaginal mucosa or vulvar skin and to determine its effect on the normal vaginal flora. Thirty women were randomly assigned to either the Reality condom or the diaphragm. Subjects were examined by colposcopy and tests were collected to identify fungal and bacterial organisms in the vagina. Both groups had intercourse with approximately the same frequency.

There was no evidence of significant trauma to the vagina with either device throughout the study. No changes were seen in vaginal flora with the Reality condom. Diaphragm users were less likely to have the normal lactobacilli and more likely to have bacteria commonly found in the colon over time. The authors mention another report which suggests that spermicide, rather than the diaphragm, may account for the increased growth of coliform bacteria among diaphragm users.

Two women in the Reality condom group had weakly positive chlamydia tests, both of which were negative on retest and were believed to be false positives. Neither woman had a history of exposure to sexually transmitted diseases. One women had cultures positive for coliform bacteria which the authors speculate may have contributed to the false positive chlamydia test. However, one wonders why there weren't more diaphragm users with positive chlamydia tests since the authors report they had more coliform growth than Reality condom users.

Speroff, L., & Darney, P. (1992). A clinical guide for contraception. Baltimore, MD: Williams & Wilkins.

This book differs from Hatcher et al., *Contraceptive Technology*, in that specific information directed toward users is not given. That is to be expected because users are not the audience. Speroff and Darney's book is aimed at health professionals: the language is quite technical. There are good discussions of studies on oral contraceptives (OCs) including the concerns that accompany OC use such as cancer and thromboembolism. Norplant is covered very thoroughly with clear illustrations on insertion and removal.

However, information on diaphragms, cervical caps, and natural family planning methods does contain several inaccuracies. The authors state that the flat spring diaphragm is for normal vaginal muscles and the arcing spring is for women with soft vaginal muscles and a shallow pubic notch when, in fact, the opposite is correct. They present the cap as if spermicide need not be used with it (contrary to FDA instructions) and as if decreasing cap odor is the reason to use spermicide. They say the cap can be left in place several days when FDA instructions are to limit cap use to 48 hours. They recommend checking cap placement by feeling for the cervix through the dome which is not even possible with the small cap and is not the best way to check any cap. And they say that only about 50 percent of women can be fitted with the cap when more than 80 percent of women can be fitted in some practices depending upon population characteristics. An error in natural family planning information includes identifying "sticky but (slippery)" as a characteristic of the clear, wet, stretchy fertile mucus. All of these inaccuracies may lead to pregnancy for some women.

Taylor, S., Pickens, J., & Geden, E. (1989). Interactional styles of nurse practitioners and physicians regarding patient decision making. *Nursing Research*, 38(1), 50–55.

This study examined interactional styles used by nurse practitioners and physicians and then examined styles used by males and females. Data were analyzed for instances of maternalism (pointing out consequences of behavior), paternalism (commanding specific behavior), and shared decision making (concordance regarding behavior). The authors found that males and physicians in solo practice used more consequence statements, and all groups used more command/consequence statements than concordance statements. Unlike concordance statements, both command and consequence statements undermine patient/client autonomy. This important piece of research emphasizes that practitioners and clients alike need to be aware of how practitioner styles of communicating may interfere with the clients' right to choose in many situations.

Thomas, D. (1991). Oral contraceptives and breast cancer: Review of the epidemiologic literature. *Contraception*, 43(6), 597–639.

This is an important review of the literature on the association between oral contraceptives (OCs) and breast cancer. All case-control and cohort studies known to the author were reviewed. He concludes that OCs may increase risk of breast cancer in young women with a history of

benign breast disease and that multiple studies have fairly consistently shown a slightly increased risk of breast cancer in women under age 45 who are long-term OC users.

Toivonen, J., Luukkainen, T., & Allonen, H. (1991). Protective effect of intrauterine release of levonorgestrel on pelvic infection: Three years' comparative experience of levonorgestrel- and copper-releasing intrauterine devices. *Obstetrics & Gynecology*, 77(2), 261–264.

This is a report on a randomized multicenter comparison of two intrauterine devices (IUDs). There were 937 women with the Nova-T copper-releasing IUD and 1,821 women with an IUD that releases 20 micrograms of levonorgestrel daily. In 36 months the cumulative gross pregnancy rate was 3.7 for the Nova-T and 0.3 for the levonorgestrel IUD. There were five ectopic pregnancies with the Nova-T and three with the levonorgestrel IUD, a significant difference.

Pelvic inflammatory disease (PID) is a long-standing concern with IUD use. For this study, diagnosis of PID required at least two of the following symptoms or signs: (1) history of lower abdominal pain and increased body temperature (over 38C), (2) increased erythrocyte sedimentation rate (peak over 30 mm/hr), (3) tenderness on pelvic exam, (4) mass on pelvic exam, and (5) ultrasound exam or laproscopy if other evidence is controversial. This study found the levonorgestrel IUD protected against PID with a 36-month PID rate of 0.5 compared with a rate of 2.0 for the Nova-T.

The disadvantages of the levonorgestrel IUD are amenorrhea and hormonal side effects. Despite these disadvantages, the low PID rate may help solve one of the major concerns associated with IUD use since the Dalkon Shield experience.

Trussell, J. (1991). Methodological pitfalls in the analysis of contraceptive failure. *Statistics In Medicine*, 10, 201–220.

As an important study for those who work in the field of contraception, it gives an appreciation of the difficulties encountered in attempting to determine contraceptive effectiveness rates for the widely different methods. The study comes from a critical review of the literature done to prepare a reference book on contraceptive effectiveness for family planning practitioners. In his review, the author found that understanding of the relative efficacy of contraceptive methods is quite limited because of defects in research design and in the analytic tools used by investigators. He discovered hundreds of mistakes in arithmetic, fraud, loss of follow-up numbers so large that the study results had little meaning, and frequent use of the Pearl index which does not control for duration of contraceptive use, rather than life table analysis which does. He discusses experimental design, problems with those designs, consequences of deviating from the ideal design, and the numerous problems in analysis of the research study. He ends with several "minimal" recommendations for researchers studying contraceptive methods.

Trussel, J., & Grummer-Strawn, L. (1990). Contraceptive failure of the ovulation method of periodic abstinence. *Family Planning Perspectives*, 22(2), 65–75.

Data from a World Health Organization clinical trial of the ovulation method of periodic abstinence were used by the authors to determine method and user effectiveness for this method of contraception. The probability of pregnancy during the first year is 3.1 percent with perfect use (method failure) and an astounding 86.4 percent with imperfect use (user failure). There are three rules that should not be broken: (1) no intercourse during mucus days, (2) no intercourse within 3 days after the day of ovulation, and (3) no intercourse during times of stress. Breaking these rules results in a 28 percent risk of pregnancy per cycle.

Vessey, M., Villard-Mackintosh, L., McPherson, K., & Yeates, D. (1989). Mortality among oral contraceptive users: 20-year follow-up of women in a cohort study. *British Medical Journal*, 299, December 16.

The authors followed 17,032 white women recruited from 17 large family planning clinics in England and Scotland for an average of 16 years to see whether oral contraceptive (OC) use influences mortality. At the time of recruitment, the women ranged in age from 25 to 39 and were put into one of two groups based on being either a current OC user or a current diaphragm or IUD user who had not previously used the pill. During the follow-up period 238 deaths occurred. This is considerably less when compared with the general population because 417 deaths would be expected based on overall death rates in England and Wales in 1980. The overall relative risk (RR) of death in OC users was 0.9%. In individual disease categories the RR in OC users was 4.9% for cancer of the cervix, 3.3% for ischemic heart disease, 1.5% for circulatory disease, and 0.4% for ovarian cancer. Death rates from breast cancer (RR 0.9) and suicide (RR 1.1) were similar in the two groups. The authors concluded there was no significant evidence of any overall effect of OC use on mortality. However, since there were only a small number of deaths in the study period, a significant adverse or beneficial effect might emerge in the future.

Winikoff, B., Wymelenberg, S., & Editors of Consumer Reports Books (1992). *The Contraceptive handbook: A guide to safe and effective choices.* Yonkers, NY: Consumer Reports Books.

This guide, published by Consumer Report Books, is definitely directed toward consumers. It is easy to read, interesting, and instructions are directed to the reader. It addresses women's concerns and answer women's questions. A unique feature of the book is that it has method costs so that one may comparison shop in one's living room. Methods discussed are the diaphragm, cervical cap, condom, sponge, spermicides, oral contraceptives, Norplant implant, intrauterine devices, male and female sterilization, fertility awareness, breastfeeding, withdrawal, morning-after contraception, abortion, and the new contraceptive options of female condoms, vaginal rings, and injectables.

Chapter 5

Childbearing

Patricia A. Geary
Marie Hastings-Tolsma
Dianne Voytko
Amgad Wahba
Thelma Patrick

INTRODUCTION

The literature about childbearing is as always bewilderingly, multitudinous and difficult to reduce to manageable size. Since the reduction also reduces the perspective which can be gained from the literature as a whole, there is some inherent danger in the selection process. Therefore, articles were selected that might either positively or negatively influence the care offered to women. The subcategories used for organization of the literature have been changed to reflect the literature itself and the message the literature contains. The categories of "Teen Pregnancy" and "Pregnancy, Health and Illness," continue to receive much attention as they reflect societal attention and change. In a 1988 review, the authors introduced "Impact of Technology" to provide a focus on the growth of technology (Leppa & Miller). The literature continues to demonstrate an increasing use of technology which intrudes on the whole childbearing experience in various ways. Therefore, the articles reviewed for this chapter were categorized more traditionally into "Pregnancy, Health and Illness," "Intrapartum" and "After Birth," reflecting the usual stages of the childbearing experience. Articles relating to technology, psychosocial aspects, medical intervention, and childbearing alternatives have been integrated into those three categories. A number of reports about the care of women with various health problems who are choosing childbearing appeared during 1989–1992. Therefore, a category, "Women with Special Needs," was created to focus attention on the choice for childbearing which is being made by women experiencing various problems as well as to sensitize health providers to this group of women. Cesarean section and breastfeeding have been singled out for attention in categories of their own. And finally, a major new category has been created for this review, "Issues in Childbearing."

ISSUES IN CHILDBEARING

After any extensive review of the literature, it is important to sit back and ask what are the impressions gained from this review. Such reflection is a more inductive thought process, typically used in feminist analysis. Following this review of the literature, the image of competition and conflict was that which arose. In an earlier publication, the authors reviewed in the area of Psychosocial Aspects, Balin's (1988) article "The sacred dimension of pregnancy and birth." A re-review and re-attention to her framework seems important now. She emphasized that pregnancy was a social status in which everyone feels a right to advise and participate, both with the individual woman and in the whole area of childbearing. Balin emphasized pregnancy as not just an individual but also a social experience. It seems that at the current time pregnancy is, in fact, a social issue which reflects all of the conflicts and problems present in our society. It probably should be no surprise that an event which is so important to a society should reflect all the concerns of society.

It is this construction of pregnancy as a social event which lead to *Issues in Childbearing*. This section has been further subdivided into four sections: legal and ethical dimensions, research, services, and professional interests. It seems that these represent the major polarities in the field. The discussion of whom to consider and why in treatment decisions continues and fuels consideration of legal and ethical dimensions. The article by Halbreich and Carson is encouraging in that it does give a model for including women in some very important studies from which they have been traditionally excluded. The research articles were spotlighted because research can fundamentally affect the care offered to women. Some research articles imply that there is only one method of research, one that is, in fact, reductionist and dampens the experiences and voices of women. The other research articles reviewed provide deferring viewpoints. Services were included in this category to underscore the tug of war in this country regarding who will pay for health care. The payment issue seems to be settled by paying for less and less hospitalization and making minimal provision for community-based services and prevention. In fact, in reality health care most likely is being paid "invisibly" by the services of female caretakers in the home. Yet the articles in this section show the need for services in relationship to cost, both financial and human. Therefore, some articles which discuss cost analysis are included. Of particular concern is research that presents data bases used to evaluate hospital care. Items not included in a data base cannot be considered. Such exclusion has the potential of leaving out much that is of importance to women themselves and retaining that which is of importance to the medical and health care establishment.

Authors that discuss the need for prenatal care focus on prematurity and the cost of prematurity; however, little is said about the impact of absent or minimal prenatal care on pregnant women. Balin's point about the sacred nature of pregnant women as a *container* for life must be remembered in an analysis of the problems with prenatal care; then, absence of concern about women unfortunately makes a great deal of sense. Although our society has a high regard for life, seldom are both the mother's life and the fetus' life considered at the same time. Even the fetus' life does not seem to be particularly regarded in this struggle for services and the finance of services. Finally, professional interest was included because more and more professionals are proclaiming an interest in pregnancy. This may be either positive or negative for childbearing women. It certainly is a trend to watch. In addition, an article published in England bemoaning the problems of maternity leaves for pregnant nurses was included as a warning. As women are more and more involved in the workforce, such reactions may become more common.

WOMEN WITH SPECIAL NEEDS

Whether the choice for pregnancy is becoming more common among women with health problems or whether we are simply paying attention to that choice, articles relating to such problems are more frequently occurring in the literature. In addition, the issues around the loss of a child are gaining attention. Such occurrence within the literature is positive in that it both emphasizes that there are more choices for women and that the health care system must be able to respond to those women. Childbearing has many more aspects for consideration than the progression through three trimesters of pregnancy and all aspects must be considered including the inability to conceive (Sandelowski, et al., 1991). This section contains one of the few articles examining the experience of childbearing women with impaired mobility (Kopala, 1989). The message of this section is that pregnancy is an individual experience with a need for individualized attention, and increasingly, women who may not have felt free to choose that experience in the past are choosing it now. The question is whether health professionals will be ready for this choice. The presence of these articles in the literature is positive and gives importance, weight, and visibility to those choices.

PREGNANCY, HEALTH, AND ILLNESS

This section illustrates what may be a continuing dialectic throughout childbearing, the struggle between advancing technology and the need to provide care tailored to the experiences and needs of women. Technology has its own demands and its own life, and if not guarded against, technology can dictate care rather than allow for care which is planned with the woman herself. To make matters worse, we are only beginning to look at the expectations of childbearing women regarding technology. The increasing stress on prenatal diagnosis mirrors its increasing emphasis in practice and a dichotomy which exists around its use. While prenatal diagnosis may give women more choices, it also imposes an expectation of good care. The tension between high technology and low technology is perhaps best expressed by prenatal diagnosis versus such things as using acupuncture for nausea in pregnancy and offering for supportive provider visits throughout pregnancy.

TEEN PREGNANCY

The interest in teen pregnancy continues. Perhaps it is in this area where pregnancy as a social concern is most visible. The issue of services is consistently and repeatedly addressed. Articles seem to focus not on prevention, as has been the case in the past, but on identifying the needs of and services for teenagers who become pregnant in order to help them have more successful lives.

INTRAPARTUM

The tension between high technology and low technology is reflected in this section as well. Technology and technologic interventions are increasingly being questioned. Not only are new applications of technology discussed, i.e., Knorr, "Relieving fetal distress with amnioinfusion," but there is also a questioning of the technology which has been taken for granted in the past. For example, Rockner questions the common wisdom that episiotomy prevents tears. In addition, there are articles discussing new childbirth alternatives such as waterbirths as well as reviewing outcomes from more long-standing alternatives such as freestanding birth centers and birthing rooms. The evidence is mounting that the less technologically oriented sites for childbirth are no more dangerous and provide a more woman-centered and positive birth experience with no greater risk than hospital births. In addition, the issue of finances is raised by Eakins, et al., noting that fees for service at an alternative birth center were two-thirds those in a hospital. Given the high expense of hospital care and the move toward reducing the amount of time the woman is kept in the hospital, one cannot help but wonder if women would be better served by delivering in a birthplace or at home with thorough postpartum follow-up.

AFTER BIRTH

The "bottom line" in the birth experience should be the experience of the woman—positive outcomes both physical and psychological for her, the infant, and family. Increasingly, the "bottom line" is the financial one imposed by third-party payers which severely restricts in-patient admissions. Unfortunately, limiting hospitalizations is not offset by home follow up. Despite this diminished hospital time, birth practices continue to result in more physical problems. Changes in care delivery must take into account women's preferences, their need for control and a careful evaluation of their readiness for professional intervention.

CESAREAN SECTION

Despite national concern about the rising Cesarean section rate, the increase has not abated. This section contains some of the same tensions which occur in "Intrapartum." The debate about when and whether Cesarean sections must be done continues. The rising rate certainly cannot be accounted for simply by an increasing incidence of complications in pregnant women. The Cesarean section rate again brings into focus pregnancy as a social phenomenon in which there are other factors at work besides the physical and physiological. As Porreco indicates, there are many factors operative in Cesarean section decisions including the physician's education, the role of the physician in labor, as well as reimbursement. We have a situation in this country where physician education is essentially technology training. When labor becomes a high technology experience, Cesarean section is much more likely. Cesarean section is endorsed by society since it is reimbursed at a higher rate than a vaginal delivery. For women who must have a Cesarean section, the opportunity to have more control over the experience can be positive. This increased control is reflected in the article by Bucknell and Skiorski on patient-controlled anesthesia. Finally, a thought provoking article by Perez explores the contributing factors that lead to Cesarean sections.

BREASTFEEDING

The choice of breastfeeding as a way to provide nutrition for a newborn should be one that any woman is free to make. This selection of articles reflects the various factors that impact on those choices from a mother's social network to the practices of the institution in which she delivers.

CONCLUSIONS

The struggle to enhance the childbearing experience is now an old one. There have been many changes and alternatives over the years. Yet the struggle is never done; it simply moves laterally to other points in the continuum of the childbearing experience. Concerned women are making changes in their own arenas. These articles seem to reflect changes in local areas, yet women still must surrender a great deal of freedom in childbearing. What will it take to curb the rampant use of technology and allow women more choices? Individual education can have only limited impact. Sustained, coordinated national strategy and vigilance may be necessary to broach the real issues of money and power.

REFERENCES

Balin, J. (1988). The sacred dimensions of pregnancy and birth, *Qualitative Sociology*, vol. 11, pp. 275–301.

Leppa, C. J., & Miller, C. (1988). *Women's Health Perspectives: An Annual Review*, vol. 1. Phoenix: Oryx Press.

BOOKS AND ARTICLES

Issues in Childbearing

Legal and Ethical Dimensions

Bushy, A., Rauh, J. R., & Matt, B. F. (1989). Ethical principles: Application to an obstetric case. *Journal of Obstetrical, Gynecologic and Neonatal Nursing, 18,* 207–212.

A case study involving a pregnant woman and treatment decisions in a high risk 25-week pregnancy is presented. The author defines the ethical principles of double effect versus consequentialism, autonomy, beneficence, utility and justice. Each principle is discussed in conjunction with the case to illustrate the guidance its acceptance would give to the medical decision. The discussion shows that ethical decision making is neither clear cut nor are the factors which would guide the selection of a particular principle. The impact of societal forces and norms on such decision making is obvious. The authors suggest interdisciplinary ethics committees as a means to facilitate ethical decision making. The authors do not come to grips with the pressures on women which come from societal expectation in such decision making. The authors also rule out application of the principle of autonomy in the case based on the grounds that there are two patients, the woman and the 25-week fetus. Thus, the tension between the rights and needs of the woman and her fetus create a complex ethical dilemma not easily resolved.

Field, M. A. (1989). Controlling the woman to protect the fetus. *Law, Medicine & Health Care, 17,* 114–129.

This is an excellent, well-documented discussion of both the potential controls which could be placed on women to protect the fetus, such as forced prenatal screening for to actual court-mandated Cesarean sections. A discussion of whether the government should regulate pregnancy is included. The author argues that government controls on pregnant women not only intrude on their lives and rights but also fail to achieve the goal of improving the health of newborns. The author makes excellent points including a discussion of the class issues underlying who is forced into treatments. A strong case is made for education of women, free prenatal care, and provision of substance abuse programs as better ways to improve the health of newborns. The tendency to view women as special cases with rights not equal to those of men is glaringly evident in the cases presented. This trend is troubling enough by itself, but the fact that the legal system and legislative bodies are comprised of predominantly males compounds the concern.

Halbreich, U., & Carson, S. W. (1989). Drug studies in women of childbearing age: Ethical and methodological considerations. *Journal of Clinical Psychopharmacology, 9,* 328–333.

The authors conducted a study of lithium (a drug used to control depression) in childbearing-age women whose protocol included the use of normal women as a control group. Because of the potential of lithium to cause birth defects, the human subjects review board requested further information and actual solutions to potential problems before approving the study. The authors discuss the proposed solutions and the physiological and pharmacological background which led to their development. Their approach to ensuring the safety of both the women and any potential pregnancies provides a model for drug studies in childbearing-age women. The ethical dimension of advising abortion in the case of pregnancy is discussed. A paucity of studies exists which include women. Hence, the potential benefits of such research are not accessible to women. The article demonstrates that drug research with childbearing-age women is difficult, but not impossible. A well-informed population of women giving truly informed consent is essential. Both researchers and women subjects assume a greater burden regarding the risks, but with careful guidelines research can be done.

Research

Anderson, G. C. (1991). Current knowledge about skin to skin (kangaroo) care for preterm infants. *Journal of Perinatology, 11,* 216–226.

Kangaroo care is a variant of the care generally offered to premature infants. The infant is held skin to skin against the mother and breastfeeding is self regulated by the infant. The article provides an excellent summary of current knowledge about these practices and includes in a tabular form a superb review of all of the English language studies available at the time of the compilation of the manuscript. The author has created four categories relating to time of initiation of kangaroo care which are used in the summary table for comparison purposes. Outcomes appear better both for the infants and for their mothers and fathers in kangaroo care. This approach to care of premature infants is being implemented widely in European countries and is being initiated on the West Coast in the United States. The positive aspect of this excellent review is that it enables the reader to compare multiple studies and supports kangaroo care as a potential modification of care of the premature infant. One potential concern, however, is the rush to cost containment which often places the burden for cost containment on the provider. Kangaroo care has the potential for being demanded of women rather than offered to them thus allowing them less control over their perinatal experiences.

Beck, C. T. (1989). Maternal-newborn nursing research published from 1977 to 1986. *Western Journal of Nursing Research, 11,* 621–626.

Beck, C. T. (1989). Fundamentals of obstetric, gynecologic, and neonatal nursing research: Part I. *Journal of Obstetric, Gynecologic and Neonatal Nursing, 18,* 216–221.

Beck, C. T. (1989). Fundamentals of obstetric, gynecologic and neonatal nursing research: Part II. *Journal of Obstetric, Gynecologic and Neonatal Nursing, 18,* 288–294.

Beck, C. T. (1989). Fundamentals of obstetric, gynecologic and neonatal nursing research: Part III. *Journal of Obstetric, Gynecologic and Neonatal Nursing, 18,* 385–389.

These four articles represent a significant contribution to the childbearing literature. The author reviews ten years of literature, offers a methodologic critique, and in the last three articles methodological recommendations are made. The first article covered three nursing research journals and categorized the articles by: stage of childbearing and topic studied, use of a theoretical framework, design and methods and recommendations. Results were compared with a larger study of nursing research. A discussion of theoretical frameworks, validity and reliability of research instruments, and research problems was presented.

This series of articles is both excellent and unsettling. The attention to research in childbearing and the excellent synopsis of deductive research methodology are exciting. However, the fact that the articles ignore inductive methodology and suggest, by implication, that non-experimental, experimental and quasi-experimental designs are the only valid approaches to research is of concern. Feminist and inductive research methodologies which can add to what is known about women without the imposition of predefinition are ignored.

Berkowitz, G. S., Skovron, M. L., Lapinski, R. H., & Berkowitz, R. L. (1990). Delayed childbearing and the outcome of pregnancy. *The New England Journal of Medicine, 322,* 659–664.

The widespread belief that advancing maternal age poses increased risk for pregnancy complications and neonatal outcomes was investigated in this large ($n = 3,917$) retrospective survey of primiparous women age 20 or older. Participants were private patients who were largely white, married, and college-educated. Findings suggest that advancing maternal age does not appreciably increase the risk of an adverse outcome in singleton gestations. However, mothers who were older were more likely to have antepartal and intrapartal complications, Cesarean births, and infants admitted for neonatal intensive care. Control of covariates and the sample size make findings particularly noteworthy. The growing proportion of American women who chose to delay birth of their first child is a well-documented trend. This study provides women with information about the risk of delayed pregnancy—important in timing pregnancy consistent with personal capability and ability.

Bright, M. A. (1992). Making place: The first birth in an intergenerational family context. *Qualitative Health Research, 2,* 75–98.

The author used a grounded theory methodology to study three families including a nuclear family and both sets of grandparents over 15 months. The study reveals the complexity of the major family process identified by the study, "making place," which included physical and social changes in order to welcome the new infant. This study broadens the usual definitions of family often used in childbearing to include the grandparent generation and emphasizes the complexity of introducing a new member into the family group. The results suggest that our current conceptualizations may be limiting and that a broader inclusion of family members could be positive both for the new child and the new parents.

Roberts, J. (1992). Practice based research in maternity nursing: Issues and examples from studies of labor and birth. *Applied Nursing Research, 5,* 93–100.

A two-part discussion of practice based research in maternity nursing is presented. The first is a review of research methods presenting them as a pyramid moving from clinical observation at the base to experimental designs at the peak of the pyramid. The author utilizes her own research to present problems which can arise in clinical experimental studies. Reviewing her own work with single subject and comparison designs, she outlines problems with experimental clinical trials including non-acceptance by subjects, infrequent occurrence of the problem being studied, and a tendency for practicing clinicians to adopt the research treatment with all patients, not just those in the treatment group. The author provides some very illuminating discussions of problems in clinical research which offer alternatives in the design of maternity nursing research. Based on the author's attempt to operationalize experimental

designs in practice settings, she recommends more descriptive ethnographic approaches to clinical problems. While her preference is for inductive structured designs, the realities of the practice situation have swayed this author to consider the more inductive research designs. These designs have the advantage of involving rather than distancing their participants.

Services

Brooks-Gunn, J., McCormick, M. C., Gunn, R. W., Shorter, T., Wallace, C. Y., & Heagarty, M. C. (1989). Outreach as case finding: The process of locating low-income pregnant women. *Medical Care, 27,* 95–102.

Donovan, P. (1989). Providing prenatal care services at family planning clinics: Problems and opportunities. *Family Planning Perspectives, 21,* 127–130, 144.

McCormick, M. C., Brooks-Gunn, J., Shorter, T., Holmes, J. A. H., Wallace, C. Y., & Heagarty, M. C. (1989). Outreach as case finding: Its effect on enrollment in prenatal care. *Medical Care, 27,* 103–111.

These three articles discuss ways of increasing the numbers of women receiving prenatal care. Brooks-Gunn, et al., and McCormick, et al., report on two different facets of the same study which employed outreach workers to enroll women in prenatal care. The authors imply that the results of using outreach workers were not as positive as expected. However, only two workers were used for one year and two others six months, which may not have been sufficient time to test the efficacy of the model. The authors suggest this program was expensive (although certainly not as expensive as care for low birth weight infants). They speculated that the clients attracted through outreach were not enrolled significantly earlier in prenatal care than other clients.

Donovan summarizes experiences of family planning clinics across the country which added prenatal care to their services. Financial issues, physician availability for delivery, malpractice insurance and well-child services are included in the discussion.

Given the real concern in this country for the limited access to prenatal care, these articles are important because they report on efforts to try new things and expand established services to reach more women. These represent positive, non-punitive, and creative attempts to address a national problem.

Gates, M., & Shelton, S. (1989). Back transfer in neonatal care. *Journal of Perinatal and Neonatal Nursing, 2,* 39–50.

Samson, L. F. (1989). Perinatal outreach education: Linking hospital and community in the care of high risk infants. *Journal of Perinatal and Neonatal Nursing, 2,* 51–57.

Troiano, N. H. (1989). Applying principles to practice in maternal-fetal transport. *Journal of Perinatal and Neonatal Nursing, 2,* 20–30.

These three articles provide excellent individual discussions of their various programs. The article on fetal transport not only discusses personnel, guidelines, equipment, referral and documentation but also presents the results of one program. The article on back transport is exemplary in the broad-ranging discussion of all the issues involved in transferring a child back to the home community. Each of the programs discussed is complex but needed. Outreach education of community health nurses to care for perinatal patients is an idea whose time has come. These articles include recommendations for change in a complex perinatal care system such as improving collaboration between institutions or agencies that provide perinatal and neonatal care.

Norr, K. F., Nacion, K. W., & Abramson, R. (1989). Early discharge with home follow-up: Impacts on low-income mothers and infants. *Journal of Obstetric, Gynecological and Neonatal Nursing,* March/April, 133–141.

Sadler, C. (1989). Unconditional discharge? *Nursing Times, 85,* 18.

Both articles deal with early discharge of high risk mothers and infants. The first article studied women in three groups to determine whether early discharge could be shown to have negative outcomes. Strict criteria were used to select women eligible for early discharge. Although there was a high incidence of both maternal and infant physical problems, there was no difference between the early and usual discharge groups nor the third group where the infant remained in the hospital after early maternal discharge. Attachment scores differed significantly between mothers discharged early with their infant and those discharged early without their infant. An attempt was made to compare cost of care. Women discharged early did receive nurse visits. The second author discusses problems midwives in England are seeing with early discharge (4.1 days!) of high risk women. Together these articles are thought provoking. Economics has forced early discharge. In most cases there is no nurse follow-up. It is possible that hospitals should be used only for birthing, and that post partum care be provided in the home. This would require a drastic revision in our reimbursement structure.

Savinetti-Rose, B., Kempfer-Kline, R. E., & Mabry, C. M. (1990). Home Photo Therapy with the Fiberoptic Blanket. *Journal of Perinatology, 10*(4), 435–438.

With early discharge, hyperbilirubinemia and increased bilirubin levels in the newborn, now occur at home and may be reason for rehospitalization of the infant. The authors describe a fiberoptic blanket which has the advantage of covering only the infant's torso, thereby avoiding eye and scrotal complications resulting from light treatment. The authors also describe a home photo therapy program which provides helpful information for instituting such a program. While this article gives more technical aspects of such care, the authors also discuss the potential for anxiety and concern on the part of the families and present specific interventions. This article is one more example of the increase in management of acute problems in the home environment which should emphasize the need for skilled home follow up by health practitioners. Health providers must enter into the discussion about health care policy and reimbursement for the sake of patients.

Schroeder, M. A., & Carter, J. (1989). Development of a database management system for an obstetrics unit. *Computers in Nursing*, 7, 112–118.

Increasingly data will be managed electronically and decisions regarding this process are critical to women. The authors describe a collaborative process for selecting software for an obstetrics unit and deciding upon the categories of data to include for retrieval. The article contains an excellent description of the software itself. The reasons for its choice are applicable whenever a software package is considered: number of fields (categories) it can handle, a tutorial system, excellent support from the vendor, and in-house experience with the software. Such systems have the capability of allowing the easy retrieval of data for staffing and programmatic decisions and research. What is disturbing about this article is that the authors, both of whom had maternity clinical background, chose to include only the classic medical and health care systems data long included in birth logs in hospitals. It seems little or no consideration was given to items important to women such as: birth plan, birthing room, prepared childbirth. Without the presence of such items on a data base they cannot be considered in research or decision making. Women are again forced into a medical model that limits their choices. Attention to the software selection processes and the categories of data which will be collected in such systems is important to consider before developing a data based management system.

Swartz, R. M. (1989). What price prematurity? *Family Planning Perspectives*, 21, 170–174.

This study sample looked at 28 perinatal centers representing over a third of all births in urban hospitals during 1985. Costs were quantified to suggest the savings that would occur if the birth weight distribution for three categories of birth weight changed so that 20 percent of all cases in each birth weight category shifted

to the next higher weight category. Centers were randomly selected from all urban tertiary hospitals. By conservative measures, savings for all groups were $73–96 million. The author estimated the cost of preventive care, subtracted it from the savings and found there would still be a $9–28 million savings. The author discusses why these would be "real" savings, as well as makes the case for expecting that this change in birth weights is possible. It is suggested that these data support a national policy change which would allow broad-based preventive maternity care for high risk women. This article makes a clear economic case for such a policy. However, there are other factors to take into account to institute such a policy including who gains, who loses, and who saves in such a shift of resources. These factors may yet force the politicization of those who would provide better services for women as hospitals and third-party payers could well lose if prematurity declined.

Professional Interests

Affonso, D., & Mayberry, L. (1989). Challenges in the perinatal clinical specialist role. *Clinical Nurse Specialist*, 3, 99–101.

This article scratches the surface in identifying some of the changes which may be necessary in the role of the perinatal clinical specialist. Its strength lies in the discussion of the need for participation in legislative and political processes. The underlying message in the article is the need to broaden the role. Lacking is a suggestion of linkages with other health colleagues and clinical specialists. The need for and impact of home care is suggested.

Eglee, K. R. (1989). No one nurses our patients but us. *RN*, August 1989, 13–14.

An anecdotal account of the process used to create a "closed" obstetrical unit in which nurses were neither floated in nor floated out is the focus of this article. The author's description of the actual staffing pattern is valuable. It is apparent from the description that the factors which provide for good care, an experienced knowledgeable staff, also create job satisfaction, patient satisfaction, and cost savings.

Hulme, J. B., Mayfield, H., & Hulme, R. (1989). Obstetrics—gynecology in the physical therapy curriculum. *Physical Therapy, 69*, 264–267.

McIntosh, J. M. (1989). Women—The captive audience. *Physiotherapy, 75*, 10–13.

These two articles illustrate the increasing interest in childbearing by various professional practice disciplines. The first article compares two surveys of content in physiotherapy programs. In the five-year interim between the two questionnaires, content had increased but practice time diminished in obstetrics and gynecology. This could be viewed positively and negatively. While physiotherapists may have more knowledge and interest in childbearing, they may have less skill.

McIntosh, in a well-documented article, presents some of the practice roles of the obstetric physiologist including pre- and post-natal classes, teaching relaxation and pelvic floor exercises, and community classes. The article is solid factually but paternalistic in tone from the title right on through. It conveys a case for an expanded role for the physiotherapist but a controlling means of obtaining it.

To have more health professionals develop skill and interest in childbearing is important. Childbearing women deserve access to knowledgeable professionals. It is important, however, that skill accompany interest and that both be developed in a context which will allow individualized care and a partnership with women.

Jacobs, B. B., & Jacobs, L. M. (1989). Transport of obstetric/gynecologic and neonatal patients. *Emergency Care Quarterly, 4*, 48–65.

Trauma has become the major cause of death in pregnancy. This article was written for emergency medical personnel. It carefully reviews physiology, assessment and interventions for selected obstetric, gynecologic and neonatal emergencies. The information is accurate and

thorough. However, the only recognition that the individuals being transported are either a pregnant, worried woman, or a mother and an infant who may need some other considerations than accurate blood pressures and management of hypovolemia, is mentioned in a single sentence, "The uncomplicated, on-scene delivery can be a heartwarming and sensitive experience for all involved." No effort is made to suggest ways to assist in assuring that such an experience occurs or even suggest sources which would provide an understanding of how to make it "heartwarming." If all that is understood by emergency personnel is the contents of this article, the transport experience could be a stressful one indeed.

Jones, I. H. (1989). The pregnant pause. *Nursing Times, 85*, 36–37.

In two pages the author decries the problems of maternity leaves for nurses from the viewpoint of the nurse manager. While there is some attempt to state positive aspects of maternity leaves both for individual nurses and the profession in general, the overall tone is a negative moan. Since the case is made that most nurses are women, these same negative arguments of difficult coverage, etc., can be made for other similar positions such as teachers or secretaries. Such attitudes prevent better leave policies for women. It is not possible to rest on the laurels of our progress. Why does no one ever stop to realize what women add to the economic base rather than worry about what they take away?

Reed, K. S. (1992). The effects of gestational age and pregnancy planning status on obstetrical nurses' perceptions of giving emotional care to women experiencing miscarriage. *Image: Journal of Nursing Scholarship, 24*, 107–110.

The researcher surveyed obstetrical nurses (n = 292) to determine the influence of gestational age (10, 15, or 20 weeks) and pregnancy planning (planned or unplanned) on nurses' emotional care for women who have experienced pregnancy loss. The study evolved from the growing recognition that patients who miscarry perceive nurses and physicians to be cold, indifferent and uncaring. The study was designed to determine if there were factors related to the miscarriage experience that might influence emotional care delivered by nurses. Both gestational age and whether the pregnancy was planned or unplanned had a significant effect on the nurses' perceptions of emotional seriousness and priority of care. Planning status was significant in the nurses' perception of emotional support. While 27 percent of the respondents had themselves experienced a miscarriage, this factor did not influence the nurses' response. Findings underscore the need to develop creative strategies for meeting the health care needs of childbearing women beyond physical care. As time in the health care system decreases, nurses will need to carefully plan ways to meet comprehensive health needs of women, responding to individual needs of women rather than stereotypes.

Women with Special Needs

Alderson, M. K., Hill, W. C., & Theesen, K. (1989). Managing depression in pregnancy. *Patient Care, 23,* 187–190, 195, 198.

Zucherman, B., Amaro, H., Bauchner, H., & Cabral, H. (1989). Depressive symptoms during pregnancy: Relationship to poor health behaviors. *American Journal of Obstetrics and Gynecology, 160,* 1107–1111.

These two articles discuss depression during pregnancy, an area to which little attention has been given in the literature. Alderson's article suggests that the use of antidepressants during pregnancy involves risks to the fetus, but may be justified when psychotherapy or hospitalization has failed. Small doses of tricyclic antidepressants are known to be associated with fewer side effects. Tapering anti-depressant therapy 2–3 weeks before delivery helps to minimize the drug's adverse effect on the fetus.

Zucherman's article examines the relationship between depressive symptoms during pregnancy, and maternal health behaviors and infant outcome. Findings suggested that women living in poverty or experiencing stress and lowered social support may develop depressive symptoms which will influence health behavior and in turn influence infant outcome. Counseling and supportive relationships with behavioral strategies can help women master the feelings of helplessness associated with depression. Given the stress of today's society, it is important to consider pregnant women's affective state, social context, and mental health. These articles have a definite contribution to the literature in the area of antepartal depression. Zucherman in particular attempts to examine some of the intricate connections between social conditions, depressive symptoms, and health habits.

Brown, L. S., Mitchell, J. L., DeVose, S. L., & Primm, S. L. Female intravenous drug users and perinatal HIV transmission. (letter) *The New England Journal of Medicine, 320,* 1493–1494.

Cohen, J. B., Hauer, L. B., & Wofsy, C. B. (1989). Women and IV drugs: Parenteral and heterosexual transmission of human immunodeficiency virus. *The Journal of Drug Issues, 19,* 039–056.

Kurth, A., & Hutchison, M. (1989). A context for HIV testing in pregnancy. *Journal of Nurse Midwifery, 34,* 259–266.

Prince, N. A., Beard, B. J., Ivey, S. L., & Lester, L. (1989). Perinatal nurses' knowledge and attitudes about AIDS. *Journal of Obstetric, Gynecological and Neonatal Nursing, 5,* 363–368.

Woleske, M. (1989). Antenatal HIV screening. *Neonatal Network, 8,* 7–13.

Each of these articles discusses some aspect of the growing population of HIV positive childbearing women. With the exception of the first, a letter to the editor, all are sensitive to the complexity of the issues. The letter asserts that female intravenous drug users are less effective users of contraception. They suggest birth control services be available on site in drug treatment programs. While this is laudable from a convenience and service viewpoint, it does not take into account that pregnancy and contraception involve more than the women themselves.

Cohen, et al., stress the difference in needs and service approaches for women who are HIV positive. They underscore the need for services which look at the unique needs of heterosexual women and lesbians and discuss research and policy implications.

Kurth and Hutchison present an excellent review of serological tests, the ethics of testing, psychological reactions to testing and counseling pre- and post-testing.

Woleske discusses the incidence of AIDS, the characteristics of the virus itself, indicators of HIV infection, laboratory findings consistent with negative findings for HIV infection, and screening recommendations.

Prince explores the level of knowledge, fear and attitudes about AIDS in perinatal nurses. Strategies to help nurses with this important change in the constellation of their practice are necessary.

Burke, M. E. (1989). Hypertensive crisis and the perinatal period. *Journal of Perinatal and Neonatal Nursing, 3*(2), 33–47.

Daddario, J. B. (1989). Trauma in pregnancy. *Journal of Perinatal and Neonatal Nursing, 3*(2), 14–22.

MacMullen, N. J., & Brucker, M. C. (1989). Pregnancy made possible for women with cystic fibrosis. *MCN, 14*(3), 196–198.

Reece, E. A., & Winn, H. N. (1989). Caring for the pregnant diabetic. *Patient Care,* (June 15), 177–184.

Walsh, S. (1988). Cardiovascular disease in pregnancy: A nursing approach. *Journal of Cardiovascular Nursing, 2*(4), 53–64.

Advanced medical technology has benefitted the general outcome of mothers and infants when pregnancy is complicated by an existent disease process or altered health state, such as cardiovascular disease or trauma.

The physical effects of the disease process or altered health state during pregnancy are reviewed in each of these articles. Medical management of the pregnancy to maintain the established health state of the mother and the well being of the fetus until delivery is the primary focus in each. Increasingly, women who were once advised to forego pregnancy are being able to use advances in medicine in planned pregnancies. This increase in choice is important for women. Also important is attention to pregnant women with needs other than those which are disease related. This attention is variably represented in these articles.

Reece makes a categorical statement which should be carefully questioned—any pregnant woman who exercises should be watched for signs of intrauterine growth retardation.

Catlin, A. J. (1989). Early pregnancy loss. *Nursing, 89,* November, 43.

Johannsen, L. (1989). As birth and death coincide. *MCN, 14,* 89–92.

Null, S. (1989). Nursing care to ease parents' grief. *MCN, 14,* 84–89.

Wilson, D. (1989). Unexpected miracles. *American Journal of Nursing, 89*(2), 306.

While none of these articles reports results of research, as a unit they make use of the available research and call attention to a group of women easily overlooked, those whose babies are stillborn or dying. Catlin gives a brief series of hints on how to help women facing a loss early in pregnancy. Johannsen's article is a thought-provoking discussion of the issues and problems that arise when only one child of a multiple gestation survives. Null describes a program offered by a hospital for women who lose a fetus or a newborn. The editorial by Wilson shows how individual a woman's perspective can be when facing a life-threatening birth defect like anencephaly. Together these articles convey a welcome message: the importance of paying attention to the experience of the individual woman and of shunning avoidance in the face of tragedy. They all emphasize the importance of sharing information and the existing need in the health care system to pay more attention to supporting the woman's decision making.

Fekety, S. E. (1989). Managing the HIV positive patient and her newborn in a CNM service. *Journal of Nurse Midwifery, 34,* 253–258.

Harvey, S. M., Carr, C., & Bernheine, S. (1989). Lesbian mothers. *Journal of Nurse Midwifery, 34*, 115–119.

Theroux, R. (1989). Multiple birth: A unique parenting experience. *Journal of Perinatal and Neonatal Nursing, 3*, 35–45.

Each of these articles considers an important group of women who approach childbearing with special needs. Two articles discuss the range of needs over the pregnancy for two special groups: HIV infected women and women with twins. The article on lesbian mothers provides comparative data on pregnancy and satisfaction with care of a group of lesbian women in an earlier study group. Each article provides a wealth of information, useful for health professionals who provide care to women with special needs. So often pregnant women are lumped together stereotypically and care provided according to trimester and cultural prescription. However, each woman is an individual with an infinite variation in needs. This variation is expanded when the woman also has some special category of needs related to life style or physical condition. Given the changes in society and the increase in the number of choices available to women, it is important to keep abreast of the changing knowledge base necessary to provide sensitive, individualized care. These articles assist in that effort.

Fox, G. N., & Strangarity, J. W. (1989). Varicella-Zoster virus infections in pregnancy. *American Family Physician, 39*(2), 89–98.

Varicella-Zoster Virus Infections, commonly known as chicken pox and herpes zoster infections, can cause life-threatening maternal illness, fatal neonatal infarction, or a congenital syndrome. This article reviews the history of the disease identification, the nature and action of the virus, and the pathophysiology of infections caused by the virus. Suggestions for treatment of the mother, fetus, or newborn are limited to those surrounding medical management of the infection, such as isolation or administration of vaccine. No attention is given to the psychosocial implications for the women of such an infection. While these infections are rare, women

should be aware of their potential and be assessed for immunity.

Kent, A. (1989). Home is where the fear is. *Nursing Times, 85*, 16–17.

This brief article is thought provoking as it deals with the tie between battering and pregnancy. The questions which are raised about services are no less relevant because they deal with the British health care system. It is troubling that a mother and unborn child are so vulnerable and unprotected—whatever the reasons and societal ramifications.

Kopala, B. (1989). Mothers with impaired mobility speak out. *MCN, 14*, 115–119.

This summarizes discussions regarding childbearing and childrearing which the author had with seven disabled women. Seven categories arising from the discussions are reviewed: conflicts around the decision to parent, adoption, childbirth, necessary adaptations for child care, satisfactions, effects on the children, and use of resources. The article performs an important function in sensitizing the reader to the perspectives and needs of these women. Since the discussion was based on interviews with women, emphasizes a supportive role on the part of nurses, and suggests a willingness to help women with impairments achieve their goals, this article is strongly positive from the viewpoint of feminist philosophy.

McKeon, V. A., & Perrin, K. O. (1989). The pregnant woman with a myocardial infarction: Nursing diagnosis. *Dimensions of critical care nursing, 8*, 92–100.

Troiano, N. H. (1989). Cardiopulmonary resuscitation of the pregnant woman. *The Journal of Perinatal and Neonatal Nursing, 3*, 1–13.

Both of these articles contain a wealth of information that has relevance to cardiac complications during pregnancy. McKeon and Perrin discuss management of myocardial infarction (heart attack) in pregnancy. This is a rare occurrence during pregnancy and necessitates skilled care. The authors present a case study in which a woman, 14 weeks into a pregnancy, had a myocardial infarction. The woman decided to continue her high risk pregnancy against medical advice. She gave birth to a four-pound, seven-ounce female. The case study depicts good, sensitive care in which the nurses were guided by the woman's desires. The article includes a review of cardiovascular changes during pregnancy and discusses care in relation to nursing diagnoses and patient anxiety.

Trioano reviews cardiovascular and respiratory changes during pregnancy and their relationship to cardiopulmonary resuscitation (CPR). The process of CPR dysrhythmias and their management and the drugs used in CPR in pregnancy are discussed. The authors assert that the life of the mother takes precedence over saving the life of the fetus when both are at risk.

These articles impress upon the reader the impact of emergency situations in pregnancy.

Sandelowski, M., Harris, B. G., & Holditch-Davis, D. (1990). Pregnant moments: The process of conception in infertile couples. *Research in Nursing and Health, 13,* 273–282.

Using grounded theory methodology, these authors study the experience of becoming pregnant in two groups of couples: those experiencing infertility treatment and those who are fertile. The descriptions of the experiences of the infertile couples are particularly poignant and well worth reading. This is an excellent example of information obtained through focus on the actual experiences of women and provides rich information which can be transferred to clinical practice.

Weitzman, B. C. (1989). Pregnancy and childbirth: Risk factors for homelessness? *Family Planning Perspectives, 21,* 175–178.

This article reports on relationships between homelessness and pregnancy and number of children in a family. It used data collected as part of a larger study on homelessness. The author used a weighting procedure to determine

that pregnant women receiving welfare have an 18 percent probability of homelessness versus 2 percent for those not pregnant. Women having a child before their 18th birthday were more likely to be homeless. The author discusses possible explanations for the findings. The actual reasons are unclear. However, it is a provocative commentary on social values when pregnancy places women at risk for homelessness.

Pregnancy, Health, and Illness

Crowe, K., & vonBaeyer, C. (1989). Predictors of a positive childbirth experience. *Birth, 16* (2), 59–63.

Possible predictors of a positive or negative childbirth experience are: the woman's knowledge of childbirth, fears about pregnancy, locus of control, anxiety, expectation of pain, and confidence in ability to control pain. Self reports of 30 primiparous women related to these factors were examined. Twenty-one subjects completed the study; all were in their last trimester. Measurements used were: the McGill pain questionnaire (MPG), the State-Trait Anxiety Inventory (STAI), the childbirth education review which was constructed for this study, the pregnancy research questionnaire (PRQ), the pregnancy attitude index (PAI), and the expectations form which was made up of visual analog scales (VAS). The VAS measures pain during labor and delivery, and confidence in ability to control pain. The components of prenatal classes which were identified as predictors of a positive experience were knowledge of childbirth, and confidence in ability to control pain. Two unexpected findings were: a less anxious childbirth was predicted for those who had high levels of fear before prenatal classes, and a less painful childbirth could be predicted for those who had a high level of anxiety after classes.

Farrell, C. D. (1989). Genetic counseling: The emerging reality. *Journal of Perinatal and Neonatal Nursing, 2,* 21–33.

Morgan, C. D., & Elias, S. (1989). Perinatal diagnosis of genetic disorders. *Journal of Perinatal and Neonatal Nursing, 2,* 1–12.

Williams, J. K. (1989). Screening for genetic disorders. *Journal of Pediatric Health Care, 3,* 115–121.

Each of the articles discusses the importance of genetic counseling in the preconceptual and perinatal period. Farrell's article clarifies the multifaceted nature of the genetic counseling process as it relates to reproductive concerns. It discusses indications for prenatal diagnosis, the techniques themselves, and the role of the nurse as educator in prenatal diagnosis. The emphasis is on providing clients with information and letting them make their own decisions, a very empowering strategy. The other two articles provide an update on the techniques and screening programs used for perinatal diagnosis which has expanded with the availability of genetic screening. The nurse's responsibility in educating clients about genetic screening tests is emphasized. All three articles emphasize the importance of information sharing, voluntary testing and the need to support the client's decision making process. The authors approach women as capable, decision-making people who are able to use information about their situation.

Fox, N. L., Sexton, M., Hebel, J. R., & Thompson, B. (1989). Brief report: The reliability of self reports of smoking and alcohol consumption by pregnant women. *Addictive Behaviors, 14,* 187–195.

Self reports of pre-pregnancy smoking and drinking (alcohol) were compared for over 700 women in a randomized clinical trial of a smoking cessation intervention. Agreement was compared using the Kappa statistic to compare early and late pregnancy reports. Reliability was moderate to substantial. A saliva test verified the reports of smoking. However, women were told the purpose of the saliva test only if they asked. The authors suggest that this may have increased the reliability of the self-reports. Both treatment and control groups were similar in their reliability. This article provides an excellent review of the issues involved in self-reports of smoking and alcohol consumption. It also helps to substantiate that women can be reliable

in such reports and their word can be trusted. It is worth reading from both treatment and clinical perspectives.

Frentzen, B. H., Dimperio, D. L., & Cruz, A. C. (1988). Maternal weight gain: Effect on infant birth among overweight and average-weight low-income women. *American Journal of Obstetrics and Gynecology, 159,* 1114–1117.

Minimal weight gain for overweight women has been questioned as a clinical strategy on the basis of the results of a study of women who were white and middle or upper class. This study examined the relationship of pre-pregnant weight, weight gain, and outcome in low-income women. Average weight and overweight women were compared. Gain during pregnancy affected birth weight in the average weight group but not the overweight group. Infant outcomes were similar. The authors note that significant prepregnancy overweight (≥ 135%) must be present for this to be the case and suggest that dietary recommendations be varied by the degree of overweight. This study attempts to look at differences among women and make recommendations based on evidence of differences rather than stereotype or assumption, a positive step. How this information is used, imposition or education is critical.

Harmon, J. S., & Barry, M. (1989). Antenatal testing, mobile outpatient monitoring service. *Journal of Obstetric, Gynecologic, and Neonatal Nursing,* 21–24.

This article described a means for improving care for antepartum, high-risk pregnant women on restricted activities in their homes. A mobile outpatient monitoring service was provided by home care nurses with expertise in antepartum care who conducted necessary maternal and fetal assessments and gave emotional support and education. The program proved to be cost-effective. Clients better adhered to bed rest and fewer were re-admitted to the hospital for increased uterine activity. Caring for pregnant women at home provided more control for the women than prolonged hospitalization would afford. This article describes a well thought out service which was able to close at least one of the gaps in the services offered to women.

Hyde, E. (1989). Acupressure therapy for morning sickness. *Journal of Nurse Midwifery, 34,* 171–178.

This study examined the efficacy of acupressure wristband therapy for morning sickness of early pregnancy using a two-group random assignment, crossover design. Of the 16 subjects who completed the trial, 12 felt that the use of acupressure therapy was helpful in relieving morning sickness. Findings indicated that early intervention with acupressure wristbands produced less nausea, vomiting, anxiety, depression, hostility, and behavioral dysfunction. The author emphasizes the implications of this study for nurse midwifery practice by evaluating acupressure as a safe, easy intervention based on a good theoretical rationale and uses the woman's own body mechanism to restore homeostasis. While this study is limited in numbers it does contribute a potential means of control of nausea during pregnancy which the woman herself can control. The author does note the tendency to explain morning sickness in ways which are unfriendly to women. This work certainly suggests a more physiological basis.

Johnson, F. (1989). Assessment and education to prevent preterm labor. *MCN, 14,* 157–160.

A preterm labor prevention program is described, including assessment, services and educational interventions. Inservice education on preterm labor is delivered to all health team members. The author suggests screening all women for risk of preterm labor each prenatal visit and educating all women about preterm labor, not only those at risk. Over one half of premature labors occur in women not identified as at risk. The author does mention family thus acknowledging that there are more factors at work than the woman herself. The woman herself is educated to recognize premature labor thus putting much of the control in her own hands.

Loos, C., & Julius, L. (1989). The client's view of hospitalization during pregnancy. *Journal of Obstetric, Gynecological and Neonatal Nursing, January/February,* 52–56.

The study examined the meaning of hospitalization to pregnant women. Eleven hospitalized pregnant women were administered a questionnaire developed for the study and interviewed 48 hours later. Both questionnaires and interviews were analyzed together. Loneliness, boredom and powerlessness were the prevailing themes. The authors identify this as a phenomenological study. The methodology is not consistent with phenomenology; however, it is an inductive study which does describe the women's own feelings and contributes to an understanding of their situation. The authors provide an excellent discussion of the implications of their findings.

Lopez, E. I. (1989). Prenatal diagnosis by ultrasound. *Journal of Perinatal and Neonatal Nursing, 2,* 34–42.

Myhre, C. M., Richards, T., & Johnson, J. (1989). Maternal serum fetoprotein screening: An assessment of fetal well being. *Journal of Perinatal and Neonatal Nursing, 2,* 13–20.

Rhoads, G. G., et al. (1989). The safety and efficacy of chorionic villus sampling for early prenatal diagnosis of cytogenetic abnormalities. *The New England Journal of Medicine, 320,* 609–617.

These articles discuss three current methods of fetal diagnosis. Lopez's article describes the many fetal diagnoses that can be made with the assistance of diagnostic ultrasound, the relationship between diagnostic ultrasound and genetic counseling and the role of the nurse in prenatal diagnosis. Myhre's article describes the purpose and procedures of maternal serum alpha fetoprotein (glycoprotein) testing as well as a voluntary screening program in the state of California, its cost, procedures, test interpretation and following. A case study is presented. The Rhoads, et al., article examines the safety and effectiveness of chorionic villus sampling as a method of prenatal diagnosis in the first trimester of pregnancy.

The authors feel it is safe but slightly less so than amniocentesis. Parental anxiety is a significant issue for any prenatal screening method. Extensive education of both care providers and parents is an important component in reducing parental anxiety and assisting decision making. Knowledge of management protocols and use of an interdisciplinary approach is imperative for proper assessment of fetal well being. Keeping clients informed of findings, including client and family in management decisions, supporting difficult decisions and psychological reactions and counseling clients for future pregnancies is crucial. The first two articles discuss those issues. The last article raises the important issue of training and the necessary commitment of resources at a center to provide for the development of skill and therefore good success rates.

Moore, Jr., R. M., Jeng, L. L., Kaczmarek, R. G., & Placek, P. J. (1990). Use of diagnostic ultrasound, X-ray examinations, and electronic fetal monitoring in perinatal medicine. *Journal of Perinatology, 10*(4), 361–365.

Care of the pregnant woman involves technology which includes electronic fetal monitoring (EFM), diagnostic ultrasound, and X-ray examinations. The sample included a pretest of 575 women, and a survey of 20,000 pregnancies (10,000 live births; 4,000 fetal deaths; 6,000 infant deaths). Findings indicated that nearly 80 percent of pregnancies received diagnostic ultrasound with most women receiving two or more. The most common reported indication for ultrasound was for gestation age or to establish dates. Further, approximately 15 percent received X-ray examination (for reasons both related and unrelated to the pregnancy), and approximately 75 percent were monitored with EFM (which included both external and internal methods) during the birth process. Evidence from this investigation suggests that diagnostic ultrasound and EFM are nearly standard interventions during pregnancy. Other studies have provided little support for use of these techniques on a routine basis. Their use results in an increasing technologization of a natural process. Conversely, the hazards of prenatal exposure to X-rays has been documented and provides evidence that low-dose prenatal irradiation may increase the risk of childhood cancer. The substantial use of X-ray noted in this investigation raises serious concerns. It is not surprising that the researchers question the disparity between scientific information and clinical practice. It may well be that professional practice issues related to potential litigation, etc., may be the key determinants of the use of these technologies. Consideration of the safety and effectiveness of these technologies is critical in meeting needs of pregnant women and their offspring.

Oakley, A., Rajan, L., & Grant, A. (1990). Social support and pregnancy outcome. *British Journal of Obstetrics and Gynaecology, 97,* 155–162.

The authors report the results of the study which provided a relatively simple "low tech" social intervention given by four mid-wives to a high risk population of women. Pregnancy outcomes were compared using delivery records for two groups assigned randomly to a support group and a control group. Women in the control group were significantly more likely to be admitted to the hospital while the intervention group was more likely to have a spontaneous labor and vaginal delivery as well as lower incidence of epidural anesthesia. The treatment group particularly appreciated the fact that the mid-wife listened to them. Both mothers and babies receiving the intervention were reported to be significantly healthier. This study supports the belief that women should have supportive care during pregnancy, and such supportive care is ultimately less costly to society and to the women themselves in terms of the women's health and the outcomes of their births. This study should be widely read, particularly in our current era of cost containment.

O'Connor, A. M., Davies, B. L., Dulberg, C. S., Buhler, P. L., Nadon, C., McBride, B. H., & Benzie, R. J. (1992). Effectiveness of a pregnancy smoking cessation program. *Journal of Obstetric, Gynecologic and Neonatal Nursing, 21,* 385–392.

This clinical investigation examined two approaches to promoting smoking cessation among pregnant women ($n = 224$) using a quasi-experimental design. Participants were less than 31 weeks' gestation, reported smoking at least one cigarette per day, and were confirmed by urinary cotinine levels. Experimental treatment consisted of an evening class providing guidance on a self-help program for 2 hours on a group basis or 20 minutes on an individual basis during the prenatal appointment. The control group received the usual care which consisted of a brief discussion, a pamphlet, and the option of attending a self-help cessation program, although none did so. Of the experimental group, those receiving immediate intervention at the time of the first prenatal visit had 2–3 times higher rates of cessation at 1 month post-intervention, and at 36 weeks gestation and 6 weeks post-partum. Use of these findings with women who smoke during pregnancy may combine to produce significant change in the smoking behavior of women. The risks associated with smoking for both the mother and fetus, as well as the favorability for smoking cessation during pregnancy make the findings particularly important.

Osborn, M. R. (1989). Selective reduction of multiple gestation. *Journal of Perinatal and Neonatal Nursing, 3,* 14–21.

Price, F. V. (1988). The risk of high multiparity with IVF/ET. *Birth, 15,* 157–163.

Advances in technology such as in vitro fertilization and embryo transfer and gamete intrafallopian transfer have allowed many women to become pregnant who previously were unable to do so. Such technologies do result more frequently in multiple gestations which has led to the question of what to do to decrease the risks of such gestations. Selective reduction (selective termination of one or more fetuses in a multiple gestation) in multiple gestation is one approach to the problem and has been the subject of controversy in lay and professional literature. Osborn's article examines the issue of selective reduction in multiple pregnancies, describes selection criteria, clinical procedures, ethical issues, and nursing implications

associated with selective reduction. Osborn suggests nurses' knowledge of available options, parental support in decision making, and acknowledging the actual and potential emotional impact of the procedures is essential. She includes a sensitive discussion of the multiple and complex issues involved. Price's article emphasizes the importance of providing information to pregnant women with multiple embryos which may include the statistical risks and associated complications. High multiparity puts extraordinary demands on caretakers and the risks extend far beyond individual cases to the wider social ramifications and financial burdens. Price's discussion of the complexity of the issues is well worth reading. She includes consideration of selective reduction within this context.

Page, S. (1989). Rh hemolytic disease of the newborn. *Neonatal Network, 7,* 31–41.

Remich, M. C., & Youngkin, E. Q. (1989). Factors associated with pregnancy-induced hypertension. *Nurse Practitioner, 14,* 20, 22, 24.

Sever, J. L. (1989). The latest on TORCH infections. *Patient Care, 23,* 155–174.

These three articles deal with three different types of obstetrical complications. Page's article discusses Rh hemolytic disease of the newborn, the various treatment approaches and their underlying rationale, and the nurse's role including physical assessment, certain precautions for infants undergoing phototherapy, and nursing care during exchange transfusions. Advances over the last twenty years and the role of prevention are mentioned. Remich's article reports the correlation between pregravid weight to ideal weight, prenatal weight gain, maternal age and the subsequent development of pregnancy induced hypertension (PIH). Low maternal age was significantly related to the development of PIH. Although the factors of gravid weight and prenatal weight were not found to be associated with the development of PIH in the study, data revealed that a significant relationship existed between women whose mean arterial blood pressure did not decrease in the second trimester and the subsequent development of PIH. Sever's article updates the reader on the latest on TORCH (toxoplasmosis, rubella, cytomegalic inclusion disease, and herpes) infections. It also includes new information on parvoviral infections and AIDS which are of growing importance. The article discusses advances in antibody testing which can help determine when infection has occurred and thus aid in counseling women. All of the articles provide excellent background information on these problem areas. However, as a group they do not give much attention to how this information should be used with women, although in two cases there is some brief comment on education.

Phelan, J. P., Park, Y. W., Ahn, M. O., & Rutherford, S. E. (1990). Polyhydramnios and perinatal outcome. *Journal of Perinatology, 10*(4), 347–350.

Polyhydramnios (amniotic fluid volume of > 2000 mL) has been associated with significant perinatal mortality and morbidity. The use of ultrasound has enabled clinicians to conduct a quantitative assessment of the amniotic fluid volume (AFV) which may be excessive. Researchers conducted a retrospective survey of 72 patients, determined to have evidence of polyhydramnios by sonography, to ascertain fetal outcome. Increased AFV was associated with a higher incidence of fetal macrosomia, fetal anomalies, diabetes mellitus, and premature births. In addition, in these patients, the likelihood of a nonreactive stress test was increased. Data provides empirical evidence useful in appropriately counseling women regarding additional fetal surveillance and potential outcomes.

Reis, J., Sherman, S., & Macon, J. (1989). Teaching inner-city mothers about family planning and prenatal and pediatric services. *Journal of Pediatric Health Care, 3,* 251–256.

This article is interesting in that it reports on a method, a videotape, created to advise about the availability of health care and practices of a specific clinic. The videotape was positively evaluated by 135 women. What is most encouraging is that this was an attempt to reach a group of women in a way which would appeal to them rather than standard written publications. The film was presented both at clinics and an alternative high school, thus providing some outreach to those not enrolled in the clinics. One can imagine television and supermarket viewings as a way to advise more women of the services available to them.

St. Clair, P. A., & Anderson, N. A. (1989). Social network advice during pregnancy: Myths, misinformation, and sound counsel. *Birth, 16,* 103–107.

One hundred and eighty-five low income, inner city women participated in this study which asked them to name up to 30 network members and identify the advice received from them during their pregnancy. Women participants were interviewed on the second postpartum day which does raise the question of the accuracy of their recollections. Mothers, sisters, and partners were the most frequent advice givers. Advice was wide ranging and often conflictual. Most advice was good but the actual reasons for the advice were not necessarily understood by those giving it. This study emphasizes the amount of advice women may receive during pregnancy from other than health care providers. It suggests that a healthy pregnancy may be more likely in this population if network members as well as pregnant women are taught new information about pregnancy. That pregnancy is a social event is emphasized by these findings. No one health professional working alone can have the impact they could have by joining forces with the network.

Villar, J., Farnot, U., Barros, F., Victora, C., Langer, A., & Belizan, J. M. (1992). A randomized trial of psychosocial support during high-risk pregnancies. *The New England Journal of Medicine, 327,* 1266–1271.

This study involved a large (n = 2,235), randomized multicenter trial of structured psychosocial support during the high-risk pregnancy. Data was collected at four sites throughout Latin America and included high-risk women who began prenatal care during weeks 15–22 of a singleton pregnancy. Eligibility for the study included the presence of one or more of the following risk factors for delivering a low-birth-weight (LBW) infant: previous delivery of a LBW infant; previous fetal/infant death; under 18 years of age; body weight ≤ 50 kg, height ≤ 1.5 m; low family income; less than 3 years of school; smoking or heavy alcohol consumption; and residence apart from the child's father. Participants were assigned into the control ($n = 1,120$) or treatment ($n = 1,115$) group. Treatment consisted of four-to-six home visits by a nurse or social worker, in addition to routine prenatal care. Findings revealed no differences between groups on any of the outcome measures. The fact that intense formal psychosocial support did not improve the biologic outcomes of the pregnancies raises important questions regarding the intervention model. Most interventions empirically evaluated to-date have been based on a medical model of care. The above investigation may be of greatest value in documenting the need for new models based on differing philosophies of care for medically and socially disadvantaged women. Care should be used in comparing these results with those obtained from North American or European populations.

Teen Pregnancy

Furstenberg, F. F., Brooks-Gunn, J., & Chase-Lansdale, L. (1989). Teenaged pregnancy and childbearing. *American Psychologist, 44*, 313–320.

An overview of what is known about teenaged pregnancy—the process of pregnancy itself, paternal involvement and the results for the mother, father, and children—is presented in this review article. While teenaged mothers do poorly initially, there is some evidence that many are able to recover later in their lives. However, they do not fare as well as women who did not commence childbearing so early in their lives. Life success is dependent on control of fertility, education and/or satisfactory marriage. Fewer studies provide knowledge about fathers but it is known they are more likely to drop out of school and some do not admit their fatherhood. While there is not a great deal of evidence of the long term effects of being born to a teenage mother, differences in cognitive skills which, although

small, continue into grade school and adolescence where school achievement is lower have been shown. The last part of the article provides a review of the effects of prevention. Contraception has the greatest effect; programs aimed at reducing sexual activity have yet to be adequately evaluated. The effects of contemporary paradoxical attitudes about sexual activity are mentioned. Few of the services for girls who become pregnant seem to have more than modest impact with the exception of alternative school programs. Services to the children of teenaged mothers are discussed. The need for applying knowledge about needs to the provision of adequate services is concluded. The stark reality of teenaged pregnancy as a social problem while not extensively discussed is clearly implied. This is a problem which demands a national conscious evaluation and solution rather than the patchwork, value laden programs and approaches which now exist. Coordinated action by women will be necessary to gain coordinated programs.

Korenbrot, C. C., Showstack, J., Loomis, A., & Brindis, C. (1989). Birthweight outcomes in a teenage pregnancy case management project. *Journal of Adolescent Health Care, 10*, 97–104.

The Teenage Pregnancy and Parenting Program (TAPP) was a case management program established to provide services to pregnant teenagers. A prospective study was completed on 411 mothers enrolled in this program. Birth weights for TAPP babies and general city teen births were significantly different when race, infant gender, parity and age were controlled. Even with adequate prenatal visits by both TAPP mothers and general city teens, TAPP participation predicted better birth weights. TAPP counselors worked hardest to provide services to teens with greatest needs. TAPP services encouraged better health habits and health outcomes were better. This program can serve as a model for health care for pregnant teens. It demonstrates that the solutions to teen pregnancy and pregnancy outcomes are not simple. They demand coordinated care which takes into account more than just the girls' pregnancies.

Moore, M. L. (1989). Recurrent teen pregnancy: Making it less desirable. *MCN*, 14, 104–108.

Social exchange posits that people will avoid behavior which they perceive to be costly and chose behavior which has the best outcomes given their perception of the resultant rewards and costs. The author argues that subsequent teen pregnancy will be prevented in greater numbers by programs which teens can see offer them better outcomes. The author then discusses programs which seem to offer better results to teens. While the repeat pregnancy rate of these programs is better it is by no means stunning. She also discusses ways to implement programs for pregnant teenagers. The article is useful as a means to stimulate thinking about social exchange theory as a potential model for delivery of services to teens. It does recognize the individual teen as capable of thought and analysis and suggests that services which assume likewise are more likely to succeed with this population. It does not give an adequate base in social exchange theory to allow its use.

Rosenwald, P. R., & Porter, G. (1989). Wee care: Reaching teenage mothers and changing their lives. *Children Today*, 18, 28–30.

The authors describe the founding of a program aimed at breaking the cycle of teen pregnancy and poverty. They hired counselors who themselves had "made it" out of the cycle. The authors discuss six tasks which they believe an adolescent must achieve in order to be successful in moving out of the cycle of poverty and welfare. These tasks make sense but seem to be an enormous step—and perhaps that is why only twenty-five percent of teens achieve it. The authors also discuss the societal vacuums present for teen fathers. If only for the six tasks, a compelling recasting of what a pregnant adolescent faces, this article is worth reading.

Stevens-Simon, C., Fullar, S. A., & McAnarney, E. R. (1989). Teenage pregnancy. *Clinical Pediatrics*, 28, 282–283.

The authors make a case for seeing both the adolescent mother and her child in the same pediatric health setting. A brief listing of maternal and infant problems is included. The major rationale provided seems to be enhanced pediatric resident training although an increase in the quality of pediatric care is discussed. At best, such combined visits seem to provide some scheduling convenience for the teenage mother. No consideration is given to how easy or difficult it might be to be both mother and patient at the same time. This article demonstrates the self-serving nature of decisions which are made around the provision of care.

Intrapartum

Andrews, C., & Chrzanowski, M. (1990). Maternal position labor and comfort. *Applied Nursing Research*, 3, 7–13.

This is a report of a study involving 40 women assigned randomly to two different groups for laboring positions, recumbent and upright. Women were assessed hourly for labor progress and comfort level using a tool designed specifically for this study. The group assuming upright positions had a significantly shorter maximum slope in labor but no significant difference in comfort level or apgar scores. Woman in the upright position group had more frequent, intense and longer lasting contractions leading to a more rapid delivery. Utilizing the comfort tool, woman in the upright position were no less comfortable than woman in the recumbent positions. The author does suggest upright positions may give the woman more feeling of control and therefore be psychologically more comfortable. This study is laudable in that it compares different positions in labor and attempts to determine outcome variations. The problem with relying on the information regarding comfort level is that the tool developed for the study had (at least as presented in this article) no reported validity and reliability. Only interrater reliability data was presented. The author does note that the nursing staff remarked that women in the upright group seemed to be more comfortable. This would suggest that perhaps the tool was not sensitive to all the dimensions of comfort that might have been assessed. In fact the upright position may not only be equal to but better than recumbent in comfort. This is a refreshing article in that it does attempt to compare more traditional medically supported procedures with less traditional and more client-focused procedures to determine outcomes.

Bergstrom, L., Roberts, J., Skillman, L., & Seidel, J. (1992). "You'll feel me touching you, sweetie": Vaginal examinations during the second stage of labor. *Birth, 19,* 10–18.

While sterile vaginal examinations are a routine procedure in births, this is one of the first investigations designed to describe this care practice in second stage labor. A qualitative, ethnographic research design was used to identify the patterns of behavior and rules governing the performance of sterile vaginal examinations during second stage labor, as well as the caregivers' actions and discussions. Participants were 23 laboring women, 18–36 years of age, of mixed parity, with low- to moderate-risk term pregnancies. Participants and their caregivers were from one of four settings: a tertiary care university hospital, a community hospital, an out-of-hospital birth center, and private homes. Researchers videotaped the second stage of labor and were in the observer role. Transcripts of the videotapes were transcribed and coded for analysis. Two themes were reported: examinations were ritualized with personal disembodiment of the caregiver, and the procedure reinforces the power of the caregiver over the laboring woman. Researchers suggest that the frequency of the procedure be decreased, that laboring women be clearly involved in the procedure, and that they be informed about possible pain during the procedure. The investigation underscores the fact that repeated vaginal examinations are not only intrusive and of questionable value, but need to be further investigated. This study is of particular value, not only because it encourages reconsideration of a procedure that may have questionable clinical value, but it also details actions for empowering women during labor.

Boylan, P. C. (1989). Active management of labor: Results in Dublin, Houston, London, New Brunswick, Singapore, and Valparaiso. *Birth, 16* (3), 114–118.

This article describes in detail organizational and medical components of active management of labor, emphasizing the heavy involvement of nurse-midwives. This article presents a different view to the involvement of physicians in labor and should be required reading for those who equate physician involvement with high technology and an aggressive approach. The purpose of active involvement is to humanize the process of childbirth allowing the woman to deliver her baby safely with a minimum of intervention.

Cahill, C. A. (1989). Beta-endorphin levels during pregnancy and labor: A role in pain modulation? *Nursing Research, 38* (4), 200–203.

A convenience sample of 10 pregnant women, 16 nonpregnant women, and 18 men participated in this study which described changes in plasma beta-endorphin-like immunoreactivity (substances involved in the central nervous system pain relief process) during labor and delivery, and its association with self-reports of pain. There was no statistical association between reported pain levels and plasma beta-endorphin-like material. Analyses of the data suggest that beta-endorphins did not eliminate the labor pain, but may have blunted the woman's perception of it. The results suggest that acute pain may be more effectively controlled than continuous pain, and that endorphins play a part in the regulation of gonadotropic hormones. Although this article is very technical, the discussion of the role of endorphins in relation to pain in labor, and as a possible regulator of reproductive function, should be of interest to all who deal with women.

Carty, E. M., & Tier, D. T. (1989). Birth planning—A reality-based script for building confidence. *Journal of Nurse Midwifery, 34* (3), 111–114.

A two-stage family centered birth plan is discussed in detail. The two-stage approach to birth planning includes: (1) scripting a birth plan, and (2) enacting that plan during a rehearsal of the birth. Both stages of this highly individualized plan are formulated in the family's home at approximately 28 weeks and 36–38 weeks gestation, respectively. During this time the family is encouraged to be assertive about their needs in discussing their expectations of the birth experience, the midwife, and the place of birth. The written plan becomes the script for the rehearsal of the birth as well as a reference during labor and provides a framework for a review of the birth experience. This is a sensitively written article, which although it stresses couples (and we know couples are not always the norm in childbearing), does suggest both the multiple factors which may influence a childbirth and a means for providing a mechanism which would allow those factors expression and impact on what is, after all, the woman's experience, not that of the birth place, hospital, or birth attendant.

Church, L. K. (1989). Water birth: One birthing center's observations. *Journal of Nurse Midwifery, 34* (4), 165–170.

Daniels, K. (1989). Water birth: The newest form of safe, gentle, joyous birth. *Journal of Nurse Midwifery, 34* (4), 198–205.

Jackson, V., Corsaro, M., Niles, C., Stange, C., & Haber, B. (1989). Incorporating water birth into nurse midwifery practice. *Journal of Nurse Midwifery, 34* (4), 193–197.

Kamayani, D. C. (1989). Water birth: A European perspective. *Journal of Nurse Midwifery, 34* (4), 190–192.

These papers all discuss the use of water immersion during birth. Water birth is presented as a safe, positive intrapartum intervention which should not be denied to those women who want it. Women are empowered through taking control of their body's functions during birth. These articles should be required reading for those who deal with women. They emphasize low technology and returning control of and participation in the birth experience to the laboring woman.

Duchene, P. (1989). Effects of biofeedback on childbirth pain. *Journal of Pain and Symptom Management, 4* (3), 117–123.

This study was conducted with 40 primiparas, low-risk women, to determine the effects of biofeedback on pain during childbirth. The subjects were randomly assigned to either an experimental group or a control group. The experimental group participated in training sessions on biofeedback and used biofeedback equipment during labor. All subjects were monitored for their reports of pain during labor and delivery by using the Visual Analogue Scale (VAS) and the Verbal Descriptor Scale (VDS). After delivery, only the biofeedback group was interviewed to assess the degree of satisfaction with biofeedback during labor and delivery. A lower level of pain was reported in the biofeedback group; they used 30 percent fewer medications than the control group. Labor for the biofeedback group averaged 2 hours less than the control group. The results of this study suggest that biofeedback, which is easily learned and maintained, should be an alternative available to any pregnant woman. This study does give a feeling for the multiple factors which may influence a childbirth as well as a mechanism for allowing those factors individual expression and impact on what is, after all, the woman's experience not that of the birth place, hospital, or birth attendant.

Eakins, P. S., O'Reilly, W. B., May, L. J., & Hopkins, J. (1989). Obstetric outcomes at the Birth Place in Menlo Park: The first seven years. *Birth, 16* (3), 123–129.

This study reviewed maternal and neonatal outcomes over a seven-year period at a freestanding birth center in California. During that period 898 women registered for childbirth services; 690 were admitted in labor. The remaining 208 were not admitted for various reasons, including medical risk factors. Eighty-two percent of the women admitted delivered at Birth Place, 18 percent were transferred to the hospital during labor for reasons such as prolonged labor and/or meconium staining. Ninety-seven percent of the babies born at Birth Place were normal; there were complications in only 3 percent. Overall the results were positive, reflecting similar findings in other free-standing birth centers in California. Several points brought out in this study should be of interest to all consumers of childbirth care. During the time of this study, fees for service at Birth Place were about two-thirds of those of the hospitals in the area. Women at Birth Place were encouraged to deliver in the position most comfortable for them: none chose the lithotomy position (supine, legs in stirrups). Five hundred of the 563 women delivered without an episiotomy. Ninety-nine percent required no pain medication during labor.

Hodnett, E. D., & Osborn, R. W. (1989). Effects of continuous intrapartum professional support on childbirth outcomes. *Research in Nursing and Health, 12,* 289–297.

One hundred-three low risk women participated in this study to determine the effects of one-to-one professional support on childbirth outcomes. All subjects attended one of two types of prenatal education programs, Lamaze or "General." Lamaze emphasized breathing and relaxation techniques in labor, while the General placed more emphasis on information of hospital routines and newborn care. Of the 49 experimental subjects, 27 were in the General and 22 in the Lamaze programs. In the control group (54), 29 were in the General program and 25 in the Lamaze. The psychological variables of anxiety, control, and commitment to unmedicated birth were measured with reliable instruments. The experimental group received continuous professional support during labor and delivery. Professional support included: emotional support, information giving, tangible support, and advocacy. Findings indicated the type of prenatal education, anxiety, and commitment to unmedicated birth had little effect on childbirth outcome. The women who had continuous supportive care were less likely to need pain relief medication. Those subjects who did not have pain medication during labor had shorter labors and perceived themselves to be in control. The results are not surprising in this low risk group. It would be interesting to see this study applied to a high risk group of women whose agenda for the childbirth experience is quite different.

Hutti, M. H., & Johnson, J. B. (1988). Newborn Apgar scores of babies born in birthing rooms vs. traditional delivery rooms. *Applied Nursing Research, 1* (2), 68–71.

Concern of staff members regarding the newborn outcome in birthing rooms versus traditional delivery rooms was the impetus for this study. Data were collected via a retrospective review of the medical records of 272 (75.3%) patients delivered in the traditional delivery rooms, and 89 (24.7%) delivered in the birthing rooms. Results of the study indicated there were no significant differences in the Apgar scores of infants born in the birthing room or the traditional delivery room. The Apgar scores of infants born in either of the delivery accommodations were not affected by the demographic characteristics of age, race, gravidity, parity, and smoking. This represents another way of questioning the assumptions upon which birthing practices are decided.

Knorr, L. (1989). Relieving fetal distress with amnioinfusion. *MCN, 14,* 346–350.

Infusion of warmed lactated ringer's solution into the uterus of women with decreased amniotic fluid volume during labor is described as a means of decreasing fetal variable decelerations (a pattern obtained by fetal heart rate monitoring). While the author does stress calming the mother, telling her what to expect and why it is being done, listening to her concerns and reassuring her realistically, nothing is said about obtaining her informed consent for a new procedure. The author implies this procedure may reduce emergency cesarean sections and allow vaginal delivery. That is the good news. The bad news is that this is one more invasive procedure which may potentially foisted on a laboring woman.

Liu, Y. C. (1989). The effects of the upright position during childbirth. *Image, 21* (1), 14–18.

Sixty-eight women participated in this study designed to clarify and verify an earlier study (Liu, 1974) investigating the effect of the angle of position during labor. Women were assigned to three groups. Analyses of the management of the second stage of labor among the three groups revealed that women who delivered in the upright position with no bearing down instruction had a shorter labor (42.25 minutes) in comparison to those women in the upright and recumbent position who received bearing down instructions (68.64 and 90.41 minutes respectively). These findings confirm the author's previous research which indicated that labor and delivery is greatly influenced by the angle of position during labor and delivery. In view of the findings, the author suggests a reassessment of the traditional method of instructing the woman to bear down and hold her breath during the second stage of labor. This is fascinating not only from the viewpoint of the angle of delivery but also the bearing down instructions. Once again the positions prescribed by medical intervention do not seem to be the best for women.

McKay, S., & Mahan, C. (1988). Modifying the stomach contents of laboring women: Why and how; success and risks. *Birth*, *15* (4), 213–221.

This paper presents a comprehensive review of studies which looked at the gastric emptying time in laboring women. The studies encompassed the various means used to ensure an empty stomach to prevent aspiration of vomitus. Although there is evidence that fasting does not decrease the gastric volume below 25 ml, the currently used standard, the "nothing by mouth" policy is still used in most traditional labor situations, presumably because the woman may require general anesthesia. It is distressing that in the face of evidence which indicates that a delay in the gastric emptying time in laboring women rarely occurs, women are still being denied fluids and nourishment during labor in the traditional hospital setting. This article should be required reading for all women. Some of the controls placed on laboring women by physicians (anesthesiologists in particular) are examined. Strong arguments for oral hydration and nourishment during labor are made. That information should be of benefit to the woman planning her birth experience. It should

help her to make choices about the birth place and birth attendant.

McNiven, P., Hodnett, E., & O'Brien-Pallas, L. L. (1992). Supporting women in labor: A work sampling study of the activities of labor and delivery nurses. *Birth*, *19*, 3–8.

As the birth experience becomes increasingly technologic, increased attention is focused on the impact of support during the labor and birth process as in this study. Prior investigations have demonstrated that birth outcomes are positively influenced by a support person during childbirth. This study was designed to obtain baseline data concerning the actual amount of time labor nurses spend in support activities using a work sampling measurement method. Observations were categorized under "supportive direct care activities," or under "all other activities." Data collection took place in the labor and delivery unit of a teaching hospital. Nurses ($n = 18$) were randomly observed for a total of 616 observations. The proportion of time that nurses spent providing supportive care (emotional, physical comfort, instruction/information, or advocacy) was 9.9 percent of the time. While a work sampling methodology may fail to capture some aspects of support provided by the nurse, the study clearly demonstrates that supportive care measures are not a priority focus by the nurse. The researchers suggest that this aspect is devalued and that caring behaviors are often considered low status and generally unimportant. The impact of this behavior by the labor and delivery nurse is of concern. The laboring woman is particularly vulnerable and further research is mandated, not only to replicate findings from this study, but also to provide data useful in providing supportive care to women.

Olson, R., Olson, C., & Cox, N. S. (1990). Maternal birthing positions and perineal injury. *The Journal of Family Practice*, *30*, 553–557.

This is a report of a retrospective descriptive study of the post delivery condition of women's perineums in a family physician's obstetrical practice. Records of 335 patients were reviewed for three birthing positions: delivery table, birthing bed, and birthing chair. Delivery positions were analyzed in relationship to perineal outcomes. A Fowler's or semi-sitting position in a birthing bed was the most used delivery position in this practice. While a significant relationship between the birthing position and perineal outcome was found, further analysis, taking into account parity demonstrated no statistically significant relationship between the birthing position and perineal outcome in first births. Women having second or more pregnancies experienced a significant difference in positive perineal outcomes when using the birthing bed. The authors mention their episiotomy rates were lower than those usually found in the United States but higher than those of midwives. The positive aspect of this article was that women were offered options as well as the support of their physicians for those options. The article leads one to wonder why midwives have lower episiotomy rates, particularly women experiencing first births. It would seem that a comparative study of birthing practices of midwives and family practice physicians would be in order. It is particularly interesting that the woman having her first birthing experience is most subject to episiotomy or perinatal trauma. In one sense it is understandable because the perineal musculature has not been previously challenged. However, if midwives can lower the rate of perineal injury in this group it can be diminished in all first time births. As the authors themselves note, reducing perineal injury is important for all groups of women no matter what their choice in birthing position.

Owen, J., Hauth, J. C., Williams, G., Davis, R. O., Goldenberg, R. L., & Brumfield, C. G. (1989). A comparison of perinatal outcome in patients undergoing contraction stress testing performed by nipple stimulation versus spontaneously occurring contractions. *American Journal of Obstetrics and Gynecology, 160* (5), 1081–1085.

Eight hundred forty-eight high-risk patients were studied over a five and a half year period to examine the perinatal outcome in contraction stress testing (CST) (a means of examining fetal response to maternal contractions) performed by nipple stimulation versus spontaneously occurring contractions. Contractions for the last test before delivery were induced by nipple stimulation in 615 patients; the remaining 233 had spontaneous contractions. In comparing both methods there was no significant difference in the incidence of low Apgar 5-minute scores, small for gestational age babies, fetal distress in labor, and fetal death rate. The contraction stress test performed by nipple stimulation compared favorably with the oxytocin infusion induced contraction stress tests in perinatal outcome. The management of the high-risk woman's pregnancy and delivery is controlled by the attendants. She is given little, if any chance to participate in that management. Knowledge that the nipple stimulation CST is reliable, less expensive, less time-consuming, and more comfortable makes it a viable option to the oxytocin induced CST. Being able to choose how she wants her pregnancy to be monitored would return some sense of control and participation to the high risk woman.

Rooks, J. P., Weatherby, N. L., Ernest, E. K. N., Stapleton, S., Rosen, D., & Rosenfield, A. (1989). Outcomes of Care in Birth Centers. *The New England Journal of Medicine, 321,* 1804–1811.

Data obtained from a study of 11,814 women in 84 free standing birth centers are analyzed. Outcomes for both the women and their infants are considered including transfer from birth centers to hospitals and the four weeks post delivery. This was a national prospective descriptive study of the care of women admitted to free standing birth centers obtained from a list of the National Association of Childbearing Centers. The article includes information on prenatal care, characteristics of the women, birth weight and gestational age, practitioners, interpartum care, complications, transfers, cesarean sections, and patient satisfaction. Results from this study of birth centers are compared in tabular form to outcomes of five other studies of low risk *hospital* births. Total mortality rates were similar. There was a higher incidence of interpartum still birth but a lower incidence of neonatal death in the birth centers. Cesarean section rates in the birth center patients were half that of the hospital studies reporting those rates. In a summary comparison of five studies of low risk hospital births, these authors found that the birth centers had similar outcomes yet they provided fewer invasive procedures including cesarean sections and more comfortable and supportive care to women. The lower cesarean section rate is important as those rates continue to rise nationally. The authors note the cost savings. This article is important in that it supports the safety of birth centers thus removing one of the arguments for allowing women a choice in the place in which they give birth. Birth centers traditionally allow more control on behalf of the woman herself. This article provides a positive step in making available quality supportive care to birthing women.

Rockner, G., Wahlberg, V., & Olnad, A. (1989). Episiotomy and perineal trauma during childbirth. *Journal of Advanced Nursing, 14,* 264–268.

The medical records of 807 primiparas in Sweden were studied to examine the frequency of episiotomy and spontaneous tears. Fifty percent (403) of the subjects had an episiotomy, 22 percent (177) had spontaneous tears, and 28 percent (227) delivered with an intact perineum. There was a greater incidence of episiotomy in women who received epidural anesthesia. The episiotomy group had a higher rate of vacuum extractions and forceps deliveries, and an increased risk for second and third degree tears. The authors conclude that there is little evidence to support that episiotomy prevents tearing. They suggest a re-evaluation of the use of episiotomy in normal deliveries. Episiotomy has become a routine part of delivery in the traditional hospital setting, usually for the convenience of the attendant. Few women are given a choice. This article questions prevailing assumptions which tend to regiment or decrease birth choices, a positive step for women.

Shannahan, M. K., & Cottrell, B. H. (1989). The effects of birth chair delivery on maternal

perceptions. *Journal of Obstetrics, Gynecological, and Neonatal Nursing, 18,* 323–326.

A 21-item questionnaire was given to 55 primiparous women in this study comparing the psychological responses of women who delivered in a birth chair to those who delivered on a standard delivery table. Thirty-three of the women delivered using a birth chair, 22 used the delivery table. Other data obtained from hospital charts included demographics, participation in prenatal classes, duration of first and second stage labor, medications, mode of delivery, and infant outcomes. Women in both groups reported positive perceptions of their childbirth experiences and perceived a similar amount of control over the experience. Women using the birth chair reported greater comfort, but more women in the delivery table group said that their experiences were what they expected. The subjects were not randomly assigned to groups, therefore, factors such as maternal age and attendance at prenatal classes were not equivalent in the two groups. The questionnaire was given after delivery and it is quite possible that the favorable outcome influenced the woman's retrospective perception of her childbirth experience.

Thorpe, J. A., McNitt, J. D., & Leppert, P. C. (1990). Effects of epidural anesthesia: Some questions and answers. *Birth, 17,* 157–162.

This article is written in an interview format with a segment for each of the three authors. The abstract presents the results of a study on the effects of epidural anesthesia completed by the three authors. Their findings suggested that epidural anesthesia may increase the incidence of cesarean section. The discussion however ranges from the study itself to complications of epidural anesthesia, the alarming rise in cesarean sections in the United States, the loss of "coaching" skills of nurses due to the heavy reliance on epidural anesthesia and necessary conditions for a woman in labor including the presence of a sympathetic caretaker. This article is well worth reading because it includes in the discussion consideration of the needs of laboring women and raises consciousness regarding the effects of interventions in labor including epidural anesthesia.

After Birth

Epperly, T. D., Fogarty, J. P., & Hodges, S. G. (1989). Efficacy of routine post partum uterine exploration and manual sponge curettage. *The Journal of Family Practice, 28,* 172–176.

Kearney, M., & Cronenwett, L. R. (1989). Perceived perinatal complications and childbirth satisfaction. *Applied Nursing Research, 2,* 140–141.

Morales-Mann, E. T. (1989). Comparative analysis of the perception of patients and nurses about the importance of nursing activities in a post partum unit. *Journal of Advanced Nursing, 14,* 478–484.

Seguin, L., Therrien, R., Champagne, F., & Larouche, D. (1989). The components of women's satisfaction with maternity care. *Birth, 16,* 109–113.

Satisfaction with the care received is an important component of the post partum experience. Each of these studies provides information about satisfaction with care and illustrates how multifactorial and complicated it is. Sequin et al. determine five dimensions to satisfaction: the delivery, medical care, nursing care, information received and involvement in decision making and physical surroundings. They make an excellent point regarding timing of data collection vis-à-vis validity of findings. Pain was one of the variables which influenced satisfaction with the delivery. Epperly et al. demonstrate that one routine post partum procedure shows no difference in outcomes but does make a difference in perception of pain. Both Morales-Mann and Kearney and Cronenwett share data in which patterns are different from those usually assumed. Morales-Mann shows discrepancies between patient and nurse perceptions of need and Kearney and Cronenwett show that women interpret the presence of complications in their birth very differently from health professionals. Together these articles provide thought provoking information for those who would provide a better experience for women

delivering their infants. Clearly the answers are not as clear as many would have them. The major contribution of these articles is that they shatter the clarity we think we have on the issue and call for rethinking.

Hampson, S. J. (1989). Nursing interventions for the first three post partum months. *Journal of Obstetrical, Gynecological and Neonatal Nursing, 18,* 116–122.

Drawing on a thorough and critical review of the literature related to initial parenting, this article discusses interventions in the first three months post partum. The author makes cogent comments on the state of the research in this area. This discussion points out the multiple potentials for assisting the adjustment to parenting, the need to focus more on the marital relationship, and the changes in society which result in changing patterns of needs.

Hill, P. D. (1989). Effects of heat and cold on the perineum after episiotomy/laceration. *Journal of Obstetric, Gynecological and Neonatal Nursing, 18,* 124–129.

LaFoy, J., & Geden, E. A. (1989). Postepisiotomy pain: Warm versus cold sitz bath. *Journal of Obstetrical, Gynecological and Neonatal Nursing, 18,* 399–403.

The use of heat and cold on episiotomies has long been prescribed by policy and physician's order. The articles are reports of two studies each of which attempts to answer the question which is better, heat or cold? The upshot is: we still don't know. The articles are worth reading together. Although their methods are different each has something to offer. Hill suggests the use of a standardized measurement tool which she used in the study. However, the instrument has not been subjected to validity and reliability testing and basically is an exacting measurement tool, useful but certainly not proven. Both studies were time limited and so could not measure longitudinal changes. LaFoy interprets her results as reason to give women choices since heat is not clearly better than cold. Hill suggests that her results corroborate the greater tissue trauma resulting from laceration than episiotomy. While greater tissue trauma may result from laceration, it should not be construed that episiotomy is therefore necessary. An intact perineum would be even better than episiotomy but requires more patience to produce.

Holz, K., Cooney, C., & Marchese, T. (1989). Outcomes of mature primiparas in an out-of-hospital birth center. *Journal of Nurse Midwifery, 34,* 185–189.

Lerum, C. W., & LoBiondo-Wood, G. (1989). The relationship of maternal age, quickening and physical symptoms of pregnancy to the development of maternal-fetal attachment. *Birth, 6,* 13–17.

The message from these two studies to older women planning pregnancy and those who care for them is once again that age does not count significantly in pregnancy outcomes. Older women can deliver in non-hospital settings. Age alone is not a significant enough risk factor to preclude women from this choice. While Holz and Marchese found more older women were transferred to the hospital from the birth center other outcomes were no different. In Lerum and LoBiondo-Wood's study of attachment, age was not a significant factor although frequency of fetal movement, income, ultrasound, and planning of pregnancy were. Such research is welcome as it shakes the foundations of the foregone conclusions on which professional choices for women (certainly not with women) are made.

Pridham, K. F. (1989). Mothers' decision rules for problem solving. *Western Journal of Nursing Research, 11,* 60–74.

This is a carefully done, longitudinal, descriptive study of mothers' decision rules for problem solving based on information processing theory. Two simulated problems were read to mothers over the phone twice in the first three months of their infants' lives. It appears that maternal responses were analyzed using a pre-set, theoretically based code. Few relationships were found. The write up is not particularly clear. However, it seems that given that the author states how little is known about maternal problem solving, the mothers' responses could be analyzed inductively to see what patterns of decision making emerge in that analysis. The mothers' descriptions then could be used to frame some understanding of this complex process rather than imposing a theoretical analysis.

Ament, L. A. (1990). Maternal tasks of the puerperium reidentified. *Journal of Obstetric, Gynecologic and Neonatal Nursing, 19,* 330–335.

Ruben's framework of taking in and taking hold was tested in this descriptive study which used a repeated measure design with 50 women in a suburban midwestern hospital. The authors administered a self-designed instrument containing 22 statements in a closed ended format for which they had content validity. However, no other psychometric data are shared. The article is worth reading since the author's results did support Ruben's framework. However, the changes took place in a compressed period of time. Nevertheless, these women were not taking in until at least 24 hours after delivery. This must be considered in light of current practice of discharging women often 24 hours after delivery. Nurses presently seem to be working frantically to "stuff" women full of information that they need in order to go home with their infants in a time when these women clearly cannot absorb the information. Our economic times may be severely disadvantaging women and may call for very different models of care.

Green, J. M., Coupland, V. A., & Kitzinger, J. V. (1990). Expectations, experiences, and psychological outcomes of childbirth: A prospective study of 825 women. *Birth, 17,* 15–24.

This excellent report of a study involving 825 women in a mixed population in the United Kingdom should be mandatory reading for all those interested in bettering the experience of childbearing women. While the study used standardized questionnaires it did cover a variety of variables including fulfillment, satisfactory emotional well being and women's descriptors of their babies. This study offers new insight into the importance of women having control over their labor, further definition of control, and questioning some of the stereotypes involving control. In addition it demonstrates that a woman's control over what happens to her in labor does have an impact on her emotional well being post-delivery. This study is well worth reading.

Olson, M. E., & Smith, M. J. (1992). An evaluation of single-room maternity care. *The Health Care Supervisor, 11,* 43–49.

This investigation focused on evaluation of single-room maternity care (SRMC) at a community hospital. Of the 811 women delivering at the facility during the first year of SRMC, 351 responded to a survey regarding satisfaction with the facility and whether or not they would elect to use the facility again, if indicated. Nursing staff (response rate 28 or 68.2%) were similarly surveyed and asked to indicate their satisfaction with SRMC, as well as how satisfied they believed patients were with the nursing care they received. Nurses almost unanimously preferred SRMC to traditional maternity care. Mothers delivering in SRMC were overwhelmingly satisfied with the nursing care and consistently identified private rooms as a positive feature. Patients were less satisfied with the no smoking policy, the business office, and the visitation policy in effect. Mothers responding to the survey wanted home follow-up after discharge. Findings emphasize the need to provide individualized care which is tailored to the needs of the parturient and extending beyond the hospital stay.

Watters, N., & Sparrow, B. (1990). Combined care: As good as they say? *The Canadian Nurse, Services, 86,* 28–32.

The authors supply two interesting sections within one article. First, the process of implementing combined care on a maternity unit in Canada is discussed. Then, the evaluation process utilized to decide upon the outcomes of what changed is reviewed. The evaluation component

is termed a research project. Four instruments which appear to have been developed specifically for this project were used. Validity and reliability of the instruments are not described. Various aspects of the experience were examined including a maternal questionnaire to be completed during hospitalization, maternal competence, maternal satisfaction, a mail questionnaire sent to the women a week after discharge, as well as a telephone interview and a staff satisfaction. A total of 412 women participated in the evaluative component. Interestingly, multiparas were more satisfied, competent and derived greater benefit from the combined care.

Evaluation yielded information helpful in modifying the system both for women and for staff. This article is worth reading because it presents an attempt to carefully evaluate several aspects of a change in care delivery and discusses some of the problematic aspects as well as those that were positive. It does point out that changes in care delivery impact differently on both patients and providers and need to be carefully considered and modified.

Weiss, M. E., & Armstrong, M. (1991). Postpartum mothers' preferences for nighttime care of the neonate. *Journal of Obstetric, Gynecologic and Neonatal Nursing, 20,* 290–295.

The researchers designed the study to examine the post-partum patients preference for nighttime care of the neonate. Although widely accepted as a preferential mode for delivering nursing services to the mother-baby dyad, care has received little research attention. Using a comparative, descriptive survey design, participants included a convenience sample of postpartum mothers who were receiving care as a mother-infant dyad (n = 28), or as a nondyad (traditional) (n = 77). All participants delivered vaginally and were at least one day post-partum, and completed a questionnaire ranking their preference for three options for delivering nursing care during the nighttime, as well as preference for nighttime care when assigned to multipatient rooms, and the degree to which they were bothered by environmental factors during the night. Findings suggest that mothers desire nighttime care service where their neonate remains in their room with the option to return the baby to the nursery if fatigue or other factors intervene. Study participants did not perceive environmental interruptions to be overwhelmingly disruptive. While the findings from this nonprobability sample must be interpreted with caution, it provides beginning evidence of the value of dyad care delivery systems for the patient who delivers vaginally. An array of options available in caring for the mother-baby unit will promote family attachment and parenting skills and better match parental expectations in caring for the newborn.

Cesarean Section

Bucknell, S., & Sikorski, K. (1989). Putting patient controlled anesthesia to the test. *MCN, 14,* 37–40.

The authors review the literature which shows patient controlled analgesia (pain medication delivered through a pump in small doses on patient demand) to be superior in pain control although resulting in more side effects. They describe the pump system used in one hospital and their experience with its trial use including the drugs of choice. Women with patient controlled analgesia tended to use significantly more drug than the control group, a surprising finding. Mothers were satisfied with patient-controlled analgesia and nurses found it easier. Cost was comparable to the usual IM routine.

The nicest thing about this study is that it demonstrates that control can be put safely in the hands of the patient. It allows the patient control over her own pain experience rather than keeping her at the mercy of an overworked floor staff to obtain pain relief. It shows that women are capable of directing their own care.

Crawford, M. E., Carl, P., Bach, V., Ravlo, O., Mikkelsen, B. O., & Werner, M. (1990). A randomized comparison between midazolam and thiopental for elective Cesarean section anesthesia: I. Mothers. *Anesthesia/Analgesia, 68,* 229–33.

Ravlo, O., Pender, C., Crawford, M. E., Bach, M., Mikkelsen, B. O., & Werner, M. (1989). A randomized comparison between midazolam and thiopental for elective Cesarean section anesthesia: II. Neonates. *Anesthesia and Analgesia, 68,* 234–37.

Bach, V., Carl, P., Ravlo, O., Crawford, M. E., Jensen, A. G., Mikkelsen, B. O., Crevoisier, C., Heizman, P., & Fattinger, K. (1989). A randomized comparison between midazolam and thiopental for elective Cesarean section anesthesia: III. Placental transfer and elimination in neonates. *Anesthesia and Analgesia, 68,* 238–42.

These three articles report the results of a study of 40 women receiving general anesthesia for elective Cesarean section. They are worth reading because both maternal and neonatal responses to the anesthetic agents were studied. So often results are reported only for the mother or the infant but not for both as in this case. Further, the fact that two agents are compared provides more information for use in choosing such agents. While both agents were found to be relatively similar with regard to efficacy and safety, in reading their effects one cannot help but wonder if there are not other better approaches to anesthesia. The complexity of adequately studying interventions involving two interdependent patient populations is illustrated.

Culp, R. E., & Osofsky, N. J. (1989). Effects of cesarean delivery on parental depression, marital adjustment and mother-infant interaction. *Birth, 16,* 53–57.

Shearer, E. L. (1989). Commentary: Does Cesarean delivery affect the parents? *Birth, 16,* 57–58.

Eighty married primiparas and seventy-six of their husbands participated in this longitudinal study. Data were collected prenatally and post partum. Data collectors were unaware of the delivery status of the subjects. Prenatal data included: demographic data, maternal depression and marital adjustment. Mother-infant interactions were observed on the second post partum day and three months post partum. At three months, the Bayley infant development scales were given. A maternal and child health index and a labor index were computed for the study from the medical records. Data were compared for vaginal and cesarean deliveries. The only difference between the two was in the labor risk index which the authors interpreted showing that the cesarean section was necessary and performed in a timely manner. The authors cite literature which notes potential negative effects of cesarean sections on both fathers and mothers in which cesarean section births are described more negatively than vaginal deliveries. The choice of instruments for this study suggests the authors expect lasting, clinical effects from cesarean delivery and are surprised not to find them. Why should a mother with a "good" baby from cesarean section show clinical depression? Is it not enough that whenever possible, parents are spared those negative effects of cesarean section which have been documented in the literature? Failing prevention of cesarean section, the prevention of negative sequellae would be better served through research which describes the negative effects of such intervention in childbirth.

The commentary provided by Elizabeth Shearer raises issues such as the effects of the rising cesarean section rate as well as the outcome measures employed in research. She makes important points about the influence of the timing of questions on the answers received. It is an important companion piece to the report of the study. Both should be read together.

Hangsleben, K. L., Taylor, M. A., & Lynn, N. M. (1989). VBAC program in a nurse wifery service. *Journal of Midwifery, 34,* 179–184.

The authors describe a VBAC (vaginal birth after cesarean section) program in a private midwifery setting. All women in the program have low transverse uterine scars (the entry into the uterus was in the lower segment. This scar heals well and is less likely to rupture). The women have classes or refresher classes, prepare a birth plan and are carefully checked prenatally and followed to be sure they do not deliver too long after their due dates. Careful labor management is described and noted to be crucial in such a program. The labor and delivery is reviewed post delivery with the couple. Eighty-three percent of the VBAC groups have had successful vaginal deliveries. Lowered chances of a successful VBAC (to 65%) was associated with failure to progress in labor as the reason for the first cesarean section. The study resulted in the affiliated hospital being less inclusive in its demands for blood work for these women.

This article demonstrates the safety of two more options for women: VBAC and midwifery care. In some institutions a woman attempting a VBAC could not choose a midwife as they would be considered high risk and in need of physician care. The provision of proven options for women as well as the chance to make up their own mind which this study supports is laudable and necessary.

James, C. F., Banner, T., & Canton, D. (1989). Cardiac output in women undergoing cesarean section with epidural or general anesthesia. *American Journal of Obstetrics and Gynecology, 160,* 1178–1184.

The authors used a non-invasive Doppler (ultrasound) technique to study cardiac output in 22 low risk women having an elective cesarean section. Patients chose either epidural or general anesthesia and their cardiac outputs, stroke volumes, heart rates and blood pressures were compared preoperatively and 15, 30, 60 and 90 minutes and 24 hours post delivery. Generally cardiac output increased immediately after delivery and returned to preoperative levels by 60 minutes post delivery. This study has three encouraging aspects: the attempt to describe women's responses to surgery and giving such responses their due in research, the use of a non-invasive, relatively comfortable technique, and the authors' suggestion that this information could be useful in women with cardiac problems who chose to be pregnant. Women with existing health problems who chose pregnancy often found providers had little or no information on which to base decisions about care. This study even though it has a relatively small sample provides some of that information. As such it demonstrates an important investment in women.

Ong, B. Y., Cohen, M. M., & Palahniuk, R. J. (1989). Anesthesia for cesarean section-effects on neonates. *Anesthesia and Analgesia, 68,* 270–5.

All infants delivered by cesarean section in a nine-year period, $n = 3,940$, at a Canadian hospital, were included in this study to determine neonatal outcomes of anesthesia used for cesarean section. Apgar scores (a score showing initial adjustment of the newborn to extrauterine life), need for oxygen and neonatal mortality were studied for four groups: elective without complications, emergency (including fetal distress), urgent (including failure to progress in labor and difficult labor) and elective sections due to complications. Low one-minute Apgars were significantly associated with first pregnancy, many pregnancies, antepartum complications, labor complications, fetal distress, low birth weight, prematurity, using narcotics in labor, breach presentation, non-elective section and general anesthesia. For all of the first three groups studied, neonatal outcomes were worse with general anesthesia. Multivariate analysis was used to control for maternal and intrapartal factors. Results demonstrated that general anesthesia still was a significant risk for low one-minute Apgar scores and was associated with low five-minute Apgar scores and resuscitation. Neonatal survival was not affected. While the authors do not argue that these data should be persuasive in suggesting regional rather than general anesthesia the case can be made. If only mortality is considered, as the authors finally do, then perhaps anesthesia does not matter. If maternal concern and worry, the opportunity to interact with the newborn, and the impact of positive birthing experiences are included as important data, then regional anesthesia should be the norm. The strength of this study lies in the size of the sample and the variety of reasons for cesarean section included in the sample.

Perez, P. B. (1989). The patient observer: What really led to these cesarean births? *Birth, 16,* 130–139.

Hospital records, patient interview summaries, physician summaries and nurse comments are presented for five patients randomly chosen from records the author maintained on a clientele of approximately 80 women who had a vaginal delivery after a cesarean section. This article is well worth reading and analyzing in the face of the rising cesarean section rate. The discrepancies between the hospital records and the patients' accounts are troubling despite the small number of cases. In many instances cesarean section may well result from iatrogenic conditions. These accounts bolster that school of thought as well as emphasize the helplessness of many women once admitted to a hospital. This article should lead to increased watchfulness and advocacy on the part of those committed to ensuring choices for women needing hospitalization or health care.

Porreco, R. P. (1989). Commentaries: The Cesarean section rate is 25 percent and rising. Why? What can be done about it. *Birth, 16,* 118–119.

Five individuals with a role in the care of women having cesarean sections comment on the rising rate and what changes they see as necessary to contain it. Each individual provides a different perspective but the prevailing theme seems to be the necessity for change in obstetrical practices in order to remove the impetus for cesarean section. This is important reading for any one concerned about women as it shows the economic and cultural factors which are operative, and must be addressed, including the physician's training and role in labor as well as reimbursement.

Baruffi, G., Strobino, D. M., & Paine, L. L. (1990). Investigation of institutional differences in primary cesarean birth rates. *Journal of Nurse-Midwifery, 35,* 274–281.

Concern for a rising cesarean birth rate has been evident for the past decade. In an effort to examine differences in primary cesarean birth rates, the investigators conducted a randomized, retrospective survey of patients who received antepartal care and delivered abdominally at one of two facilities: a primary care, family-centered maternity hospital staffed by CNMs ($n = 796$), and a university teaching hospital staffed by resident and attending physicians ($n = 804$). Use of 127 strata such as maternal age, education, race, and parity, facilitated samples which were demographically similar and excluded complications which would not normally be a part of the birth center population. Results indicated that the maternity center had a significantly lower rate of performing cesarean sections. The authors conclude that management of labor and delivery is a probable explanation for the differences noted between facilities. Given the increased morbidity risk for women delivering abdominally, as well as the uncertain outcome for neonates, alternate models of health care delivery which ensure positive outcomes are needed. While this research is based on data from 1977 and 1978, it provides compelling evidence that antenatal and intrapartal care of clients by CNMs in a maternity center with fundamentally different approaches in labor management from the traditional hospital setting, is a reasonable solution to lowering abdominal delivery rates.

Breastfeeding

Bernard-Bonnin, A. C., Stachtchenko, S., Girard, G., & Rousseau, E. (1989). Hospital practices and breastfeeding duration: A meta-analysis of controlled trials. *Birth, 16*, 64–66.

Nine studies of controlled clinical trials of breastfeeding were subjected to meta-analysis to integrate the findings. Studies which met three inclusion criteria were utilized: early maternal-infant contact, no supplemental feeding, support from nurses. Early mother-infant contact and nursing support with telephone contact were found to have significant effects on the duration of breastfeeding. Many demographic factors have

been shown to influence the duration of breastfeeding. This meta-analysis offers strong evidence that hospital practices can also have an influence. This finding suggests that hospital practices need to change to support this choice on the part of women. The authors also hint at the potential impact of reimbursement practices on breastfeeding due to diminished hospital stays. This meta-analysis also demonstrates the complexity of the problem; breastfeeding is subject to many influences.

Ford, K., & Labbok, M. (1990). Who is breastfeeding? Implications of associated social and biomedical variables for research on the consequences of method of infant feeding. *American Journal of Clinical Nutrition, 52*, 451–456.

It is generally recognized that breastfeeding is a superior form of infant nutrition. While several studies have sought to identify variables associated with the choice and duration of breastfeeding, this investigation identified social and biomedical variables that influence the selection of method of infant feeding in the United States. Data were drawn from a national survey of children ($n = 2,951$) conducted in 1981. Multivariate regression analysis was used to ascertain those variables which are determinants in the initiation and duration of breastfeeding: ethnicity, socioeconomic status, and health of mother and infant. Findings are important in identifying those variables which vary between specific subgroups and should be carefully considered in future lactation studies, as well as by clinicians seeking to develop strategies for fostering breastfeeding rates. Results provide evidence useful in working with ethnically diverse groups of women as selection factors for breastfeeding are reviewed to promote maternal and infant health.

Kaufman, K. J., & Hall, L. A. (1989). Influences of the social network on choice and duration of breastfeeding in mothers of preterm infants. *Research in Nursing and Health, 12*, 149–159.

One hundred and twenty-five mothers of low birth weight preterm infants participated in this study. The authors developed an Influence of Social Referents Scale (ISR) to measure the women's perception of the influence of her social network. Social network support was the total number of seven categories of the ISR which provided help or emotional support. During early post partum the 88 mothers who chose to breastfeed filled out a questionnaire to provide information on their perceptions of network members' wishes regarding breastfeeding and their willingness to comply with those wishes. Every two to four weeks mothers were telephoned to obtain information about sources of support. The ISR scores of women who breastfed were significantly higher than those who did not. Categories of the ISR were ranked by amount of influence. Support scores for breastfeeding were positively related to duration of breastfeeding. Other variables were investigated. The procedures used in this research are difficult to follow at times but the article does provide useful information. It appears that for women who chose to breastfeed, the baby's father, baby's doctor and baby's nurses were the strongest motivators. The use which is made of such information is important. The authors discuss possible ways to augment the mother's support network or intervene with her partner. The unwritten assumption in this article is that breastfeeding is better for the infant and ought to be done. What the authors do not discuss is the possible cost to the mother of persisting in breastfeeding when her natural support system is not supportive. The scenario of a mother caught between the wishes of a natural network and a professionally derived one is troubling. Such interventions must be carefully done and involve the mother in decision making.

Kearney, M. H., Cronenwett, L. R., & Reinhardt, R. (1990). Cesarean delivery and breastfeeding outcomes. *Birth, 17,* 97–103.

This study examined breastfeeding outcomes in 121 primiparas to determine the impact of cesarean birth on the timing of the first breastfeeding encounter and was part of a larger study. The sample consisted of married couples who were recruited from childbirth education classes. All participants were Caucasian, reported moderate to high incomes, with a mean maternal age of 28.7 years and a paternal age of 30.3 years, and delivered at one of four hospitals located in university communities. Twenty-three percent had cesarean delivery. Findings suggest that little evidence exists for failure at breastfeeding and cesarean birth. No relationship was found between cesarean delivery and duration of breastfeeding, nor pain and fatigue related to the breastfeeding experience. Similarly, a timing delay in the first breastfeeding encounter was not found. At a time when cesarean rates are relatively high and age of the first birth is rising, results of the investigation add important information useful in discussing breastfeeding with women.

Lethbridge, D. J. (1989). The use of breastfeeding as a contraceptive. *Journal of Obstetric, Gynecologic and Neonatal Nursing, 18,* 31–37.

A careful, beautifully done review of the literature is presented to support the limited use of breastfeeding as a contraceptive measure. The article is packed with information which must be carefully studied for utilization in practice. Contraception through breastfeeding is not easy. The women who would use breastfeeding as a contraceptive must be highly motivated, with an excellent support system, and willing to have a subsequent pregnancy in a relatively short interval. This article provides highly useful information for the nurse working with women who wish to use only natural methods of birth control as well as fascinating information for all those who are interested in the interplay between lactation, ovulation, and cultural patterns.

Moon, J. L., & Humenick, S. S. (1989). Breast engorgement: Contributing variables and variables amenable to nursing intervention. *Journal of Obstetric, Gynecologic and Neonatal Nursing, 18,* 309–315.

The authors report on the self-reports of breast changes of 54 women in the first 78 post partum hours. Women recorded breast changes on a form provided for them according to a set of operational definitions. Duration of feedings were also noted. The sample included primiparas and multiparas with both vaginal and cesarean section deliveries. Initiation, frequency, and duration of feedings, rate of milk maturation and supplementation were all correlated with engorgement levels. While the sample is relatively small, this study is interesting because it provides an empirical analysis which leads to questioning of one of the procedures accepted as a means of preventing cracked nipples—limiting feeding time. It provides data which should lead to changes in hospital procedures. It also should underscore the necessity of studying so many hospital procedures which are based on custom, practice and belief rather than data.

Morse, J. M., & Bottorff, J. L. (1989). Leaking: A problem of lactation. *Journal of Nurse Midwifery, 34*, 15–20.

This study is delightful for two reasons: it focuses on a phenomenon about which only a minimal amount is known and it does this through interview of experts in the phenomena, breastfeeding mothers. Since breastfeeding is seen as advantageous to the infant, and women wish to return to the work world, this study provides valuable information which can be shared with women to help them be able to both breastfeed and work. It is obvious that this 'little' problem (from the amount of attention paid to it in the literature) can be a very large one leading to interruption of breastfeeding. The authors discuss the mothers' perceptions and feelings and the ways women managed to control and cope with the leaking. It is time that the amount of attention paid to problems mirror women's needs. This study is a step in that direction.

Nice, F. J. (1989). Can a breastfeeding mother take medication without harming her infant? *MCN, 14*, 27–31.

This is a well written, useful article authored by a pharmacist who supports breastfeeding. He argues against automatic weaning of the infant in the case of maternal medication. Instead he suggests individual evaluation of the situation through analyzing what is known about the actual drug and assessment of infant safety based on six critical questions about the drug and another set of twelve questions which assess the maternal-infant situation. A list of unsafe drugs is included as well as a way to schedule drug doses to avoid high concentration in breast milk at feeding times. The author avoids the absolute and provides a framework for increasing options for breastfeeding women who must take medication.

Sollid, D. S., Evans, B. T., McClowry, S. G., & Garrett, A. (1989). Breastfeeding multiples. *The Journal of Perinatal and Neonatal Nursing, 3*, 46–65.

The authors have provided an excellent resource for nurses interested in assisting women to breastfeed two or more newborns. Based on careful review of the literature, the authors make suggestions for intervention in preparation for breastfeeding, establishing lactation, and post hospital concerns. Excellent material about positioning is included. The authors suggest more research in this area. Dealing with breastfeeding two or more infants is another aspect of breastfeeding which is often superficially treated. The authors contribute depth of information which can only benefit women. Although women may be free to choose to breastfeed their twins or triplets, without adequate information, it is not a real choice as the woman may not know how to be successful. This is a positive step toward making the choice a real one.

Williams, K. M., & Morse, J. M. (1990). Weaning patterns of first-time mothers. *MCN, 14*, 188–192.

One hundred primiparous women participated in this study of weaning patterns. All women were either weaning or had just completed weaning and completed a semi-structured telephone interview when they began weaning and when they completed. Monthly calls were made between beginning weaning and completion for purposes of updating. The results included: three patterns of weaning, mothers' ways of seeking information on weaning, infants' reactions, and the influence of support people in the mother's network. The authors discuss the significance of their findings for nursing practice. This study also represents a focus on the actual experiences of women, particularly a group of women who are not easily accessed in the current health care system. The design allowed the discovery of factors which were important to the women themselves and may reflect changing societal patterns, thus providing up-to-date and useful information both for breastfeeding women and health care providers dealing with them. The size of the sample is significant given the research design.

Chapter 6

Midlife Women's Health: There's More to It Than Menopause

Nancy Fugate Woods

INTRODUCTION

Midlife women account for a growing proportion of the United States population, yet their health concerns have received little attention from health researchers and clinicians. Indeed, most published work about midlife women's health focuses on menopause. The purpose of this review is to summarize what has been written about midlife women's health during the years 1980 to 1992. This review begins with definitions of midlife and a summary of women's health status as reflected in available U. S. health statistics. Next biological, personal, and social changes accompanying midlife will be addressed. Finally, a composite picture of factors affecting midlife women's health will be presented.

Citations for this review appeared in databases for Medline, Psychological Abstracts, Women's Studies Abstracts, and Studies on Women Abstracts for the period 1980 to 1992. In addition to the journal articles identified through the databases, this review contains citations from a collection of papers entitled *Women in Midlife*, edited by Grace Baruch and Jeanne Brooks-Gunn in 1984. Reading the literature of the past decades makes clear the necessity for a contemporary study of midlife women's health that is guided by an integrative perspective, one that emphasizes the complexity of contemporary women's lives and the multiple dimensions of their health. Currently, there are three integrative longitudinal programs of research in progress, directed by Patricia Kaufert (1984), Sonja McKinlay (1986), and Karen Matthews (Matthews, et al., 1990). These studies are discussed in greater detail below. Together, these efforts will help illuminate women's experience of midlife, including menopause as one important facet of that experience.

DEFINITIONS OF MIDLIFE

Midlife has been defined in a variety of ways. Some use age boundaries, such as 35 to 65 years to differentiate midlife from young adulthood and old age. Others base their definitions on women's reproductive capacity, using menopause or hormonal changes consistent with menopause as markers. Still others base their definitions on women's role patterns, using indicators such as a child leaving home or a woman's return to the workplace to designate the beginning of midlife. Another option is using women's own perceptions about whether they are in phase with the middle of their lives (Brooks-Gunn & Kirsh, 1984).

Whatever the markers might be, understanding the context for the experience of midlife for each particular cohort of women under consideration is extremely important. Anticipation of midlife by each woman's age cohort (those women born at the same time), as well as socialization for midlife experienced by these same women, will influence how women interpret the events of midlife. Moreover, awareness of health experiences unique to each age cohort of women may help us understand their health and health care needs during the middle years.

HEALTH STATUS DURING MIDLIFE

Because most United States health statistics focus on morbidity and mortality, we know most about midlife as a time of sickness and death. During midlife, many chronic illnesses become increasingly prevalent. Women between 35 and 44 years of age are most likely to die from malignant neoplasms and heart disease, with these causes persisting as major causes of death throughout the middle years. In addition, cerebrovascular disease, accidents and adverse events, suicide, chronic liver disease, and homicide account for a large proportion of deaths for women between 35 and 44 years. For women 45 to 54 years, malignant neoplasms, heart disease, cerebrovascular disease, chronic obstructive pulmonary disease, chronic liver disease and cirrhosis, accidents and adverse events, diabetes, and suicide claim the most lives. For women 55 to 64 years, malignant neoplasms, heart disease, cerebrovascular disease, chronic obstructive pulmonary disease, pneumonia and influenza, chronic liver disease and cirrhosis, and diabetes mellitus account for the most deaths (National Center for Health Statistics, 1988).

MORBIDITY PATTERNS

Acute conditions include illnesses and injuries that last less than three months and involve one or more days of restricted activity or medical attention. The incidence of acute conditions for women exceed those for men for nearly every condition except injuries. Chronic conditions are those that were noticed at least three months earlier or belong to a group of conditions that persist for a long period of time, such as heart disease or diabetes. Women 45-to-64 experience more arthritis, hemorrhoids, chronic bronchitis, and chronic sinusitis than men, but men of the same age experience more visual impairment, cataracts, hearing impairment, abdominal hernia, heart disease, and emphysema than women (National Center for Health Statistics, 1985).

CONSEQUENCES OF ILLNESS

As a consequence of illness, people may treat themselves, by restricting their activity, staying home from work or school, or using health services. Midlife women engage in slightly more illness behavior, such as staying in bed or missing work or school than their male age counterparts. Women 45-to-64 years of age make more telephone contacts with physicians than do men, but have fewer hospitalizations (National Center for Health Statistics, 1985).

PERCEPTIONS OF HEALTH

Women and men asked to rate their health as poor, fair, good, very good, or excellent, give similar ratings. About 6.6 percent of men rate their health as poor versus 5.7 percent of women, but only 24.6 percent of women rate their health as excellent compared to 29.5 percent of men (National Center for Health Statistics, 1985).

BIOLOGICAL CHANGES DURING MIDLIFE

Menopause is a nearly universal experience during midlife, with every woman experiencing the biological transition as a natural event or as a medical or surgical event. Menopause refers to cessation of menses and is said to occur when women have not menstruated for one year (Treloar, 1982). In the United States most women experience menopause during their late forties and early fifties, with the median age being 51 years (McKinlay, Bifano, & McKinlay, 1985; McKinlay, Brambilla, & Posner, 1992). Recent awareness of variable production of ovarian hormones after cessation of menses has caused clinicians and researchers to question the definition of menopause based on only the absence of menses. Indeed, some advocate classifying women's experience of menopause with respect to their continued production of ovarian hormones (Utian, 1991).

In contrast to biomedical definitions of menopause, women's definitions of being menopausal are based on their noticing changes in bleeding patterns or cyclicity prior to noticing the absence of menstrual periods. Thus, women's definitions will not always correspond to those of clinicians or researchers (Kaufert, 1986).

During the past three decades investigators have devoted significant attention to identifying ovarian, hypothalamic, and pituitary hormonal mechanisms producing changes attributed to menopause (Voda & George, 1986). How menopause, as one part of aging, does or does not affect various dimensions of women's health has been clarified by recent longitudinal studies.

During the 1980s and early 1990s, three longitudinal studies of midlife women in North America were conducted. Although the primary emphasis of these studies concerned menopause, investigators have also collected data that inform us about the nature of women's experiences with aspects of health other than menopause. The Massachusetts Women's Health Study, directed by Sonja McKinlay, included 2,570 Massachusetts women 45 to 55 years of age who were menstruating in the last three months prior to their enrollment in the study. Women participated in six telephone interviews conducted over a 5-year period. Data collected for this study includes personal factors, social factors, hormone changes, and health outcomes including menstrual changes, bone density changes, and psychiatric symptoms (McKinlay, Brambilla, & Posner, 1992). The Manitoba Project, directed by Patricia Kaufert, enrolled 477 Canadian women 45 to 55 years of age and interviewed them six times over a 3-year period to determine the relative effects of menopause and other aspects of their lives on their health (Kaufert, Gilbert, & Tate, 1992). The Healthy Women Study, directed by Karen Matthews (Matthews, et al., 1990) involved a cohort of 541 premenopausal women 42 to 50 years of age who have been evaluated clinically at baseline and followed for three years with clinical evaluations of biological factors, including those of menopause, and behavioral factors affecting coronary artery disease risk factors. Taken together, these studies inform us about the consequences of menopause as well as other dimensions of midlife women's lives on their health.

SYMPTOMS

As Neugarten and Kraines (1965) pointed out over twenty years ago, symptoms often attributed to menopause occur throughout the lifespan, including hot flashes. The longitudinal studies of the 1980s and 1990s indicate that only hot flashes and night sweats increase in incidence as women progress through menopause (Kaufert & Syrotuik, 1981; Kaufert, 1988; McKinlay, McKinlay, & Brambilla, 1987a; McKinlay, Brambilla, & Posner, 1992). Women participating in the Massachusetts Women's Health study experienced more symptoms, including hot flashes and sweats as well as other distressing symptoms, during the perimenopausal period than during the premenopausal or postmenopausal periods. Those who had a shorter perimenopausal transition were more likely to experience hot flashes than those with a longer perimenopausal transition. Although women experienced more symptoms during the transitional period, their distress was short-lived, and did not persist beyond menopause (McKinlay, Brambilla, & Posner, 1992). Women participating in the Healthy Women Study experienced few changes associated with menopausal transition, among these, an increase in hot flashes (Matthews, et al., 1990). Among Manitoba women, the prevalence of symptoms other than vasomotor symptoms (hot flashes and night sweats) was unrelated to menopause. Indeed, Kaufert, Gilbert, & Hassard (1988) suggested that researchers and clinicians consider sources of midlife women's symptoms other than menopause.

HEALTH STATUS

Self-assessed health was not related to menopausal status or to vasomotor symptoms in the Manitoba population (Kaufert, Gilbert, & Tate, 1992). Moreover, other studies do not support a relationship between perceptions of health and menopausal transition (McKinlay, Brambilla, & Posner, 1992).

The Healthy Women Study has followed 69 women who stopped menses for 12 months, and another 32 who had stopped menses and took hormone therapy for 12 months. These women were age-matched to a comparison group of premenopausal women. Natural menopause led to few changes in psychological characteristics aside from a decreased introspectiveness. An increase in LDL-C and a decrease in HDL-C was observed for women experiencing natural menopause. Hormone users, on the other hand, reported more symptoms of depression and experienced elevated trigylcerides and weight gain. Weight gain averaged 2.25 Kg over 3 years for all women in the Healthy Women Study. Women who remained premenopausal over the 3-year period experienced similar weight gain to those who experienced menopause, suggesting that menopause does not cause weight gain (Wing, Matthews, Kuller, Meilahn, & Plantings, 1991).

Premenopausal and postmenopausal women from the Healthy Women Study differed on stress reactivity. Postmenopausal women exhibited greater increases in heart rate in response to laboratory stressors relative to the premenopausal women. They were especially responsive to a social stressor, illustrating an important joint effect of their menopausal status and the type of stressor (Saab, Matthews, Stoney, & McDonald, 1990).

McKinlay and McKinlay (1989) examined the relationship between women's roles and their health, using five indicators of health: self-assessed general health, number of days of restricted activity, physical symptoms, psychological symptoms, and new chronic conditions. Prior health status predicted current health status. Education, employment, and marital status also helped account for current health. Having a recent surgical menopause was the only variable related to menopause that helped account for health status, and then only increased the days of restricted activity. Current employment reduced the impact of other roles and accompanying stress on health and utilization of health services. Education and work had positiveeffects on self-assessed health; stress related to husbands had negative effects on health, including physical and psychological symptoms.

MENTAL HEALTH

Depression, prevalent among midlife women, has been attributed to menopause as reflected in the term *involutional melancholia*. Depression was not associated with a natural menopause for women participating in the

Massachusetts Women's Health Study. Instead, depression was associated with surgical menopause and may have been responsible for women's encounters with the health care system that led to their experience of a hysterectomy. Most marked increases in depression were associated with multiple causes of worry and multiple roles among currently married women (including their paid work, parenting adolescent children, caring for ill husbands, aging parents, and parents-in-law) (McKinlay, McKinlay, & Brambilla, 1987b). Among participants in the Manitoba study, those who rated their health as poor were 17 times more likely to become depressed on subsequent study occasions than were those who rated their health as good. Arthritis or high blood pressure put women at greater risk of becoming depressed, but not allergies or thyroid problems, or having a large number of these conditions. Likelihood of depression increased for women with current stress in their lives, especially if their problems were related to husbands or children. Children leaving home did not increase the likelihood of depression (Kaufert, Gilbert, & Tate, 1992).

USE OF HEALTH SERVICES

Women's pattern of use of health services does not appear to be influenced solely by menopausal status. Instead, menopausal symptoms such as flooding (heavy vaginal bleeding) and vasomotor symptoms may account for some women's increased use of health services. Almost 30 percent of Manitoba women experiencing flooding sought help. Those in the perimenopausal and immediately postmenopausal groups were least likely to have seen a physician (Kaufert, 1986). Women in the Massachusetts study who experienced a longer transition to menopause had more physician contacts than those with shorter transitions (McKinlay, Brambilla, & Posner, 1992). Manitoba women were more likely to seek professional help for depression or distress than for menopause (Kaufert, 1980; McKinlay, McKinlay, & Brambilla, 1987a; McKinlay, McKinlay, & Brambilla, 1987b), and often used health services because of their health problems experienced prior to menopause (McKinlay, McKinlay, & Brambilla, 1987a). Women also consulted their lay networks for depression and physical symptoms and when it became necessary for them to restrict their activity (McKinlay, McKinlay, & Brambilla, 1987a).

WOMEN'S DEVELOPMENT: MIDLIFE EXPERIENCES

Women continue to grow and develop through the lifespan and midlife is no exception. Indeed, midlife is a dynamic period of development, noteworthy for the complexity of change patterns as they occur within the context of historical and cultural forces.

Gilligan (1982a) proposed restoring the missing text of women's development rather than simply replacing it with work about men's development. She sees women's middle years as a risky time due to women's embeddedness in lives of relationship, their orientation to interdependence, their ability to subordinate achievement to care, and their conflicts over competitive success. Should midlife bring an end to relationships, and with them, a sense of connection for women, then midlife may be a time of despair. The meaning of midlife events for women is contextual, arising from the interaction between the structures of women's thought and the realities of their lives. Women approach midlife with a different history than do men, and they face a different social reality with different possibilities for love and work (Gilligan, 1982b).

Rubin's study (1979) of midlife women revealed an "elusive self" for many. Nearly 25 percent of midlife women in this study could not describe themselves, that is, who and what they were. Other women described having two selves, one for home and one for work. Still others made the distinction between who they were in relation to being and doing: their internal identity represented their being whereas their work represented their doing. For these women, work was what they did, not who they were.

Rossi (1980) found that no midlife women wanted to be older than they were, but half wanted to be under thirty. Most wanted to live to at least 75 years. Women who had short lifespan preferences were those who were living with very stressful lives. Certainly, women's responses to changing appearance reflect social ideology about how a woman should look. Although most women feel positive about their appearance, some express a great desire to look younger. In this regard, women who are most vulnerable are those who are attempting to meet men or needing to find work (Berkum, 1983). Women's sexuality does not seem to suffer during midlife, with no deficit appearing in sexual desire, response, or satisfaction. Only a subset of women with low estradiol levels tend to experience problems with intercourse (Cutler, 1987).

SOCIAL CHANGES IN MIDLIFE

Several social changes occur during the course of midlife for women. These may include returning to employment, having children leave home or move back in with parents, changing marital relationships, and caring for aging parents. To date, most investigators have focused on women's roles and their relationship to health.

The balance between the rewards and concerns related to women's roles significantly affects their experience of well being. The challenge and social relationships associated with employment, in balance with the potential dullness and dead end nature of much work, together influence the mastery and pleasure women experience. Likewise, the satisfaction associated with being available to one's family, freedom from supervision, and the opportunity to do tasks fitted to one's skills in balance with boredom, isolation, and not earning money, influence the well being of homemakers. Marriage balances feeling emotionally supported and appreciated with conflict, and this balance in turn affects women's happiness. Conflict with children, along with the pleasure associated with parenting them, relate to women's experience of pleasure. Together, the complex dimensions of women's roles, and the rewards and concerns associated with each, influence women's sense of well being during midlife (Baruch, 1984).

Relationships with parents, especially mothers, have important health effects for midlife women. Rapport with one's mother is related to women's sense of mastery and happiness, and is contingent on the entire constellation of a woman's roles (Baruch & Barnett, 1983). Caretaking responsibilities for one's parents depend on the parent's health status and the extent of responsibility women assume as a function of their social class and the nature of family timing patterns and employment responsibilities (Stueve & O'Donnell, 1984). Just as it is important earlier in life, equity and dependency in parent-child relationships remains important in midlife women's relationships with their aging parents (Wood, Traupmann, & Hay, 1984).

Stressors during midlife have been linked to both psychological and somatic symptoms. Of particular importance are exit stresses or losses from a woman's social network. Vulnerability to psychological and somatic distress has been related to the loss of one's mother early in one's life, and also to the number of losses from one's current network, for example, through divorce or death (Cooke & Greene, 1981; Cooke, 1985).

The importance of women's friendship networks as a means of support during stressful periods has been emphasized (Brooks-Gunn & Kirsh, 1984). Indeed, the number of confidants available to women reduced the health-threatening effects of stressors (Cooke, 1985).

Investigators have characterized the stressors to which midlife women are exposed and described how women cope with them. Midlife women and men experienced more hassles related to finances, work, home maintenance, personal life, and family and friends than older people, but women reported more hassles having to do with environmental and social issues than do men. Moreover, women and men demonstrated different coping approaches. Compared to men, women used less self-control, sought more social support, and used more positive appraisal. Compared to older people, those in midlife used more confrontive coping and sought more social support, and used less distancing and positive reappraisal (Folkman, Lazarus, Pimley, & Novacek, 1987).

In addition to gender differences, Griffith (1983b) found that women experienced different stressors depending on their age group. Of six major stressor areas—love relationships, personal success, physical health, parent-child relationships, personal time, and social relationships—major stressors for midlife women included physical health and personal time. Women used a variety of strategies to cope with these stressors. Talking, working, and turning to religion were most commonly used by women between 35 and 64 years of age (Griffith, 1983a).

How various ethnic groups of women experience midlife remains poorly understood. Unfortunately, there is little published work about women from underrepresented ethnic groups. Studies have often focused only on how women experience menopause, although recent work with African American women and Native American women have addressed midlife and aging directly (Barbee & Bauer, 1988; Jackson, 1990; Buck & Gottlieb, 1991).

FACTORS INFLUENCING MIDLIFE WOMEN'S HEALTH AND CARE

This review supports the concept of midlife as a complex time for women with personal and social changes having health effects that are as important, if not more important, than the biological changes of menopause. Although there are probably biological changes of aging that progress in a relatively immutable fashion, women's well being during midlife appears to be inextricably linked to the fabric of their lives.

The necessity of considering women's birth cohort as an important factor in the context for women's lives has been emphasized throughout much of the literature reviewed here. The importance of considering the meaning of midlife events as a product of women's unique interpretations should be foremost in the minds of clinicians and researchers. Meaning, then, becomes central to a model accounting for midlife women's health. For some women, definitions of femininity and self are not independent of their marital and parental roles. For others, such definitions hinge on their own expectations related to multiple dimensions of their lives.

Therapists urge that women plan for their own lives and take responsibility for the risks and benefits of these choices (Barnett, 1984). Yet for many who are currently in midlife, life choices hinged on a husband's or children's needs, not only on their own. The challenge of integrating multiple life roles faces women who have not had the benefit of preparation from their mother's experiences (Notman, 1984). Affirmation of women's choices from therapists and life partners, family members, and friends may help women restructure their relationships rather than leave them.

Although significant progress can be made through studies such as those being conducted by Kaufert, Matthews, and McKinlay, many significant questions remain unanswered about midlife women's health. For example, little is known about midlife women's health promotion patterns and their consequent effects on health and longevity. Health locus of control, self-esteem, and health status seem to have important influences on women's health promoting practices, including self-actualization, interpersonal support, exercise, nutrition, health responsibility, and stress management (Duffy, 1988). Effects of these health promoting patterns on morbidity and mortality over the lifespan remain unclear.

Activity, rest, and dietary patterns among midlife women have also received little attention to date. Studies of exercise among midlife women have begun with investigations of women's unique activity patterns over the lifespan (Dan, Wilbur, Hedricks, O'Connor, & Holm, 1990). Early work with aerobic exercise demonstrates that both premenopausal and postmenopausal women achieve comparable improvements in aerobic fitness. Aerobic exercise does not appear to have direct effects on stress response (Blumenthal, et al., 1991). Among the Healthy Women Study participants, however, physical activity levels assessed over a 3-year period were associated with less weight gain over time and mitigated the drop in HDL-C (Owens, Matthews, Wing, & Kuller, 1992). Sleep studies provide a link between sleep patterns and distress in midlife women. Polysomnographic records indicating poor sleep in concert with perceived poor sleep were more prevalent among women with menopausal symptoms than among those without symptoms. Women with no polysomnographic indicators of poor sleep, but with perceived sleep problems, had more distress (Shaver, Giblin, & Paulsen, 1991). Studies focusing on nutrition and dietary patterns, exercise, and rest simultaneously could make a significant contribution to understanding the relationship between health behaviors and health among this population.

The available literature supports a multidimensional model to account for midlife women's health. Although menopause influences women's experiences of certain symptoms, such as the hot flash, women's other symptom experiences, functional status, ability to adapt to their environments, and well being are relatively unaffected by menopause. These other dimensions of health are probably a product of personal and social resources women bring to midlife, their past health experiences, socialization for midlife, past and current social demands and patterns of coping with them, and health promoting and health damaging behavior patterns (Woods, Mitchell, & Lentz, 1989).

Until there is greater information to guide health care for midlife women, we would do well to begin following De Lorey's (1984) recommendations: (1) establish priorities of health care reflecting women's experiences as well as the findings from social, behavioral, and medical sciences; (2) establish an information base considering precursors of health at midlife, for example, nutrition and exercise; (3) redefine research priorities to include non-clinical populations and prospective studies about women's experiences; (4) present a more realistic view of midlife women to health professionals in their training;

and (5) support environments in which women can develop realistic expectations about midlife health issues.

Note: Full citations for books and articles appear in annotated bibliography.

REFERENCES

National Center for Health Statistics. Current estimates from the National Health Interview Survey, United States, 1985. U. S. Public Health Service Pub. No. 8601588, Washington, D.C., U.S. Government Printing Office.

National Center for Health Statistics. Vital statistics of the United States Vol. II, Part A. Mortality. U.S. Public Health Service, Pub No 88-1479, Washington, D.C., U.S. Government Printing Office.

Neugarten, B., & Kraines, R. (1965). Menopausal symptoms in women of various ages. *Psychosomatic Medicine, 27*, 266–273.

Treloar, A. E. (1982). Predicting the close of menstrual life. In A. M. Voda, M. Dinnerstein, & S. R. O'Donnell (Eds.), *Changing Perspectives on Menopause,* pp. 289–304, Austin: University of Texas Press.

Utian, W. (1991). Menopause—a proposed new functional definition. *Maturitas, 14*(1), 1–2.

Woods, N., Mitchell, E., & Lentz, M. (1989) Midlife Women: Health and Health Seeking Behaviors. Proposal funded by National Center for Nursing Research, National Institutes of Health.

BOOKS AND ARTICLES

Ackerman, R. (1990). Career developments and transitions of middle-aged women. *Psychology of Women Quarterly, 14*, 513–530.

Ackerman studied job transition behaviors in 71 women in their middle years of professional careers who had changed jobs in the past 3 years. All were employed in a utility company in a midwestern city where 11 percent of jobs were eliminated. She classified women according to their job transition attitudes and behaviors into groups who wanted versus didn't want change, and those who planned for versus those who didn't plan for the change. She found that personal characteristics (including demographic, personality, and attitude factors), situational characteristics (intrafamily life events and outside of family life events), and person by situation characteristics (coping behaviors, job-changing strategies, and job and life satisfaction) significantly discriminated between the four groups of women. Creators, those who wanted and planned for change, were positively attuned to their change and used family, professional, and community supports. Reactors, who didn't want change and didn't plan for it, experienced the highest levels of stress, physical illness, hostile behavior, and legal problems. These women did not have support from the family or community, had lowest incomes and did not readily adapt to incorporate new skills in their job transitions. Most were single or single parents, and family needs ranked as a high priority in their lives. Maintainers (wanted change, but didn't plan for it) and Conventionalists (didn't want change, but planned for it) had intermediate levels of stress. For all groups, family priorities created tensions about changing work roles.

Alington, D., & Troll, L. (1984). Social change and equality: The roles of women and economics. In G. Baruch & J. Brooks-Gunn (Eds.), *Women in midlife*, pp. 181–202, New York: Plenum.

The authors trace the history of women's opportunities in response to economic conditions. They propose that lasting change may occur when its source is "the wellspring of human need, when it is inspired by human deprivation, and when its goal is the improvement of the human condition." Their review demonstrated how temporary change is when its source is external, when inspired by institutional necessity and based on economic exigencies. Factors affecting women's opportunities, such as economic exigencies, ultimately affect women's chances for health.

Barbee, E., & Bauer, J. (1988). Aging and life experiences of low-income, middle-aged African American and Caucasian Women. *The Canadian Journal of Nursing Research, 20*(4), 5–17.

The investigators studied the influence of life experience on perceptions of aging by interviewing 54 low-income African American and 46 Caucasian midlife women. They found that African American women reported more aging signs and symptoms, such as the condition of their teeth and weight, than white women. With the exception of attending religious services, both groups participated in few social activities. Most of the African American and Caucasian women desired to be younger (an average of 13-to-16 years). For African American women, desired age was negatively related to aging signs

and symptoms, social activities, pleasures, and positively related to their worries. Aging signs and symptoms were also related to fewer social activities and exhaustion. For white women, desired age was negatively associated with worries. Aging signs and symptoms were related to social activities, pleasure and exhaustion.

Barnett, R. (1984). The anxiety of the unknown—choice, risk, responsibility: Therapeutic issues for today's adult women. In G. Baruch & J. Brooks-Gunn (Eds.), *Women in midlife*, pp. 341–358, New York: Plenum.

Barnett considers issues that middle-class white women address in therapy. She finds women are now grappling with the need to plan for their own lives and take responsibility for them. They also face the risks (costs and benefits) of these choices. For many, choices take them down paths untraveled by their mother's generation or perhaps by anyone else in their circle of friends. Definitions of femininity independent of marital and parental roles are not yet widespread. Sexuality and new moralities cause women to confront new issues (this chapter was written predating AIDs becoming a well-recognized health problem).

Baruch, G. (1984). The psychological well-being of women in the middle years. In G. Baruch & J. Brooks-Gunn (Eds.), *Women in midlife*, pp. 761–780, New York: Plenum.

Baruch examines psychological well being of midlife women. Well being is a good or satisfactory condition of existence. In earlier studies, Baruch found that for women 35-to-55 years, eight measures of well being, including happiness, satisfaction, optimism, anxiety, depression, mastery, self-esteem, and the balance of rewards and concerns women had factored into two primary dimensions: mastery and pleasure. Citing the results of her research with Barnett and others' findings, Baruch provides evidence of little change in well being associated with age for women 35 to 55 years. Employment status was not associated with pleasure, but with a greater sense of mastery regardless of women's marital and parental status. In addition, marital status was associated with higher pleasure scores. A subset of 72 women were interviewed intensively about the rewarding and distressing aspects of their various roles and subsequently 238 women indicated to what extent each item was rewarding or distressing.

For employment, major reward factors were challenge and social relationships whereas major concern factors were dullness of the job and whether it was a dead end. Rewards and concerns here were significantly related to both mastery and pleasure with the exception of social relationships which had no effect on mastery. In addition, women asked about homemaker's rewards indicated the satisfaction of being available to one's family, freedom from supervision, and opportunity to do tasks fitting one's skills. Concerns here were related to boredom and isolation and not earning money. Again, the balance between rewards and concerns was related to both mastery and pleasure.

Like employment and homemaking, marriage and childrearing had associated rewards and concerns. Feeling emotionally supported and appreciated was the major reward of marriage, with the major concern being marital conflict. Both affected mastery and pleasure. The central concern about not being married was lack of an intimate relationship. Women who reported distress about the lack of an intimate relationship had lower pleasure scores, but not a lower sense of mastery. Marriage enhanced happiness when married women were free to choose their employment status and to end an unhappy marriage. However, a good job was the key to self-esteem and protection against anxiety and depression.

In this regard as well, the balance of rewards and concerns vis-a-vis motherhood was related to both mastery and pleasure. Conflict with children was the major concern and was related to lower pleasure. For employed women, conflict with children also implicated a sense of lower mastery.

Also important were women's relationships with their mothers. Maternal rapport was positively related to both pleasure and mastery. For divorced women, however, maternal rapport and mastery were negatively related. In the Barnett and Baruch study, employed married women who had children were the highest in well being despite their busy lives.

Baruch, G., & Barnett, R. (1983). Adult daughters' relationships with their mothers. *Journal of Marriage and the Family*, 601–606.

The authors used a three-item index of "maternal rapport" to examine perceived relationships between mothers of 171 women aged 35 to 55 years. They found that overall, relationships were seen as rewarding, especially by women who were not currently mothers. Although the age of the daughter and the mother's marital status (widowed or currently married) were not significantly related to maternal rapport scores, the mothers' health was significantly related to maternal rapport scores. In addition, psychological well being, as measured by sense of mastery and pleasure, was significantly correlated with maternal rapport, with relationships being stronger for the women who were not mothers themselves. The gratifications of adult women in the role of daughter seem contingent on their entire constellation of roles.

Baruch, G., & Brooks-Gunn, J. (1984). *Women in midlife*. New York: Plenum.

Berkum, C. (1983). Changing appearance for women in the middle years of life: Trauma. In E. Markson (Ed). *Older women*, pp. 11–35, Lexington, MA: Heath.

The author explores the effects of changing appearance on middle aged women's experience of themselves. She interviewed 60 physically and mentally healthy white suburban women between 40 and 55 years of age. Most were married or had been married, and said they had been married largely because it was the only desirable option they perceived. Most had internalized the social ideology about women's appearance. For example, 68 percent felt different without makeup, 57 percent thought they looked older without makeup, and 85 percent thought they were less attractive without makeup. For all but 3, cosmetic surgery was only a fantasy, not to be realized because of the expense and risk. Some thought middle age was frightening, but others perceived they had more self-confidence, social ease, and a better perspective on life than they had held earlier. Others pointed out the negative aspects of aging on their appearance, usually those facing a harsh social reality, such as those trying to attract men or needing to find work. For many women, changing appearance was not problematic. Only 23 percent expressed a great desire to look younger, 21 percent felt they had lost in their appearance as they aged, and 58 percent felt positive about their appearance. Berkum recommends that patterns fitting the feminine stereotype may be dysfunctional for middle-aged women. Midlife women may benefit from an educational process that involves learning new ways of thinking about themselves and their behavior and understanding that there may be no social reinforcements for these. Women who have discarded old patterns of thought and behavior may experience difficulty with others in their environment. Middle-aged women may cling to marriages regardless of their quality. Self actualization may have little meaning for middle-aged women. Perception of middle-aged and older women as valuable and attractive personally and physically will require social and political change.

Blumenthal, J., Fredrickson, M., Matthews, K., Kuhn, C., Schniebolk, S., German, D., Rifai, N., Steege, J., & Rodin, J. (1991). Stress reactivity and exercise training in premenopausal and postmenopausal women. *Health Psychology, 10*(6), 384–391.

Fifty premenopausal and postmenopausal women were given aerobic fitness evaluations and pretested for stress responses, then randomly assigned to a 12-week exercise program of either aerobic exercise or non-aerobic strength and flexibility training and re-evaluated. Postmenopausal women had lower resting epinephrine levels but greater epinephrine reactivity to a speech stressor compared with premenopausal women, but menopausal status did not differentiate women with respect to cardiovascular or catecholamine responses during the cold challenge stressor.

Both groups achieved comparable improvements in aerobic fitness, but there was no direct effect of exercise on stress response.

Brooks-Gunn, J., & Kirsh, B. (1984). Life events and the boundaries of midlife for women. In Baruch and Brooks-Gunn (Eds.), *Women in midlife*, pp. 11–30, New York: Plenum.

Midlife has been characterized as a transitory rather than a distinct life cycle phase. Midlife is more than preparation for old age and death; instead it can be a period of generativity, satisfaction, and competence. The authors stress the multidimensional and multidirectional nature of change in midlife, describing the boundaries as fluid and constructed by the society and the individual rather than chronological age. Boundaries of midlife are unclear for several reasons: (1) young adulthood is now protracted; (2) health of the midlife woman is relatively good; (3) midlife may be a period of enhanced sexuality for women; (4) midlife is believed to coincide with the children leaving home, yet later parenting and reblended families may postpone women's perceptions of being in midlife; (5) change in life expectancy alters the boundary of midlife, especially for women; and (6) being old carries a stigma that discourages women from claiming to be in midlife. There are many markers of midlife, including chronological age, parenting status, perceiving oneself to be in phase with the middle of one's life, activities that women engage in such as changes in work life events, hormonal changes occurring at midlife. Whatever the markers, the historical context for a cohort of women experiencing midlife is important in anticipatory socialization for the events of midlife. Post hoc socialization may occur in observation of role models, seeking new referent groups, asking friends for information, and being offered information. Some cohorts may anticipate one pattern for midlife, yet encounter another. The authors also examine data from two cohorts of Radcliffe College graduates, one finishing in 1947 and the other in 1962. Although more of the 1962 graduates had established careers than the earlier cohort, most of the earlier cohort were employed at the time of the study. The earlier cohort felt unprepared for social change in the norms affecting sexuality. Women in both cohorts reported finding romance and love relationships in their middle years. Friendship networks were especially supportive, particularly for the earlier cohort. Although it is commonly believed that at midlife there is no plot line left for women, or that it is completely predicated upon a woman's marital or parental status, the results of this study suggest that midlife is a time for growth and change.

Buck, M., & Gottlieb, L. (1991). The meaning of time: Mohawk women at midlife. *Health Care for Women International, 12,* 41–50.

The investigators conducted a grounded theory study of eight Mohawk women, finding four major issues related to the concept of time. These included: it is time for me, being where I should be, time for myself, and my time is spent meaningfully. Women in synchrony (those who were where they thought they should be in life) viewed their lives as following expected time pathways, whereas those out of synchrony viewed their lives as problematic. These latter women were either taking action or were stuck.

Bungay, G., Vessey, M., & McPherson, C. (1980). Study of symptoms in middle life with special reference to the menopause. *British Medical Journal, 281*(6234), 181–183.

A population of 1,120 women and 510 men were sent mailed questionnaires. Peaks for prevalence of flushing and sweating were associated closely with the mean age of menopause, either coinciding with it or occurring shortly after it. Less impressive peaks of prevalence of a group of minor mental symptoms were associated with an age just preceding the mean age of menopause. Complaints about aching breasts, irritability, and low backache diminished after menopause. The authors conclude that a cluster of symptoms occurs about the mean age of menopause, but since no measures were obtained to

determine which women had and had not experienced menopause it is difficult to make the attribution to menopause.

Cooke, D. (1985). Social support and stressful life events during mid-life. *Maturitas, 7,* 303–313.

The author explored the influence of eight social relationship variables on both psychological and somatic distress in a sample of 78 midlife women between 35 and 54 years of age residing in Glasgow. The psychological symptoms included depressed mood, panic attacks, crying spells and worrying. Somatic symptoms included faintness, dizziness, headaches and tingling, or numbness of the body. The total number of vulnerability factors was calculated based on women's situations, including: loss of or separation from mother before age 11; number of children under 15 years living at home; lack of full-time employment outside the home; extent of confiding with spouse; number of confiding relationships available. Number of children under 15 and degree of confiding in the spouse had no effects on psychological or somatic symptoms. Both loss of the mother and being unemployed had important interactive effects on both somatic and psychological symptoms. Number of confidants available had important interactive effects with total life stress to reduce both psychological and social symptoms. Although degree of involvement with children had no effect on psychological symptoms, it reduced the experience of somatic symptoms.

Cooke, D., & Greene, J. (1981). Types of life events in relation to symptoms at the climacterium. *Journal of Psychosomatic Research, 25,* 5–11.

The investigators studied life stress, social support and adjustment using semi-structured interviews with 408 women between the ages of 25 to 64 years. They found that psychological symptoms increased during ages 35 to 44 when there was also a high rate of exits, including deaths from the network. Women who experienced somatic symptoms were exposed to both a high level of miscellaneous stress as well as exits.

Cutler, W. (1987). Perimenopausal sexuality. *Archives of Sexual Behavior, 16*(3), 225–234.

An interview with 124 women during the perimenopause about their sexual responses and the results of 52 women's prospective coital records over three months with concomitant steroid analysis indicate that in general, women around 49 years do not suffer from a particular sexual deficit in sexual desire, response, or satisfaction. A subset of women with especially low estradiol levels (less than 35 pg/ml) tends to have reduced coital activity.

Dan, A., Wilbur, J., Hedricks, C., O'Connor, E., & Holmn, K. (1990). Lifelong physical activity in midlife and older women. *Psychology of Women Quarterly, 14,* 531–542.

The investigators developed a questionnaire to assess levels of lifelong physical activity with three subscales: occupation, leisure, and household. They present psychometric properties of the measure indicating its utility for studies with women and across the lifespan. The patterns of physical activity varied over the lifespan for each subscale. Total physical activity peaked between ages 25 to 39 and declined steeply after age 39 with small decreases across each subscale. This measure is unique in its inclusion of household physical activity to document lifelong levels of activity in studies of women's health.

De Lorey, C. (1984). Health care and midlife women. In Baruch and Brooks-Gunn, (Eds.), *Women in midlife,* pp. 277–301, New York: Plenum.

De Lorey challenges the assumption that menopause is the most important aspect of women's lives and health during the middle years. She reviews major health issues for midlife women, pointing out that they are not gynecological conditions. Instead, major killers are heart disease and cerebrovascular disease.

Moreover, she explores the differences in causes of death for underrepresented ethnic groups and white women. Of interest is that no women who participated in a community survey done by the author believed that menopause was the major health problem for midlife women, despite the fact it seemed a major concern for physicians. The author discusses menopause, heart disease, cancer, and occupational health concerns relevant to midlife women. She points out that coronary risk factors for women have received scant attention. Uterine, cervical, and breast cancer account for approximately 40 percent of all women's cancer deaths. De Lorey concludes her review with the recommendation that gynecologists are not the appropriate primary health care providers for many women. She recommends the following: (1) establishing priorities of health care that address women's priorities based on their own experiences, the social, behavioral, and biomedical sciences; (2) establishing an information base considering precursors of health at midlife, eg. nutrition and exercise; (3) redefining research priorities so nonclinical and prospective studies are available about midlife women's health rather than merely clinical studies; (4) presenting a more realistic and less pathological view of midlife women to health care providers; (5) supporting environments in which women can develop realistic expectations about midlife health issues.

Dennerstein, L. (1987). Depression in the menopause. *Obstetrics and Gynecology Clinics of North America, 14*(1), 33–48.

The author examines complaints of depressed mood and other minor psychological changes in women during perimenopause. She cites current evidence to support a biopsychosocial etiologic model in which underlying endocrinologic changes trigger emotional complaints in women who are vulnerable because of developmental factors, personality, psychiatric history, known vulnerability to hormonally triggered mood changes or current social problems.

Duffy, M. (1988). Determinants of health promotion in midlife women. *Nursing Research, 37*(6), 358–361.

The author gave 262 women between 35 and 65 years of age questionnaires to measure health locus of control, self-esteem, health status, and health-promoting lifestyle activities. Internal health locus of control, self-esteem, current health status, and future health status explained 36 percent of the variance of a composite of the self-actualization, interpersonal support, and exercise health promotion subscales. Age, negative chance health locus of control, health worry/concern, and negative prior health status explained 36 percent of the variance of a composite of the health responsibility, nutrition, and stress management subscales. These results support parts of the Pender health promotion model. They suggest that a combination of personal characteristics influences the combination of health promotion behaviors women perform.

Engel, N. (1987). Menopausal stage, current life change, attitude toward women's roles, and perceived health status. *Nursing Research, 36*(6), 353–357.

Engel studied the influence of menopausal stage, current life change, and attitudes toward traditional women's roles on perceived health status in 249 women 40-to-55 years of age. As women passed through menopausal stages, their perceived health status was poorer, but the difference was small. Women with more stressful life events had poorer perceived health status. There was no relationship between sex role attitudes and perceived health status.

Engel, N. (1984). On the vicissitudes of health appraisal. *Advances in Nursing Science, 7*(1), 12–23.

Engel administered the Health Perceptions Questionnaire, Affect Balance Scale, Life Satisfaction Index, and Menopause Symptom Checklist to 249 women 40-to-55 years old who lived in the mid-Atlantic region who had not yet experienced menopause, had not perceived themselves to be ill or disabled, were not pregnant, had not experienced past mental breakdown, were U.S. born, and had completed at least the eighth grade. She found a negative relationship between the scores on the Menstrual Symptom Checklist, which includes symptoms other than hot flashes and night sweats, and Perceived Health Status, a summation of scores on the Health Perceptions Questionnaire, Affect Balance Scale, and Life Satisfaction Index.

Folkman, S., Lazarus, Pimley, S., & Novacek, J. (1987). Age differences in stress and coping processes. *Psychology and Aging, 2,* 171–184.

The authors compared younger and older community-dwelling adults with respect to their experiences of daily hassles and their use of eight kinds of coping. There were clear age differences in hassles and coping. In addition, sex differences were apparent in some of the analyses. Of special interest are comparisons of women between 35 and 45 and those 65 and 74. Younger men and women experienced more hassles related to finances, work, home maintenance, personal life, and family and friends than the older group. Women reported more hassles having to do with environmental and social issues than men. Younger men reported more household hassles than younger women, whereas older men reported fewer of these hassles than did older women. Compared to the older group, younger people used more confrontive coping and sought more social support, and used less distancing and positive reappraisal. Compared to men, women used less self-control, sought more social support, and used more positive reappraisal. Detailed analyses compare both age and gender differences in choice of coping strategies for several types of stressors, including threats to family, health, self-esteem, and loved one's well being.

Gath, D., Osborn, M., Bungay, G., Iles, S., Day, A., Bond, A., & Passingham, C. (1987). Psychiatric disorder and gynecological symptoms in middle aged women: A community survey. *British Medical Journal, 294*(6566), 213–218.

Five hundred twenty-one women aged 35-to-59 were selected randomly from all patients registered in two group practices. They were interviewed at home and asked standardized psychiatric measures and gynecological history. Levels of psychiatric morbidity were within the expected range for the sample. Psychiatric morbidity and neuroticism were significantly associated with gynecological symptoms including dysmenorrhea, premenstrual tension, excessive menstruation and flushes and sweats. There was no relationship between psychiatric morbidity and absence of menses for six months or longer. Psychiatric state was significantly associated with recent adverse life events and with indices of psychiatric vulnerability including neuroticism and previous psychiatric history.

Gergen, M. (1990). Finished at 40: Women's development within the patriarchy. *Psychology of Women Quarterly, 14,* 471–493.

The author presents a review of women's adult development as chronicled in textbooks, revealing that the prevailing focus is the woman as a biological creature, especially a mother; the proposed lifecycle trajectory is one of decline for women after 40; and little attention is paid to the character of women's life narratives. These approaches to understanding adult womanhood reinforce patriarchal systems of power. She recommends a social constructionist approach to create theories that liberate interpretations of women from an exclusive focus on their reproductive roles; support feminist methodologies; emphasize relational networks over autonomous individualism; create new narrative life forms for women that are multiple and nonlinear; and support a critical function with psychology and society. The author's emphasis on the value of relational theory, rather than on developing another theory about the single self changing over time could stimulate studies of relational networks that might encompass intergenerational activities, family relations, collegial interactions, and social group performances. In addition, narratives that encompass the complexity of women's lives could account for the multiple relational patterns that characterize most women's lives. Gergen urges researchers to face the challenge of being a critic rather than accepting existing social practices as the basis for theorizing.

Giele, J. (1982). *Women in the middle years: Current knowledge and directions for research and policy.* New York: Wiley.

Gilligan, C. (1982a). Adult development and women's development: Arrangements for a marriage. In Giele, (Ed.), *Women in the Middle Years,* pp. 89–114, New York: Wiley.

Gilligan proposes restoring the missing text of women's development rather than simply replacing it with work about men's development. She proposes that the middle years of a woman's life are not simply a time of return to the unfinished business of adolescence. Instead, women's embeddedness in lives of relationship, their orientation to interdependence, their ability to subordinate achievement to care, and their conflicts over competitive success place them at risk in midlife. This dilemma is a commentary on the society more than a problem in women's development. Gilligan argues that the events of midlife can alter a woman's activities of care in ways that affect her sense of herself. For example, if midlife brings an end to relationships, and with them the sense of connection on which she relies and the activities of care through which she judges her worth, then this life transition can lead to despair. The meaning of midlife events for a woman is contextual, arising from the interaction between the structures of her thought and the realities of her life. Women face midlife with a different psychological history than men and make sense out of experiences on the basis of their knowledge of human relationships. It is as if men and women have two different languages to describe their development. Understanding the tensions between these two languages may help in gaining understanding of the concept of adult work and family relationships.

Gilligan, C. (1982b). *In a different voice. Psychological theory and women's development.* Cambridge: Harvard University Press.

Gilligan explores woman's place in man's life cycle, considering the images of relationship, concepts of self and morality, crisis and transition, and women's rights and women's judgment. Of most relevance to midlife women is the chapter focusing on "Visions of Maturity," in which the author examines models for a healthy life cycle derived from studies of men, advancing the notion that separation leads to attachment and that individuation eventuates in mutuality. Gilligan points out the fusion of identity and intimacy in women's development and emphasizes that the standard of moral judgment that informs their self assessments is a standard of relationship, with an ethic of nurturance, responsibility, and care. Morality arises from the experience of connection and becomes a problem of inclusion rather than one of balancing claims. Women find themselves approaching issues with two different moral ideologies, with separation justified by an ethic of rights and attachment supported by an ethic of care. As a result, women reach midlife with a different psychological history than men and face a different social reality with different possibilities for love and work. They also make a different sense of experience based on their knowledge of human relationships. Since the reality of connection is experienced as a given rather than as contracted, women arrive at an understanding of life reflecting the limits of autonomy and control.

Griffith, J. (1983a). Women's stressors according to age groups: Part I. *Issues in Health Care of Women, 6,* 311–326.

The author studied 579 women 25 to 64 years of age. Women indicated their personal life goals/values and satisfaction in achieving them. Six major stressors were identified: love relationships, personal success, physical health, parent-child relationships, personal time, and social relationships. Women 35 to 44 years indicated the major stressors for them were physical health, personal time, love relationships and personal success. Those 45 to 54 indicated physical health, personal time, love relationships, and parent and child issues and personal success. Those 55 to 65 years listed physical health and personal time.

Griffith, J. (1983b). Women's stress responses and coping patterns according to age groups. *Issues in Health Care of Women, 6,* 327–340.

In the study described above, the author also analyzed the relationships between women's age groups and their physical and emotional symptoms of stress and their usual coping patterns. Age-related patterns of symptoms appeared for many types of symptoms. For women 35 to 65, feeling fat and overweight and frequently nervous and tense were the most prevalent symptoms. In addition, women used a variety of coping styles. Those 35 to 44 years used talking, work, religion, and consumption of food. Those 45 to 54 and 55 to 64 used work, religion, talking, and food consumption.

Jackson, B. (1990). Social support and life satisfaction of black climacteric women. *Western Journal of Nursing Research, 12*(1), 9–27.

The centrality of women's relationships to life satisfaction was confirmed in this study of black midlife women. Women between 40 and 60 years of age (*n* = 120) responded to a mailed questionnaire regarding life satisfaction, social support. Support from husband or lover, positive relationships with children, supportive relationships with relatives, and involvement with friends had positive effects of different dimensions of life satisfaction. Relationships with husbands and lovers and with children affected current life satisfaction, while relationships with children, relatives, and friends influenced retrospective life satisfactions. Relationships with friends and organizations influenced retrospective life dissatisfaction. Involvement with institutions and voluntary social organizations demonstrated a trend toward a significant relationship with life satisfaction.

Jennings, S., Mazaik, C., & McKinlay, S. (1984). Women and work: An investigation of the association between health and employment status in middle-aged women. *Social Science and Medicine, 19,* 423–421.

The authors analyzed the results of the first large U.S. epidemiological study of 8,114 women aged 45 to 54 randomly selected from Massachusetts. Women employed for pay (69%), full time homemakers (24%) and women unemployed (5%) or living with an unemployed spouse (2%) were included in the analyses. They found the strongest associations between employment status and health status, including self-assessment of current health compared to others, the number of psychological symptoms, and use of medications designed to alleviate them. Lay help-seeking about health problems was more strongly associated with employment status than professional help-seeking. Employed women had the fewest health problems and reported the fewest illness behaviors while unemployed women reported the most health problems and the most illness behavior. Homemakers reported intermediary levels. The investigators attempted to account for the "healthy worker effect," that is, those women with poor health leaving the labor force. While it is likely that the health worker effect did influence the association between employment and good health, there still remains evidence of salutogenic effects of employment on women's health.

Kaufert, P. (1980). The perimenopausal woman and her use of health services. *Maturitas 2,* 191–205.

The author investigated whether perimenopausal women had higher physician contact rates and a more negative self-assessment of their health than nonmenopausal Manitoba women in the same age band of 40-to-60 years. In addition, she examined relationships between subjective health status, physician contact rates, and vasomotor and psychological symptoms. Kaufert found that women experienced a change in vasomotor symptoms with menopausal status, with those women who

were immediately postmenopausal and in the advanced post-menopausal years experiencing the most symptoms. Women who had experienced artificially induced menopause, e.g., by hysterectomy, had more psychological symptoms than those who had a natural menopause. Health assessments were not related to menopausal status, vasomotor symptoms, or the rate of contact with a physician. Menopausal status and physician contact within the previous two weeks and past year were related, with women in the advanced postmenopausal group having more frequent physician contact. Women in the perimenopausal and immediately postmenopausal groups were least likely to have seen a physician more than twice in the past year, but also were least likely to have had physician contact. Women with high frequency and severity of vasomotor symptoms were more likely to have seen a physician and there was a significant association between physician contact in the previous two weeks and a high score on the psychological symptom list. Of interest was that 95 percent of this Canadian sample had seen a physician during the previous 12 months.

Kaufert, P. (1984). Women and their health in the middle years: A Manitoba project. *Social Science and Medicine, 18,* 279–281.

The author describes a project focusing on the health and health behavior of women between 40 and 59 years of age. Midlife women are typified as high users of medical services and of various forms of medication, especially psychotropic drugs, and are more likely to have been treated for psychological problems and have neurotic or psychosomatic labels attached to their symptoms. Midlife women's health problems are commonly attributed to menopause or to changing family roles. Yet the balance between work and family life, changes in support and network characteristics, and occurrence of life events that affect health have not yet been addressed in this population of women. Indeed, no investigator in Canada or the United States examined the consequences for health of the coincidence of hormonal changes with a life phase marked by stress. Likewise, no one had examined whether a woman's attitudes toward and experience of menopause were moderated by characteristics of her social network, availability of social support, or level of family or workplace stress. Information to account for apparently high use of physician services, consumption of psychotropic drugs, and general physical and psychological malaise is lacking. The Manitoba project is a 3-stage project with stage 1 consisting of a cross-sectional mail survey, stage 2 a longitudinal study extending over a 3-year period in which a subset of women in stage 1 take part, and stage 3 is a series of semi-structured, in-depth interviews with 100 women, a subset of stage 2 participants. Over 2,500 responses were obtained to stage 1, with data having been collected on the health and health behavior of midlife women, including chronic health problems, symptom profiles, medication use, and patterns of physician contact. Other information included emphasizes women's employment patterns, household and family structure, women's attitudes toward the roles available to them as wives, mothers, daughters, housewives, or employees. Stage 2 will involve about 500 women who will be followed for three years, during which time most will experience menopause. Because of the longitudinal design, it will be possible to see the wider context of a woman's health over time and to see the relationship between availability of support or experience of stress in relationship to menopause. Stage 3 will emphasize the diversity of psychosocial meanings of menopause, including their status at menopause, its symbolism, the relationships between loss of fertility and identity as women, and re-appraisal of their life career as wives, mothers, and daughters. The author emphasizes her collaboration with the McKinlay study which occurred about the same time in Massachusetts.

Kaufert, P. (1986). Menstruation and menstrual change: Women in midlife. *Health Care for Women International, 7*(1–2), 63–76.

Kaufert used data taken from a cross-sectional survey of 2,500 Manitoba women 40-to-59 years of age to discuss the impact of changes in menstrual pattern on women's likelihood of seeking medical care and on their perceived menopausal status. Data from 1,254 women who had menstruated in the past 12 months were analyzed. Women's periods became less regular and lighter over the age groups from 40 to 54. Women demonstrated increased likelihood of being transitional, that is having a change in regularity and/or flow during the preceding 12 months as they became older. In addition, the likelihood of becoming perimenopausal, that is, having a period within the past year, but not the last three months, also increased with age. Only 38 percent of women who had not noticed a change in menstrual pattern had discussed their menopausal status with a physician, but 60 percent of the transitional, and 71 percent of the periomenopausal women had done so. Of interest is that only 38 percent of the transitional and 36 percent of the perimenopausal women had discussed any menstrual problem with a physician. Only 28 percent of those reporting heavy menstruation and only 16 percent of those reporting either pain or intermenstrual bleeding had discussed a menstrual problem with a physician.

Kaufert, P., Gilbert, P., & Hassard, T. (1988). Researching the symptoms of menopause: An exercise in methodology. *Maturitas, 10*(2), 117–131.

Four hundred seventy-seven women were interviewed 6 times over a 3-year period about their menstrual status, their physical, menopausal, and psychological symptoms. Analysis of variance demonstrated that only vasomotor symptoms varied across menopausal status. This important work demonstrates that symptoms other than vasomotor symptoms are unrelated to menopause. The authors suggest that researchers and clinicians should consider sources of midlife women's symptoms other than menopause.

Kaufert, P., Gilbert, P., & Tate, R. (1992). The Manitoba Project: A re-examination of the link between menopause and depression. *Maturitas, 14,* 117–126.

The authors re-examine the association between menopause and depression with data from the Manitoba study of 477 midlife women. Rather than hormonal changes, a woman's poor health, coupled with shifts and stresses of family life appear to trigger depression. Hysterectomy was associated with depression, possibly because women with depression tend to be at greater risk of surgery.

Kaufert, P., & Syrotiuk, J. (1981). Symptom reporting at the menopause. *Social Science and Medicine, 151,* 173–184.

This paper presents the summary of findings from a pilot study being conducted in Manitoba, Canada with 200 midlife women. Three problems, the use of multiple and highly diverse symptom lists in menopause research, claims regarding the presence or absence of psychological distress at menopause, and scant attention to the probable bias arising from the influence of cultural factors on symptom reporting, are addressed in this study. Psychological and vasomotor symptoms were measured using an 11-item scale from the International Health Foundation. Factor analysis of the items revealed two symptoms, hot flashes and night sweats, which varied with menopausal status. Psychological symptoms, tiredness, irritability, depression, nervous tension, and trouble sleeping, did not vary with menopausal stage. Although psychological symptoms were correlated with self-esteem levels and negative affect levels, there was no relationship between menopausal status and any indicators of mental health.

Lachman, M. (1984). Methods for a life-span developmental approach to women in the middle years. In Baruch and Brooks-Gunn, (Eds.), *Women in midlife,* pp. 31–68, New York: Plenum.

The goals of life-span research are to examine the nature and course of development and to search for antecedents and consequences of developmental change. Lachman examines development during adulthood as a multidirectional, reversible, and variable process across individuals, cultures, and historical time. Three major sets of influences that control development are normative age-graded (influenced by age), normative history-graded (influenced by one's birth cohort), and nonnormative. From a life-span view, midlife is a dynamic period of development, noted by the complexity of change patterns. In addition, midlife is part of an integrated whole occurring within the context of historical and cultural forces. The author discusses four goals for life-span research and how to attain these: adopting techniques to enable reliable measurement of change; developing and using measurement instruments valid for the age being studied; capturing complexity and diversity of change; and identifying methods for examining individual and cultural/historical patterns of change.

Long, J., & Porter, K. (1984). Multiple roles of midlife women: A case for new directions in theory, research, and policy. In Baruch and Brooks-Gunn, (Eds.), *Women in midlife,* pp. 109–160, New York: Plenum.

The authors provide an extensive framework based on role theory for understanding women's experiences of multiple roles in midlife. They emphasize the importance of asking what the latter half of life holds for women in terms of work rewards, success, satisfaction, and economic security. They consider occupations and careers, in general, and examine the concepts of dual roles and role conflict as they apply to the worlds of work and family for women. Examining the usual mechanisms for reducing role conflict, such as compartmentalization of roles, delegation of role performance, elimination of roles, and role accumulation, they conclude that application of theory based on "male roles" to women's lives is inappropriate. The authors emphasize the importance of examining women's role partners as sources of role conflict, particularly spouses and coworkers. In addition, they examine the marital and parental career at midlife, concluding there is evidence of growth during midlife and that transitions in parenting and domestic careers have minimal effects on women's lives. The authors also point out the economic consequences of women's discontinuous work life experiences and suggest policy changes to decrease the poverty which many women experience in later life.

Lopata, H., & Barnewolt, D. (1984). The middle years: Changes and variations in social-role commitments. In Baruch and Brooks-Gunn, (Eds.), *Women in midlife*, pp. 83–108, New York: Plenum.

The authors discuss concepts of role conflict and role strain as they may be relevant to women in midlife. They present data from nearly 1,000 Chicago area women who were asked to respond to the question "What are the most important roles of a woman?" Few women considered a role in which they were not involved currently as the most important. In all, the role of mother outweighed any other role, including wife, as most important for the Chicago women. Blue collar women were most apt to list the role of employee first in the absence of wife and mother roles. Work-oriented women saw themselves as leaders and successful people, and were less likely to see themselves as emotional than were women who gave first importance to other roles. The age of their children, rather than the age of the woman, was the crucial variable. Presence of small children, especially under age 6, decreased the choice of employeee as the most important role. Women who chose the wife role as most important were married to men with more education, prestigious occupations, and higher incomes. Women who chose mother as the most important role were most likely to have a child under the age of 3 at home. Also, those who had their first child at age 27 or later were more likely to list the role of mother first. Generally, child-oriented women were of lower socioeconomic background than others because they lived alone or shared a household with someone other than a husband. Women tended to see their involvement in social roles in life-course terms, with those currently involved as a mother expecting to shift from the role of mother to the role of wife more as they grew older. Those nearing 55 did not anticipate major changes in the near future with the exception of an increased involvement in roles outside the complex of wife and mother. Over the past two decades, the major shift has been in the devaluation of the role of housewife. The importance women assign to their roles may influence their sense of well being in midlife.

Luria, Z., & Meade, R. (1984). Sexuality and the middle-aged woman. In Baruch and Brooks-Gunn, (Eds.), *Women in midlife*, pp. 371–398, New York: Plenum.

The authors review past works on women's sexuality during the middle years, beginning with Kinsey's studies conducted in the late 40s and early 50s, involving birth cohorts from 1880-to-1910. Later work by Pfeiffer and Davis confirmed that the double standard, different expectations for men and women, influenced midlife women's sexual behavior. Moreover, a relationship with a man with health problems, particularly those affecting erection, reduced women's frequency of sexual practices and interest. Data from Udry and Morris' studies of contemporary women (data collected mid-70s) suggest that women have more influence on sexual frequency than in previous age cohorts. Studies of lesbians indicate that white lesbians demonstrate a decline in sexual interest (as indicated by thinking about sex and the importance of sex) as they age. These patterns are not the same for black women. The authors also point out that conceiving of sexual behaviors as outlets, with masturbation and coitus as simple variants of sexual expression, may not be accurate for women's experiences. Instead, women experience coitus as relational, whereas they experience masturbation as a solitary act. Thus, the meanings ascribed to different sexual behaviors for women is likely to be different than that ascribed by men. Although contemporary women have new freedoms, it is also clear that they are not universally comfortable in telling partners what pleases them. The authors hazard predictions about the sexuality of the baby boom generation as it enters midlife. They predict that middle-aged women will be seen as sexual rather than asexual, a function of greater acceptance of sexuality across the lifespan. In addition, they predict a growing absence of stable male sexual partners for many women because of divorce rates and shorter lifespans for men. Finally, they anticipate that labor force participation for women could have variable effects on sexual activity, interfering with sexual frequency because of increased responsibilities or enhancing it because of increased social skills development for women.

Matthews, K., Wing, R., Kuller, L., Meilahn, E., Kelsey, S., Costello, E., & Caggiula, A. (1990). Influences of natural menopause on psychological characteristics and symptoms of middle-aged healthy women. *Journal of Consulting and Clinical Psychology, 58*(3), 345–351.

The investigators studied the psychological and symptom consequences of natural menopause longitudinally in 541 premenopausal healthy women. After an extensive evaluation at baseline, women were followed for 3 years. The investigators matched 69 women who experienced menopause and another 32 who had stopped menses and had taken hormone therapy for 12 months with 101 control women of the same age. Natural menopause led to few changes in psychological characteristics with only a decline in introspectiveness and an increase in hot flashes. Natural menopause had no adverse effects on type A behavior, anxiety, anger, total symptoms, depression, public self consciousness, perceived stress, job dissatisfaction, body worry, excitability, aches in neck and skull, nervousness or difficulty sleeping. Cardiovascular risk factors changed in women who had experienced natural menopause, with LDL-C increasing and HDL-C decreasing. Hormone users reported more depressive symptoms, were more type A, and more self-conscious in public and also developed dramatic elevations in triglyceride levels and weight gain. Some of the behavioral characteristics may have been causes of hormone use rather than their effects.

McKinlay, S., Bifano, N., & McKinlay, J. (1985). Smoking and age at menopause in women. *Annals of Internal Medicine, 103*(3), 350–356.

Although women can expect to live one half of their adult lives beyond menopause, knowledge about this physiologic event and its various influences on subsequent health and quality of life remains incomplete. In Massachusetts a population-based random sample of 7,828 white women, aged 45 to 55 years (response rate, 77 percent) was conducted. The median age at last menstruation for the sample is 51.4 +/− 0.19 (SE) years. No evidence was found of a secular trend toward a later age at menopause in the last 25 years. Current smokers reach menopause an average of 1.74 years earlier than nonsmokers (t = 3.78, p less than 0.01), but the quantity smoked has a negligible effect. Other potential correlates measured—education and marital status, number of children, and urban/rural residence—have little effect on the age at menopause. The results confirm earlier, more tentative findings from clinical populations.

McKinlay, J., McKinlay, & Brambilla, D. (1987a). Health status and utilization behavior associated with menopause. *American Journal of Epidemiology, 125,* 110–121.

Prospective data gathered over 27 months on a cohort of approximately 2,500 women representative of women 45-to-55 years in Massachusetts, demonstrated the following: (1) menopause did not cause poorer health status; (2) menopause does not increase utilization of health services; (3) occurrence of a surgical menopause is the primary menopause-related change affecting perceived health status and utilization behavior, and then minimally; and (4) nearly all the explained variability in health status and utilization behavior outcomes can be attributed to prior health status of the respondents and to a lesser extent to past utilization behavior.

McKinlay, J., McKinlay, S., & Brambilla, D. (1987b). The relative contributions of endocrine changes and social circumstances to depression in mid-aged women. *Journal of Health and Social Behavior, 28*(4), 345–363.

The investigators studied 2,500 premenopausal midlife women (45 to 55 years) randomly selected from the population of Massachusetts. They found that depression was associated with a surgical menopause and may even be a cause rather than an effect of this surgery. In addition, depression was not associated with the natural changes to menopause. The most marked increases in depression were associated with multiple causes of worry and multiple roles among currently married women (including paid work, adolescent children, ill husbands, aging parents and parents-in-law).

McKinlay, S., Brambilla, D., & Posner, J. (1992). The normal menopause transition. *Maturitas, 14*, 103–115.

Data from 5 years of follow-up of 2,570 women aged 45-to-55 years in January 1, 1982 who had menstruated within the last 3 months and had not undergone removal of the uterus and/ or ovaries. Following these women revealed that the median age at menopause was 51.3 years with smokers experiencing earlier menopause by about 1.8 years when compared to non-smokers. Inception of perimenopause occurred at 47.5 years with approximately 4 years required for perimenopausal transition. Perimenopause was defined as 3-to-11 months of amenorrhea or increasing irregularity over subsequent interviews. A longer perimenopausal transition was associated with higher rates of physician consultations. Menopausal transition and symptom reporting was a time-bound phenomenon with a compensatory decrease occurring postmenopausally.

McKinlay, S., & McKinlay, J. (1986). Aging in a 'healthy' population. *Social Science and Medicine, 23*, 531–535.

In this article, the McKinlays describe their 5-year project which builds on an ongoing epidemiological study of menopause in 2,500 women. The new study includes both men and women, and will emphasize the experience of healthy individuals randomly selected from the general population. This multi-disciplinary project combines physiological measurement with psychosocial data, and uses community-based methods of collecting physiological and psychological information. Models of the studies for women, men, and couples are presented. The model for the study of women includes personal factors, social factors, hormone changes, and outcomes including menstrual changes, bone density changes, and psychiatric symptomatology.

McKinlay, S., & McKinlay, J. (1989). The impact of menopause and social factors on health. In Hammond, C., Hazeltine, F., and Schiff, I. (Eds.), *Menopause: Evaluation, Treatment and Health Concerns*, pp. 137–161, New York: Alan Liss.

The authors found that women experience more personal changes or major life events during midlife than at any other point in their lives, and the assumption has been that they are negative rather than positive. The authors studied 2,300 women randomly sampled from the general population and who were approaching menopause at the beginning of the study. During 4.5 years of follow-up, 55 percent experienced transition to natural or surgical post-menopause. Telephone interviews were conducted every 9 months, seeking answers to the questions: (1) To what extent are changes in physical and mental health associated with the occurrence of menopause? (2) To what extent do other social roles affect health, independently of menopause? (3) How do women's feelings toward menopause change as they approach and experience the event? Five measures of health status were considered: self-assessed general health, number of days of restricted activity, physical symptoms, psychological symptoms, and new chronic conditions. Current health status was explained best by a model including prior health status. Small contributions were made by education, employment, and marital status. Having a recent surgical menopause was the only variable related to change in menstrual status that contributed to the variance in health status, and then only to variation in days of restricted activity. Likewise, the Center for Epidemiological Studies-Depression (CES-D) depression score was also related to surgical menopause in the prior 3 months, with women recently experiencing surgical menopause having twice the rate of depression as other women (CES-D scores > 16). When women with surgical menopause are excluded from the analyses, poor health status, lay consultation, and use of tranquilizing medications are associated with high rates of depression, independent of menstrual status. Worry caused by a member of the immediate family also is associated with a further increase in the rates of depression. When women's roles were related to measures of health, the role of current employment reduced the impact of other roles and accompanying stress on health and utilization of medical services. For self-assessed health, education and work had positive health effects, but husbands had negative health effects. Likewise, husbands had negative effects and employment positive effects on activity restrictions and CES-D scores. In addition, education had protective effects but caregiving to a parent had deleterious effects on CES-D scores. Finally, employment reduced tranquilizer use, but parenting children increased it. The combination of women's roles and associated demands and supports had important health effects. Overall, most women reported a more positive or neutral attitude as they experienced menopause.

Mitchell, V., & Helson, R. (1990). Women's prime of life: Is it the 50s? *Psychology of Women Quarterly, 14*(1990), 451–470.

The investigators tested the hypothesis that the early 50s is women's prime of life, a time of good health combined with autonomy and relational security. Using responses from a sample of 700 college graduates studied in 1983, they found that women in their early 50s most described their lives as very satisfying. Using data from a longitudinal sample from the same college in 1989, they found women in their early 50s rated their quality of life as high. The conditions distinguishing the early 50s from earlier and later periods of the middle years included more "empty nests," better health, higher income and more concern for parents. The first three of these factors accounted for quality of life in the early 50s women. The investigators offer prime of life as a useful concept in women's adult development.

Nathanson, C., & Lorenz, G. (1982). Women and health: The social dimensions of biomedical data. In Giele, J. (Ed.), *Women in the middle years: Current knowledge for research and policy,* pp. 37–87, New York: Wiley.

The authors review mortality, illness, illness behavior and the use of health services by midlife women. They conclude that current mortality rates indicate women in midlife are relatively healthy and can look forward to many additional years of life. At the same time, midlife women use health services at relatively high rates. Women appear more sensitive to symptoms of illness and more active in their orientation toward the detection and treatment of disease than are men. The authors also investigated the influence of biological and social roles on women's health, including the relatively invariant dimension of women's roles such as those influenced by genes and the hormonal cycle. The consequences of these are very difficult to evaluate since biological processes are defined and managed within the context of American society and values, and thus subject to medicalization. The influence of variant aspects of women's roles on their health are also difficult to evaluate. Women's various combination of roles affect their opportunities for social integration, exposure to changing sex role norms, and occupational exposures to toxic substances. Moreover, women's health can be evaluated only with an understanding of the structural arrangements developed in American society for managing women's reproductive cycles and health problems.

Nolan, J. (1986). Developmental concerns and the health of midlife women. *Nursing Clinics of North America, 21*(1), 151–159.

The author focuses on two factors that have been implicated in midlife women's experience of physical and/or psychological symptoms: menopause and environmental stressors. She sorts out the symptoms most predictably related to menopause, hot flashes and night sweats, from others that have been mistakenly attributed to menopause. In addition, she examines the environmental stressors, including changes in the familial environment and work. She proposes an integrative approach to understanding and caring for the health of midlife women.

Notman, M. (1984). Reflections and perspectives on therapeutic issues for today's adult women. In Baruch and Brooks-Gunn, (Eds.), *Women in midlife*, pp. 359–370, New York: Plenum.

Notman reminds us that in confronting the finiteness of life as one comes to perceive it in midlife, one makes assessments of where one is and where one might like to be. She believes that women in therapy address questions as to how far-reaching changes in opportunities for women have been, and that social limitations may have circumscribed women's possibilities. Confusion about the chronology of life's components, such as career and childbearing, and the challenge to integrate competing roles occurs in a context of generational discontinuity. Concepts of femininity may create confusion, partly because femininity is defined differently for different women and along multiple dimensions, such as childbearing, behavioral characteristics, or the type of job a woman chooses. Affirmation in the context of relationships can help women in restructuring their relationships and adapting, not only in leaving relationships. Similarly, such assistance may help in sorting out attitudes of others from one's own feelings. Mothers may play an increasingly positive role in the lives, accomplishments, and well being of their daughters. Therapists must pay attention to patterns of needs, fulfillments, and relationships that occur in women's lives in a context of new life patterns, solutions, and options. This orientation may help therapists strengthen women's self-esteem without relying on outmoded definitions of "femininity."

Owens, J., Matthews, K., Wing, R., & Kuller, L. (1992). Can physical activity mitigate the effects of aging in middle-aged women? *Circulation*, 85(4), 1265–1270.

Participants in the Healthy Women Study were evaluated at study entry and 3 years later. Weekly physical activity level was assessed with the Paffenbarger Physical Activity Questionnaire. During the 3-year period, women increased significantly in weight, blood pressure, levels of total and low density lipoprotein cholesterol, triglycerides, and insulin and decreased significantly in levels of total high density lipoprotein cholesterol. Women who reported higher levels of activity at baseline had less weight gain over time. Women who increased their activity during the 3-year period had the smallest increases in weight and the smallest decreases in total HDL levels. Changes in lipids were independent of changes in body weight.

Parlee, M. (1984). Reproductive issues, including menopause. In Baruch and Brooks-Gunn, (Eds.), *Women in midlife*, pp. 303–314, New York: Plenum.

Parlee presents a critique of research on midlife women, emphasizing that everyday thought and language tend to impute a causal role to female reproductive biology at major transition points in the social life cycle. She points out that menopause may be the stimulus for applying a social label or stigma that triggers social interactions that will produce negative consequences for women. In addition, menopause may be psychologically significant as one marker for cessation of fertility, an event that has different meanings for different women. These two areas of research may help us learn more about the genuine psychological significance of menopause and of midlife than have earlier approaches.

Riley, M. (1985). Women, men and the lengthening life course. In A. Rossi (Ed.), *Gender and the life course*, pp. 333–347, New York: Aldine.

The author points out that the impact of unprecedented increase in longevity has altered the social structure by increasing structural complexity and the options open to individuals as they age, and has altered the aging process by prolonging the opportunity for accumulation of social, psychological, and biological experiences as lives lengthen. Family life has changed with the dramatic prolongation of the linkages between family members: because women live longer, midlife women may know their daughters for as much as two or three times the length of their childhood. Because of the prolongation of roles, there is also the possibility of varied role sequences and complexes of roles for simultaneous occupancy. Although biological aging, the accumulation of wear and tear on biological systems, probably progresses in a relatively immutable way, physiological functioning may improve due to changing risk behaviors. In addition, psychological functioning may improve in response to social stimulation. Taken together, longevity will bring new needs for health care, much of which will be led by women who will invent new forms of care. In addition, longevity will bring new flexibility in phasing over the life course of education, work, and leisure. Longevity will give women a new capacity for self-hood, through greater independence, personal mastery, and assurance.

Rosenthal, C., Matthews, S., & Marshall, V. (1989). Is parent care normative? The experiences of a sample of middle-aged women. *Research on Aging, 11,* 244–260.

Current literature on parent care asserts that modern women at some time in their lives may expect to be sandwiched between responsibilities to old parents and their other commitments. The authors studied a random sample of 163 women between 40 and 69 years of age to determine their commitments. They found that considering the multiple commitments of children in the household, husbands present, and employment, women younger than 55 are most likely to be affected by competing commitments. Although these women are most likely to have living parents, many of their parents are younger and relatively healthy. Older respondents are less likely to have living parents, but when they do, their parents are less healthy that those of younger women. The risk to midlife women of actually providing extensive parent care was estimated as less than that projected by current studies based on caregivers.

Rossi, A. (1980). Life span theories and women's lives. *Signs, 6,* 4–32.

The author begins with an exploration of major issues in developmental research, considering lifespan theories of development and their limitations, including cohort particularity and neglect of physiological factors. She presents results of her studies of women aged 33-to-56 years to illustrate women's development. Women were asked about the meanings of age and aging in several ways. None wanted to be older than they were, but half wanted to be under 30. Most expressed a desire to live to be at least 75 years. Those who wanted to be younger than they were and those who had very short longevity preferences were those with very high levels of stress in their current lives, having marital tension, difficulty with children, large family size, economic strain, or sharp increases in symptoms of aging. Family size and work both influenced women's well being. Looking ahead as women baby-boomers enter midlife requires that we consider areas of stability between age cohorts as well as areas of difference. As more women become co-earners, the increasing stability of their worklives will influence their experiences of aging. Moreover, as family size decreases in future generations, the influence of large family responsibilities for future generations of women can be mitigated.

Rubin, L. (1979). Women of a certain age. New York: Harper.

Rubin examined the issues and milestones in midlife identified in interviews with 160 women between 35 and 54 years. She found that women were not devastated by the "empty nest," the time when their children left home. Instead, she found that the elusive self was central to midlife women. Indeed, some women described themselves as having two selves, one for home and the social world she lived in and one for work. The two selves represented the difficulty of integrating the self emphasizing achievement with the self emphasizing emotional, intuitive functions central to human relations. Rubin asked women if they could briefly describe themselves in some way that would give her a good sense of who and what they were. Nearly 25 percent could not answer the question. In addition to describing themselves as physical entities, some women used words such as "warm, sensitive, kind, outgoing, considerate, caring, concerned, and responsible." In addition, most mentioned that they were wives and mothers. Although half of the women held paid jobs outside their homes, not one described herself in relation to her work. Many were surprised when this was pointed out to them. A fundamental theme found in these women's identities was the distinction they experienced between being (internal, identity) and doing (external, work). In short, their work was what they did, and not what they were.

Ryff, C. (1985). The subjective experience of lifespan transitions. In A. Rossi (Ed.), *Gender and the life course*, pp. 97–113, New York: Aldine.

The author explored the "inner" side of lifespan development, examining whether life stage models and sex differences are valid when considered in light of people's descriptions of their own development. Results of several studies which the author conducted to examine self-perceived change in the domain of values show that midlife women had a comparatively higher preference for instrumental values (for ambition, capability, courage, etc.) in the present, but anticipated a decline in this preference as they aged. In a later study, women in early adulthood and middle age (40-to-55) rated intimacy as being more salient in their self-assessments during young adulthood than during middle age. Middle aged women rated themselves higher in generativity than they would have at earlier ages. Comparing age cohorts and genders, the investigator also found that adults do have a subjective sense of changes in themselves with age, such that sex differences are less important in factors directly related to developmental scales, e.g. generativity. On the other hand, sex differences appeared in terms of perceived value changes and on certain personality dimensions. The author recommends that future work focus on both subjectively experienced developmental change with studies of actual events or critical experiences in people's

lives to more fully illuminate the processes by which one affects the other.

Saab, P., Matthews, K., Stoney, C., & McDonald, R. (1990). Premenopausal and postmenopausal women differ in their cardiovascular and neuroendocrine responses to behavioral stress. *Psychophysiology, 26*, 270–279.

Midlife women (45-to-51 years of age) performed tasks while their heart rate, blood pressure and plasma catecholamines were measured. Tasks included serial subtraction, mirror image tracing, speech, and postural tilt. The speech task was judged relevant to women due to emphasis on social skills. Fifteen premenopausal women and sixteen postmenopausal women were tested. Postmenopausal women had greater increases from baseline in heart rate during all tasks, with a pronounced increase in the speech task. Postmenopausal women exhibited greater increases from baseline in systolic blood pressure and epinephrine relative to premenopausal women only during the speech task.

Schindler, B. (1987). The psychiatric disorders of midlife. *Medical Clinics of North America, 71*(1), 71–85.

Midlife is a time for significant psychologic growth and development. Careful scrutiny of the notion that women's psychologic health and physical health are closely tied to reproductive function reveals that attributions of symptoms to the "menopausal syndrome" are inappropriate. The author advocates consideration that the menopause is only one factor along with biologic, psychologic, and sociocultural stressors, that increase the individual woman's vulnerability to several psychiatric disorders. She recommends careful attention to a woman's presenting symptoms and specific diagnostic criteria for psychiatric illness to promote accurate diagnosis and treatment of midlife women.

Shaver, J., Giblin, E., & Paulsen, V. (1991). Sleep quality subtypes in midlife women. *Sleep, 14*(1), 18–23.

Midlife women 40 to 59 years of age (82) were classified as poor or good sleepers according to both their self-reported sleep quality and polysomnographic sleep recordings. Self-reported good and poor sleepers did not differ on any of the somnographic variables, but self-reported poor sleepers demonstrated more distress as measured by the Symptom Check List-90 (SCL-90) scales. Using only sleep efficiency criteria from somnographic recordings, good and poor sleepers did not differ on psychological distress. Those who had poor somnographic recordings and were self-reported poor sleepers reported the most severe menopausal symptoms.

Spurlock, J. (1984). Black women in the middle years. In Baruch and Brooks-Gunn, (Eds.), *Women in midlife*, pp. 245–260, New York: Plenum.

The author emphasizes the diversity of black women in the middle years, pointing out that the double jeopardy of race and gender often accounts for differences when black women and white women are compared. What black women bring to midlife is a function of their earlier life experiences and how they have dealt with life. Most are part of a family unit, even if they live alone and their family members are adoptive kin. Relationships with men are varied. Black women's economic status, their involvement versus nonparticipation in the women's movement, and their approaches to coping and adaptation have significant effects on their midlife experiences and well being.

Stueve, A., & O'Donnell, L. (1984). The daughter of aging parents. In Baruch and Brooks-Gunn, (Eds.), *Women in midlife*, pp. 203–226, New York: Plenum.

The authors studied adult daughters, including 81 working women 30-to-60 years of age who had one living parent more than 70 years of age. They found that not all daughters were at the same point in their own lives. Variation among family timing patterns shaped how the daughters dealt with issues and considerations of their aging parents, for example, some framed their parent's death as their own loss versus being inevitable.

Parents' needs depended on health and life circumstances. Most instrumental support was provided by working class daughters who assumed interdependence and the necessity of helping out. Middle class, college-educated daughters had tighter boundaries around their nuclear families, and were less likely to integrate their aging parents. Middle class children were more likely to buy care from others outside the family. Daughters were more likely than sons to provide care to their parents. The authors conclude that the "caught in the middle" label assigned to midlife women is inaccurate for all women. Although employment, per se, made little difference in caregiving, features of employment, such as freedom to negotiate schedules and the number of hours worked, did affect caregiving to parents. The authors point out the need to consider the birth cohort of midlife women when considering the effects of employment on caregiving patterns to elderly relatives: employment has different meanings for different birth cohorts. In addition, those concerned about midlife women's health would consider women's involvements with other elderly kin, not just their parents, but also their in-laws. Whether women with elderly kin feel caught in the middle, and feel the competing demands of their roles can only be determined by exploring each woman's situations. Finally, consideration needs to be given to caregiving for the midlife women who are currently providing care to their elderly relatives.

Udry, J. R., & Morris, N. M. (1978). Relative contribution of male and female age to the frequency of marital intercourse. Published by the Society for the Study of Social Biology, 25(2), pp. 128–134, Madison, Wisconsin.

Discussion of age- and sex-factors in marriage in the United States.

Uphold, C., & Sussman, E. (1981). Self-reported climacteric symptoms as a function of the relationships between marital adjustment and childrearing stage. *Nursing Research, 30*, 84–88.

The authors examined the influence of role and childrearing, marital, recreational, and work role integration in 185 healthy midlife women. The number and severity of symptoms commonly attributed to the climacteric, such as depression, were related to women's participation in roles such that women involved in more roles complained of fewer symptoms. Women who participated in recreation and had good marital adjustment were less likely to have symptoms. Childrearing and work roles were unrelated to symptoms.

Whiting, B. (1984). Problems of American middle-class women in their middle years: A comparative approach. In Baruch and Brooks-Gunn (Eds.), *Women in midlife*, pp. 261–274, New York: Plenum.

The author explores five fundamental needs of human beings, including (1) the desire to reproduce oneself, (2) the need for physical contact from infancy onward to reduce anxiety and fear and provide comfort, (3) need for social, cognitive, and sexual stimulation, (4) need for support from other human beings responsive to one's overtures, and (5) need to predict events in the physical and social world. In her discussion of midlife women's situations, Whiting points out that changing family patterns have led some midlife women to opt out of parenting. In addition, the need for physical contact among aging persons is not commonly met except in sexual arrangements. The need for effectance (the interest in and effort toward acting upon the environment for change) is also not well met for midlife women, particularly those whose work is limited to the inside of the household. Need for support may also become a problem as women have less exposure to learning social skills through their mothers. Finally, the need to predict the behavior of the physical and social world may cause us to blame ourselves for our failures. Two predominant lifestyles for contemporary midlife women are (1) adjusting to the middle years by accepting their roles as wives, mothers of teenagers and grown children and grandmothers of their children and (2) women who have already embarked on careers, have never given them up during their child-rearing years, or are attempting to return to careers or initiate new

ones. Whiting discusses the consequences of these lifestyles for meeting basic human needs.

Wilbur, J., & Dan, A. (1989). The impact of work patterns on psychological well being of midlife nurses. *Western Journal of Nursing Research, 6,* 703–716.

Midlife nursing alumni were studied about their work patterns, presence of children at home, menopausal status, and well being and physical symptoms. Perimenopausal women who had interrupted and unstable work patterns had the lowest scores on the Bradburn positive affect scale. Not surprisingly, women with multiple roles reported the most fatigue.

Wing, R., Matthews, K., Kuller, L., Meilahn, E., & Plantinga, P. (1991). Weight gain at the time of menopause. *Archives of Internal Medicine, 151,* 97–102.

Participants in the Healthy Women Study gained an average of 2.25 kg over 3 years of follow up. Twenty percent gained 4.5 kg or more. Only 3 percent lost 4.5 kg or more. Menopausal status did not differentiate women who gained weight. Weight gain was associated with increases in blood pressure and levels of total cholesterol, low density lipoprotein cholesterol, triglycerides, and fasting insulin.

Wood, V., Traupmann, B., & Hay, J. (1984). Motherhood in the middle years: Women and their adult children. In Baruch and Brooks-Gunn, (Eds.), *Women in Midlife*, pp. 227–244, New York: Plenum.

Although research focusing on the mother-child relationship has emphasized the early years, these authors consider dependency and equity as two important dimensions of mother-child relationships for midlife and older women. Dependency refers to situations in which one member of a dyad receives more from the other than she gives in return. Dependency becomes salient when the child is an adolescent and striving for it, and again when the mother is old and attempting to maintain her independence.

During the mother's middle years, both the mother's and child's autonomy seems unthreatened, with both capable of reciprocating care and assistance. Equity, a fair balance between giving and receiving, was explored in a study of 187 mothers aged 50-to-93. Respondents were asked how they thought things stacked up for themselves and their children, including whether the children got a much better deal or whether they got a much better deal than their children. In addition, they were asked to consider what they had done for their parents, and how things had stacked up for them and their parents. The respondents were then classified according to whether they: felt their children got a better deal, felt the deal was equitable, or felt they got a better deal than their children.

Nearly two-thirds of the women felt they had an equitable relationship with their children and with their parents. Most of those who perceived their relationships were inequitable believed their children got a better deal than they. Those who were overbenefited as children tended to repeat that pattern with their own children, but those who were underbenefited reported undoing that pattern with their own children. In addition, women were asked about the division of their responsibility for their aging parents. Those who were underbenefited as children were more likely to be caring for their parents than those who were overbenefited. The happiest and least stressful relationships were the equitable relationships, followed by the overbenefited and the underbenefited relationships.

Chapter 7

Women and Weight Control

Amy Olson

INTRODUCTION

L osing weight for women, is not a simple process, in fact, it's surprisingly difficult. To determine how serious the problem of obesity is for women four factors must be considered: (1) the number of people who are obese; (2) the number of people dieting; (3) the amount of money we spend to treat obesity related problems; and (4) the amount of money spent on obesity research.

One-third of all Americans are overweight; 57 percent of adolescents age 13–17 are overweight, and 22 percent of children under age 12 are overweight. Currently, there are approximately 34 million adults ages 20–74 in the United States affected by obesity. Forty percent of all US women and 25 percent of men are currently trying to lose weight and 20 percent of the population is estimated to be currently enrolled in a weight loss program (Berg, 1993). In 1992, we spent $39.3 billion on obesity related health problems. More money was spent on the complications of obesity than for diabetes and stroke combined (ADA report, 1992; Colditz, 1992). Another $35 billion per year was spent on quick weight reduction methods. This adds up to more than $74 billion spent annually treating obesity. In sharp contrast, only $35 million has been spent on obesity research and there is only one Obesity Research Center (Bray, 1992a). Obesity appears to be a significant problem that is not taken seriously.

DEFINITIONS OF OBESITY

Obesity is an excess of body fat. For a woman, when her body fat exceeds 30 percent of her weight she is considered obese (Griffen, 1992). However, measurement of body composition requires sophisticated techniques and equipment, and in the obese population, accurate determinations are very difficult. Consequently, most studies estimate obesity using a weight-for-height measurement (Bray, 1992a). Typically the most accepted definition of obesity is a body weight (as opposed to fat) which is 20 percent or more above one's ideal body weight (we assume the excess weight is fat and not muscle mass). The standard for ideal or desirable body weight is estimated by: (1) the Metropolitan Life Insurance Height and Weight Table, or (2) for women using the equation: 100 pounds for 5', plus 5 pounds for every additional inch of height. Therefore, if a woman is 5' 4" tall, medium frame and weighs more than 144 pounds (her ideal weight calculated as 120 pounds) she would be classified as obese. Surprised? A potential problem with ideal weights is while they can be adjusted for frame size, neither standard estimates body composition or the distribution of body fat, both of which affect risk and influence interpretations of data. The effects of body composition and fat distribution will be addressed in a later section.

Body mass index (BMI) is perhaps the most consistently used descriptor in research literature to determine degrees of obesity. BMI is calculated by dividing the body weight in kg by the height in meters squared. This is a simple method and correlates well with other measures of fatness such as skinfold thickness. However, BMI is not a precise measurement and cannot estimate the percent body fat of an individual or distinguish between adiposity, muscularity, and/or edema. Consequently an individual with an unusually large muscle mass or an individual who is short may be misclassified; additionally, the association between BMI and obesity may not be the same for all ages, particularly in the young (Kissebah, Freedman, Peiris, 1989).

The most appropriate use of BMI is to classify individuals into mild, morbid or superobese groups, or estimate the incidence of obesity in large populations. This categorization is essential since obese individuals experience different health risks and responses to therapy which are influenced by their original body weight (Brolin,1992). In fact, decisions regarding the appropriate choice of treatment are determined to a great extent upon the individual's degree of obesity (Bray, 1992a).

Unfortunately, there are many different definitions for obesity and different definitions of success in terms of weight loss in the medical literature which contributes to the confusion. Determining a classification system to describe the obese population has been the subject of considerable discussion. The two major points of emphasis are to avoid language or descriptors for the obese population which are pejorative and to develop universal definitions so the results of research can be accurately compared (Kuczmarski, 1992; Bray, 1992a).

Table 1 (below) is provided to allow comparisons between BMI and body weight and percent of ideal body weights. The table represents one classification system; there are other classification models in the literature, for

Table 1. Descriptions of Obesity

Definition— Woman 5'4"	BMI	Weight kg (pounds)	Percent of Ideal Body Weight
Ideal weight	20–24	55–65 kg (120–143 pounds)	< 120%
Mild obesity	25–32	66–87 kg (144–191 pounds)	120–159%
Morbidly obese	33–46	88–123 kg (192–269 pounds)	160–225%
Super obesity	> 46	> 124 kg (> 270)	> 225%

Source: Adapted from Mason, E. E., Renquist, K. E., & Jiang, D. (1992). Perioperative risks and safety of surgery for severe obesity. *American Journal of Clinical Nutrition, 55*, 573S–576S.

Table 2. Classification System (Bray)

Class	BMI	Risk
0	20–24.9	Very Low
I	25–29.9	Low
II	30–34.9	Moderate
III	35–39.9	High
IV	> 40	Very High

Source: (Bray, 1992a).

example Bray (1992a) divides obesity into four categories distinct from normal body weight (see Table 2). Data reported in this chapter will reflect the different classifications used by the various authors.

GENDER DIFFERENCES

Women between the ages of 18–49, with higher than average incomes, represent the largest consumer group of weight loss products and programs (Berg, 1993). Women seek treatment for their obesity 4–5 times more often than men. Furthermore 85 percent of patients having surgical procedures to treat obesity are female and when men do seek treatment, they are on the average 20 percent heavier than the women seeking treatment (Grace, 1992; Mason, Renquist, & Jiang, 1992).

As depicted in Table 3: (1) nearly equal percentages of men and women with BMI < 27; (2) more men than women are mildly obese (BMI 27–30); and (3) more women are found in BMI categories > 30, 16.8 percent for women relative to 12.2 percent for men. When the races are separated, a

Table 3. Comparison of Weight in United States Men and Women by Body Mass

BMI*	Males Percent	Females Percent
BMI < 27	69.9	71.0
BMI > 27–30	18.0	12.2
BMI > 30–35 (13 million)	9.8	10.3
BMI > 35–40 (4 million)	1.9	4.3
BMI > 40–45 (1 million)	0.35	1.4
BMI > 45 (558,000)	0.1	0.8

* BMI—Body Mass Index is calculated by weight in kg divided by height in meters squared.
Source: (Kuczmarski, 1992).

different pattern emerges. Equal percentages of white women and men fall within the mild obesity category (BMI 27–32); however, slightly more white women (9.6%) than men (7.8%) are in the morbidly obese category (BMI > 32). Among blacks, there are nearly twice as many black women as black men in both the mild and morbidly obese categories. Significantly more women than men are in the mild and morbidly obese categories for Mexicans and Puerto Ricans, and slightly more Cuban women than Cuban men were mildly obese (Kuczmarski, 1992).

RISK FACTORS

There are serious health risks associated with obesity for those individuals who demonstrate a BMI > 30. The risks are dependent upon the duration of obesity (years individual has been obese) and its progression, (whether the individual is actively gaining weight or is weight stable). Weight gain creates a greater risk for cardiovascular disease than unchanging obesity. Gender is also an important risk factor; women demonstrate less risk than men at the same level of obesity. For example, a woman must be 20 kg heavier to acquire the same health risk as a man (Bray, 1989).

It is not possible to predict the exact point where serious health risks associated with excess weight begins. The relationship between body weight and relative risk does not follow a straight line, but rather demonstrates a J-curve pattern. The curve begins to sharpen at a BMI of 30; with BMI 30–35 demonstrating moderate risk, BMI of 35–40, high risk, and BMI > 40 very high risk of mortality associated with obesity (Bray, 1992a).

Most of the large epidemiological studies of body weight have not provided data for women > 40 percent above ideal weight. Subjects studied are predominately male, white, middle-income, and middle-aged and yet the population undergoing obesity surgeries is predominately female and lower-income (Brolin,1992). The limited data that is available for women reveals some trends.

When research data on women is separated by age groups, the greatest risk appears to be for younger women with the risk decreasing for older age groups at the same percentage of ideal body weight. The relative risks of excess weight are very different when separated by disease. (See Table 4.)

Predicting risk would seem to be a simple process; however, conflicting reports in the literature complicate interpretations. In some studies the presence of other risk factors were not considered. For example:

1. In one study, 80 percent of underweight persons smoked, whereas only 55 percent of those at > 140% IBW, smoked.
2. Underweight individuals may have an existing disease contributing to their lower body weight which might explain a lack of health benefits associated with lower body weights in some studies.

3. Obesity may be a coexisting symptom for some health problems but the direct cause of increased risk may be physical inactivity or excessive dietary intake of saturated fat.

4. A long follow-up period (15–20 years) is required to observe some risks of obesity; studies failing to collect long-term data may miss critical connections.

5. The timing of obesity appears more important than the actual degree of overweight. Excess weight gained in adulthood is localized in the trunk and demonstrates a greater health risk of cardiovascular disease than carrying the excess weight since childhood. Often this type of detail (onset of obesity) is not collected in many studies.

6. Misclassification of subjects has created confusion. Many studies categorize their populations using BMI exclusively, which fails to consider body composition and distribution of body fat. This is particularly a problem when young muscular individuals are studied.

(Kissebah et al.,1989; Sjostrom, 1992a; Sjostrom, 1992b).

Body fat distribution is a particularly important variable when determining the risk associated with excess weight. Women typically deposit a greater proportion of body fat in their hips, buttocks and upper thighs (pear shape). This is referred to as a gynoid pattern of fat distribution, while males deposit more excess fat in the torso and upper abdomen, the android pattern (apple shape) (Markman, 1987). This distribution is easily determined by measuring the ratio of the waist (at the narrowest point) to the hip (at the widest point). When the waist-hip ratio is greater than 0.8 for women or 1.0 for men there is an associated increased risk of hypertension, diabetes mellitus, and atherosclerotic cardiovascular disease (Seidell, Deurenberg, & Hautvast, 1987).

Why is there increased risk with larger waist-hip ratios? Fat cells from different areas of the body demonstrate different characteristics and within one body area, subcutaneous fat is different from deep fat. The following excerpt demonstrates the difference between abdominal fat cells compared to peripheral fat cells as well as the tendency for accumulation of fat in the abdominal area in later life.

Table 4. Risk in Women by Weight and Disease

Disease in Women	120% IBW	140% IBW
Diabetes	3.3	8.0
Coronary heart disease	1.4	2.0
Cancer—overall	1.2	1.6
Digestive diseases	1.6	2.3

* IBW—Ideal Body Weight.
Source: (Berg, 1993; Kissebah, 1989).

A slim young girl severely burned her hand and received a full thickness skin graft from her abdominal wall to her hand. As an adult she gained an excessive amount of weight which accumulated around her waist. The graft on her hand also became obese, developing a grotesque boxing glove appearance. Even though the tissue was removed from the abdominal region, the metabolic characteristics of those cells persisted. The ability of abdominal cells to selectively store fat relative to peripheral fat cells is clearly evident (Seidell, Deurenberg, & Hautvast, 1987).

Fat cells from the waist and abdominal area are more active metabolically and more responsive to nutritional or hormonal factors than those cells from the thigh and buttocks (Markman, 1987). Similarly, intra-abdominal or omental fat cells are more responsive to the lipolytic (fat mobilizing) effects of epinephrine and norepinephrine and less responsive to the antilipolytic effect of insulin than subcutaneous fat cells. In response to epinephrine (hormonal stress) large amounts of free fatty acids (FFAs) are released from the deep intra-abdominal fat cells into the portal vein which directly supplies the liver. The liver converts these FFAs into triglycerides and very low density lipoproteins (VLDLs). The high influx of FFAs inhibits the liver's uptake and degradation of insulin resulting in hyperinsulinemia. This leads to insulin resistance and glucose intolerance which together with the elevated serum lipids increases the risk of diabetes, atherosclerosis and hypertension (Seidell, Deurenberg, & Hautvast, 1987). When subcutaneous stores are stimulated, the FFAs are released into the general systemic circulation rather than the portal system. The FFAs are diluted and taken up by tissues other than the liver; consequently, the biochemical effect is greatly reduced. The bottom line: the more fat stored intra-abdominally, the greater the potential risks.

Women with the gynoid pattern of fat distribution and a waist-hip ratio of 0.7 or less do not demonstrate increased risk in spite of excess fat. Additionally, women store more of their fat subcutaneously, while men store more fat intra-abdominally; therefore, women experience less risk. Even with matching body weights, males have higher serum triglycerides (VLDLs), blood glucose and insulin levels and blood pressure than women, and when women do have metabolic complications, they typically have an increased waist circumference (a more android pattern), and a relatively large amount of intra-abdominal fat (Markman, 1987; Staff, 1985a).

On the other hand, fat from the gluteal region (femoral fat), hips and thighs, is more difficult to mobilize. Additionally, women with the gynoid pattern have a significantly lower resting metabolic rate (RMR) than those with an android pattern. Individuals with a lower RMR are calorically more efficient and will have a greater tendency to gain weight and more difficulty trying to lose weight (Westrate, Dekker, Stoel, Begheijn, Deurenberg, Hautvast, 1990). Many women already know this fact; they have observed that even with successful weight loss, inches seem to come off more readily from their waist with much smaller changes occurring through their hips and thighs. This unique effect of gynoid fat is mediated by both hormonal and enzymatic differences. Fat cells from the hips and thighs demonstrate higher levels of lipoprotein lipase, an enzyme which facilitates fat storage. In the nonpregnant woman fat is preferentially stored; post-partum, the hormone pattern changes allowing mobilization which suggests a biological mechanism to ensure adequate energy to support lactation (Markman, 1987; Seidell, Deurenberg, & Hautvast, 1987; Kissebah, et al., 1989). Also, chronic dieters, women who repeatedly lose and regain weight, increase their waist to hip ratio, i.e., shift their distribution of fat to more abdominal fat and women who gain weight rapidly or later in life gain more in the abdominal region (Berg, 1993).

The significance of this finding for women is that it is literally safer for moderately overweight women with a gynoid pattern to stay obese. These women will have difficulty effectively reducing their body weight and if they become chronic dieters repeatedly losing and regaining weight they will greatly increase their health risks (Markman, 1987; Staff, 1985b).

In addition to the consequences affecting health, the obese must deal with losses in normal body functions: shortness of breath, disordered sleep, pathological hunger, sexual impairment, excessive perspiration, urinary incontinence in women, inability to cleanse oneself, and limited mobility (Kral, 1992). Simple pleasures such as sitting in a seat at a theater to watch a movie, taking a bus downtown to a museum, shopping for and finding clothes that fit, being able to sit at a picnic and get up unassisted, are denied the obese. Quality of life can be drastically affected. For example in one study, a woman whose bathroom was on the second floor of her home, was unable to go up the stairs for two years due to her obesity (Olson, 1974).

The health risks and physical losses are truly significant, and yet, the obese population perceives the discrimination and prejudice against them as their heaviest burden. Discrimination against the obese occurs on both social and economic levels and is more severe for obese women than obese men. The employment barriers and costs in terms of reduced earnings associated with obesity are significant. It's been estimated that each pound of fat costs executives $1000/year in reduced income. Employers are reluctant to hire the obese; 44 percent of employers would not hire obese women except under special circumstances and another 16 percent of employers would not hire obese women under any circumstances. Sixty percent of employers would not choose an obese woman as an employee given any other choice.

Social discrimination is also evident; obese women are twice as likely to move down in social class when they marry as non-obese women. Prejudice begins at an early age. Studies have demonstrated that even six-year-olds describe pictures of obese children as "lazy, dirty, stupid, ugly, cheats, and liars," and rate obese children as "least likable" when compared to children with severe disabilities such as facial disfigurement or missing hands. Ironically, this same prejudice is demonstrated by the obese themselves (i.e., the obese are highly critical of other obese individuals) and regrettably, also by the medical profession. The obese frequently have negative experiences with the medical profession. Nearly 80 percent reported that they are "always" or "usually" treated with disrespect by the medical profession because of their weight. This perception is apparently accurate; surveys of physicians have described their obese patients as "weak-willed, ugly, and awkward" (Stunkard, Stinnett, Smoller, 1992).

An alarming observation is that 62 percent of the women trying to lose weight, are not overweight according to their self-reported heights and weights. For teenagers, dieting seems to be a way of life and even girls as young as nine-years-old demonstrate negative attitudes about their body size and potentially dangerous weight loss practices (Berg, 1993). The desire to diet and lose weight obviously extends beyond the concern for the health risks and is an unhealthy reflection of our society.

METABOLISM OF WEIGHT LOSS

Why is losing weight so difficult for women? In theory, losing weight seems simple; decrease the number of calories consumed, and/or increase the number of calories burned by activity, and lose weight. The caloric equivalent of one pound of adipose (fat) tissue is 3500 calories; therefore, if we decrease the calories consumed for a week by 3500 calories, or increase our activity by the equivalent of 3500 calories, we should lose one pound of fat. If weight is stable, the calories consumed equals the calories burned.

The reality of losing weight is not simple. To understand why weight loss is not merely balancing "calories in and calories out," we must recognize that many of the assumptions being made with this simple logic are incorrect.

First, we assume that all the weight lost is fat. Actually, the composition of the tissue lost is water, protein (from lean tissue), and glucose, in addition to fat. The rate (i.e., how fast the weight is being lost), and the duration of dieting (i.e., length of time weight is being lost) will affect the actual composition of the tissue lost. The faster we lose weight, the greater the percentage of protein (lean tissue) lost. In order to lose mostly fat stores (and not protein), we must lose weight slowly for a minimum period of three–four weeks. Shorter durations of weight loss result in mostly water, protein, and glucose being lost.

Second, we assume that the resting metabolic rate (RMR) does not change with dieting. However, when we fast or consume a very low calorie intake, our resting metabolic rate drops rapidly within days. The decrease in RMR observed in dieting women ranges from 10–30 percent, with the greatest effects observed in obese women who are chronic dieters. Since RMR represents the largest component of our energy expenditure, decreases can have a sizable impact on the rate of weight loss.

Third, we assume that physical activity does not change during the period of dieting. This assumption is inaccurate. Careful observations and videotapes made of individuals during periods of caloric restriction reveal subtle but significant decreases in activity. Individuals become more efficient with motion and decrease their expenditure of calories without being consciously aware of the change, i.e., they may report the same level of activity as during non-dieting periods. Additionally, as the individual loses weight, the energy required for a given activity decreases; consequently, even if the hours of exercise are kept constant, as their body weight decreases they burn less calories. The energy expenditure of physical activity has been reported to be 25 percent less during dieting periods when compared to pre-diet expenditures. Clearly, the caloric cost of activity during dieting does not continue at pre-diet levels.

Fourth, we assume the thermic effect of food does not change. The thermic effect of food is the energy required to process and assimilate nutrients. On the average, about 10 percent of our caloric intake is used to process our food to convert nutrients to a usable form. For 2000 calories the cost of processing food is approximately 200 calories. If, however, the caloric intake is 400 calories per day, the cost to process now drops to approximately 40 calories (deBoer, van Es, Rovers, van Raaij, Hautvast, 1986).

If we try to correct for these assumptions in our original equation, we can obtain a more accurate understanding of the process of weight loss. For example, if a woman whose weight is stable and typically consumes 2400 calories/day, then decreases her intake to 420 calories/day for 16 weeks, a weight loss of approximately 64 pounds would be expected. [This change in intake represents nearly 2000 calories/day deficit or 14,000 calories/week deficit. Each 3500 calorie deficit is the caloric equivalent of one pound of adipose tissue. Therefore, 14,000 caloric deficit per week $\times$ 16 weeks = 224,000 total calories $\div$ 3500 calories/pound = 64 pounds.] However, if there is a drop in RMR associated with the low calorie intake of approximately 20 percent, this woman would burn 280 calories less than expected each day (assumed RMR of 1400). Instead of losing 64 pounds, the weight loss will be only 55 pounds. If we factor in a decrease in the thermic effect of food (only 42 calories instead of her typical 240 calories) and an estimated reduction in physical activity of 25 percent, the weight loss would be only 45 pounds instead of our original estimate of 64!

It is no wonder that so many women feel like failures at weight loss. The loss achieved hardly seems worth the sacrifice endured. If these women go off the diet and regain the lost weight, they are getting caught in the yo-yo syndrome. This is the cycle of losing and regaining weight (Wadden, Foster, Wang, Pierson, Yang, Moreland, Stunkard, VanItallie, 1992; Blackburn, Wilson, Kanders, Stein, Lavin, Adler, Brownell, 1989). What causes this pattern to perpetuate? In the previous example a woman experienced a 45 pound weight loss through dieting. However, if she goes back to her original caloric intake of 2400 calories, she will rapidly gain weight. Her energy requirements are now less due to her reduced body weight and her energy expenditure is less due to her lower RMR, so more of the calories consumed are in excess of her needs. In many cases women regain weight equivalent to the amount lost and may exceed their original weight (George, Wilson, Sanders, Stein, Laving, Adler, Brownell, 1989). When this pattern repeats over and over, there can be shifts in body composition. Weight gain is predominately fat; however, when weight loss is rapid, the composition of the tissue lost has a higher percentage of lean tissue.

The seriousness of the yo-yo syndrome may not be obvious. As long as the original body weight is achieved what difference does body composition make? Our basal metabolic rate is largely determined by the amount of lean tissue in our body. When we fast there is a temporary drop in RMR; when we resume eating, the RMR returns to normal, that is, if there has been no significant change in body weight or composition. In those individuals who experience weight regain, the associated higher body fat and lower LBM results in a reduction in resting metabolic rate; and, less calories are needed to support energy needs at rest.

Another study which examined the weight loss of obese women following VLCDs found that when these women transitioned from 420 calories/day to 800 calories/day for five weeks of "refeeding," weight loss did not continue. The average RMR pre-diet for these women was 1692 calories/day; 800 calories/day should have easily resulted in continued weight loss according to the simple "calories in = calories out" equation. This unexpected finding was in part ascribed to increased noncompliance, the reduced RMR, and lower energy cost of activity at the lower body weight (Barrows & Snook, 1987b).

Do we have a set point, that is a weight which our bodies defend? There has been speculation in the literature about a mechanism which carefully regulates body weight. Weight stays within an amazingly narrow range for most individuals in spite of wide fluctuations from day to day in activity and dietary intake. Individuals who lose a significant amount of weight often regain back to within pounds of their original weight. No clear mechanism has been proven to explain these observations; however, evidence is accumulating that fat cell size may play a role.

Fat cell size increases with weight gain until a maximum size is reached. This critical size stimulates the conversion of preadipocytes to mature adipocytes contributing to the development of hypercellular or hyperplastic obesity. Hypercellular obesity is observed in individuals who are 75 percent above normal weight, BMI > 35 kg/m^2, and is associated with an increase in lipoprotein lipase (LPL) which continues with increases in weight up to BMI of 50 kg/m^2 (Bray, 1992a). When an individual loses weight the number of adipose cells remains the same, but the size of cells decreases and the levels of lipoprotein lipase and lipoprotein lipase messenger RNA increase. The increased activity of LPL may potentially enhance lipid storage and make further weight loss more difficult and perhaps even enhance weight regain. This increase in LPL is significantly correlated with the initial body mass but not consistently with the amount of weight lost. This suggests that individuals with hypercellular obesity may have greater difficulty maintaining a weight loss; when the adipocytes shrink, lipoprotein lipase levels increase. The more cells that shrink the greater the stimulation of LPL. This propensity to maintain the size of adipose cells is suggestive of a set point mechanism (Kern, Ong, Saffari, Carty, 1990).

Additional research in animals reveals that increased levels of LPL also stimulate feeding behavior. Although it is not known whether LPL has a similar role in humans (Kern, 1990), it is recognized that a significant percentage of morbidly obese individuals have problems with binge eating approaching 40 percent of individuals in BMI 34–42 category. Also, there is evidence in the literature that suggests that restrictive eating results in bingeing (Stunkard & Wadden, 1992). Consequently, an individual struggling to lose weight by following a very restrictive diet may be driven physiologically to go off the diet and binge. To avoid these consequences of the yo-yo syndrome or weight cycling, we must understand the metabolism of dieting.

What happens metabolically when we lose weight and why is weight loss initially fast, then slower and slower? There is a short answer and a long answer to this question. First, the short answer. The change in the rate of weight loss is largely due to the change in the tissue being used to meet our energy needs. When we fast, most of the initial weight loss is water (caloric value zero), and hydrated glycogen (caloric value 1 cal/g). Once the glycogen is depleted, the body utilizes fat which provides approximately 8 cal/g. Since the caloric value of each pound of fat is approximately 8 times higher than a pound of hydrated glycogen, it takes 8 times longer to lose each pound.

Now, the long answer. The initial weight loss is predominantly water due to glycogen and muscle breakdown, and urea and sodium excretion. Glycogen is a glucose polymer, which is stored with 3–4 grams of water for every gram of glycogen. Maximally, we store about 2000 grams of hydrated glycogen or about 4.4 pounds. As glycogen is being broken down for energy, the water is released. Therefore, in the first day of a fast, if one's caloric expenditure was approximately 2000 calories, glycogen would be completely utilized and an individual could lose over 4 pounds in the first day (Kreitzman, 1992; Alpert, 1988).

Once glycogen is depleted, usually after one day, the body must make glucose to maintain essential levels of glucose in the blood. Most of the glucose is made through gluconeogenesis from amino acids derived from protein. Excess protein is not stored in our bodies so the supply of available circulating amino acids is small and rapidly utilized. If fasting continues, muscle, which is nearly 80 percent water and 20 percent protein, is targeted. When muscle protein is broken down to amino acids, water is again liberated. Additionally, the amino acids must be deaminated in order to make glucose. This ultimately yields urea which must be excreted in the urine which increases urine output and water excretion. Also, in the absence of dietary carbohydrate, the kidneys fail to conserve sodium. As sodium is excreted, water is drawn into the kidney tubule further increasing water excretion. On day three of a fast we might lose 2 pounds; however, 66 percent of this two pounds is water, 24 percent fat and 10 percent is protein (Kreitzman, 1992; Alpert, 1988).

Fatty acids derived from adipose stores are being utilized but do not become the major fuel until nearly two weeks into the fast. As the level of circulating fatty acids increases, ketones, a breakdown product of fatty acids are produced. Ketones are small and can cross the blood-brain barrier allowing ketones to replace part of the brain's requirement for glucose. This reduces the need for protein breakdown and its conversion to glucose, so the rate of lean tissue loss slows, which is a highly desirable adaptation to the fast. Our initial 10 percent of weight loss as protein, decreases to approximately 5 percent (Kreitzman, 1992; Alpert, 1988).

Once glycogen (caloric value 1 cal/g) is depleted, the body utilizes adipose stores with an approximate caloric value of 8 cal/g; consequently, the caloric value of each pound lost increases. For example, a pound of fat yields 3500 calories; whereas, a pound of hydrated glycogen or protein yields only 450 calories. If an individual has reduced her caloric intake to achieve a daily deficit of 2000 calories per day and hydrated glycogen is her only fuel, she could theoretically lose 30 pounds in one week (assuming unlimited stores of glycogen); however, if she burns fat exclusively, the amount of weight lost in one week would be only 4 pounds! Fortunately we do have limited stores of glycogen, and excess calories are stored as energy dense fat. To illustrate, suppose we stored the same number of calories in 10 pounds of fat as glycogen, we would be 78 pounds heavier since glycogen is less calorically dense (Kreitzman, 1992; Alpert, 1988).

TREATMENT APPROACHES TO OBESITY

Most women who are trying to lose weight reduce their caloric intake; about one-third increase their exercise as the primary method, and less than one-fourth increase their exercise and reduce their calories. Typically, women who desire to lose weight make five attempts per year (*Obesity & Health*, 1989, October). This suggests problems, either there was insufficient weight loss at each attempt, or the weight lost was regained, or these women may not really need to lose weight.

Achieving weight loss is easy but losing weight safely and permanently is very difficult. Most experts select a treatment approach which takes into consideration the person's initial body mass and the health problems related to their obesity. The benefits of treatment for the individual must exceed the treatment risks. Therefore, riskier treatments should be reserved for individuals with more serious health risks. The following model has been proposed as a basis for selecting appropriate treatments.

Individuals in Class 0 (BMI 20–25.9) and Class I (BMI 25–29.9) because of the low risk associated with this weight class should only use exercise and conservative diet approaches to weight loss (calories > 800/day). Those in Class II (BMI 30–34.9) may benefit most from medically supervised very low calorie diets (VLCDs) and perhaps exercise and/or drug therapy. Class III (BMI 35–39.9) individuals demonstrate high risk which suggests prompt treatment such as VLCDs and drugs, but are sufficiently overweight that exercise is of limited value. Class IV (BMI > 40) individuals are at very high risk often demonstrating serious comorbid conditions necessitating aggressive treatment such as surgery, VLCDs, and/or drugs (Bray, 1992a).

How do we achieve an acceptable weight loss? The trick here is to not lose lean body mass. The composition of the weight we lose ideally should be the same composition as the weight when we gain. Weight gain in adults is mostly a gain in energy stores (fat) not muscle (unless the individual is engaged in a weight training program); however, it is not 100 percent fat, but rather is only 65 percent fat, 25 percent lean tissue and 10 percent fluids. Therefore, losing weight of approximately the same composition is not considered detrimental.

DIETS

Conservative diets which are not overly restrictive are appropriate for individuals in Class 0 and Class I. Low calorie diets such as those typical of very low calorie diets (VLCDs) (300–600 calories) are too low for women who are not at least 50 pounds over their ideal body weight. When obese women dieted for periods of two months or longer using VLCDs, approximately 25 percent of the lost weight was lean tissue (fat-free mass). However, non-obese individuals lose more lean tissue per kilogram of weight lost, 20 g nitrogen/kg of weight lost as opposed to 10 g nitrogen/kg in the obese. Children and adolescents are particularly susceptible to loss of lean tissue; weight loss may approach 50 percent lean tissue (Gelfand & Hendler, 1989).

Each gram of nitrogen (N) lost reflects the breakdown of 6.25 grams of protein. The obese lose 3–6 g of nitrogen/day after a period of stabilization (weeks) on a VLCD; this represents a loss of 20–40 grams of body protein or 100–200 grams lean tissue since lean tissue is 20 percent protein by weight (Gelfand & Hendler, 1989). These protein losses can be reduced if during the fast the individual receives a supplement providing high-quality protein at a level of 1–1.5 gram/kg ideal body weight [e.g., a female who is 5'4" would have an ideal body weight of 55 kg (120 pounds) and should receive according to this guideline 55–83 g of protein.]. While women in general seem to conserve nitrogen better than men, losses vary considerably among dieters, some individuals continue in negative nitrogen balance even while receiving as much as 100 grams of protein/day (Fisler & Drenick, 1982).

Women comprise 70 percent of the individuals who enroll in medically supervised VLCDs. Most (80%) use a moderate-involvement hospital program costing about $1000; 20% select high involvement costing $2400–$6000 (Berg, 1992).

Very low calorie diets (VLCDs) typically are semi-synthetic formulas composed of high quality protein which provide between 300–600 calories per day and are used as the total food replacement (Lerman & Cave, 1989). VLCDs are designed to promote fat loss and minimize lean tissue loss so that metabolic rate is preserved and weight loss sustained. VLCDs provide rapid weight loss and the anorexic effects similar to total fasting but produce less hyperuricemia and negative nitrogen balance than fasting (Barrows & Snook, 1987a).

It is recommended that VLCD programs provide: a team approach (physician, dietitian, psychologist); a diet of 1.2–1.5 g of good quality protein/kg ideal body weight, with vitamins and minerals; weekly or biweekly monitoring of electrolytes and other pertinent lab tests; 12–16 weeks of semi-fasting, 3–6 weeks of careful refeeding, and long term follow-up; and a multi-disciplinary approach which includes nutrition education, exercise, and behavior modification (ADA Report, 1990). In the last decade, 12–15 million people have used VLCDs. A renewed interest in VLCDs is associated with Oprah Winfrey's successful weight loss using a commercially well-known weight loss plan. VLCDs are popular because they work; people do lose weight. There are reports of remarkable weight losses; for example, a woman weighing 506 pounds reduced to 218 in 18 months. During the first week, weight loss is 10–15 pounds due to the diet induced diuresis (water loss). After the initial rapid rate, weight loss is typically 3–5 pounds/week. A weight loss of 40 pounds is achieved by 80 percent of the individuals while the average weight loss is 85 pounds, representing 20–35 percent of their initial weight (Lerman & Cave, 1989). The rapid successful weight loss provides a psychological benefit and motivation to continue with the diet and many individuals experience a significant reduction in their appetite which makes compliance easier for longer periods of time (ADA report, 1990).

VLCDs are appropriate only for individuals with BMI > 30 or are > 140 percent of their ideal weight to ensure proper composition of weight loss. Nonobese persons placed on a fast lose predominantly LBM rather than fat, nonobese lose 37 percent fat, 63 percent LBM, obese lose 76 percent fat, 24 percent LBM. VLCDs are most appropriate for individuals who face higher risks, e.g., men who have an abdominal fat distribution. Individuals preparing for surgery, persons with diabetes or arthritis, or having a family history of cardiovascular disease, and those rapidly gaining weight approaching grade III (BMI > 40) should be considered for VLCDs (Pi-Sunyer, 1992; Wadden, Van Itallie, Blackburn, 1990).

Persons > 65 years old should not use VLCDs; their decreased growth hormone, insulin and growth promoting factors cause them to lose unacceptable amounts of lean tissue with hypocaloric diets. VLCDs are inappropriate for children, adolescents, and pregnant women. Also individuals with heart disease and gallstones should be excluded due to a high risk of complications (Pi-Sunyer, 1992). Other groups which should not use VLCDs are airline pilots and heavy equipment operators since they may experience blackouts. Individuals on medications such as lithium and diuretics should consult their physician to prevent drug toxicities or adverse reactions while following VLCDs (ADA Report, 1990).

VLCDs are not for everybody. The drop-out rate for VLCDs can be as high as 69 percent, and non-adherence, 20–80 percent (Laporte and Stunkard, 1990). Some individuals experience a severe dieting depression which develops abruptly one-to-three weeks into the diet (Stunkard, Stinnett, & Smoller, 1986).

VLCD diets should not be used for longer than 12–16 weeks. The longer the individual follows the VLCD the greater the nitrogen losses, the tendency to develop gallstones, and risk of cardiovascular complications. VLCDs are a radical program that enhances diuresis and electrolyte loss, and may disturb acid-base balance. Unsupervised VLCDs are the most dangerous. The potential for abuse of certain commercial products is great. These products are intended as a replacement for one or two meals per day, with the third meal, consisting of "reasonable" amounts of normal food. When used as a total food replacement (against manufacturer's directions) weight loss is rapid; since these individuals are obviously not monitored, serious problems go unrecognized and untreated. Without medical supervision, there is a strong tendency to binge eat during the refeeding process, which can be dangerous and set the cycle in motion for weight regain (*Obesity and Health*, 1990, March).

Today's VLCDs are different from the first liquid protein diets which were introduced in 1976. One early formula resulted in 58 deaths. In one year, 1977, 98,000 American women between the ages of 25–52 used "liquid protein" as their sole or primary source of food for at least one month and 37,000 used it for two months or longer. The deaths were due in part to atrophy of the cardiac muscle; 17 otherwise healthy obese died of ventricular arrhythmias during or shortly after completing rapid massive weight reduction. The VLCD was a collagen hydrolysate (poor quality protein) used for 2–8 months. This demonstrates that the heart muscle is not protected from the accelerated protein breakdown associated with a very low calorie diet in spite of its vital role. A correlation between pre-diet body mass index and the duration of survival on the VLCD was noted, but the deaths were not caused by individuals becoming underweight as 7 were still obese at the time of their death (Van Itallie & Yang, 1984).

Lessons learned from the early experience with VLCDs include: the less obese die sooner than the more obese, and a maximum safe period exists for some individuals for this mode of weight reduction. Severely obese who lose 30 percent of body weight rapidly are at risk. Less obese individuals who reduce rapidly, lose as little as 10–15 percent, and could develop ventricular arrhythmia with 2 months of dieting (Van Itallie & Yang, 1984). Obesity per se is associated with cardiovascular changes including left ventricular hypertrophy and prolongation of the QT interval. With weight loss, the mass of the heart and left ventricle decrease. ECG abnormalities depend upon diet duration and whether protein and mineral nutritional status is maintained; copper, potassium, and magnesium deficiencies may promote an unstable heart (Fisler, 1992).

Other complications are loss of body protein and calcium, dehydration, hypoglycemia, hypokalemia, hyperuricemia, hair loss, anemia, postural hypotension, cold intolerance, halitosis (bad breath), water retention, fatigue, constipation and gallstones (ADA Report, 1990; Fisler & Drenick, 1987; Lerman & Cave, 1989). Individuals who demonstrate unusually rapid weight loss or experience ongoing fatigue should be monitored with periodic measurements of 24-hour urinary creatinine and urea nitrogen excretions. These measurements can provide an estimate of the lean tissue lost. If losses of lean tissue are greater than the acceptable 25 percent of weight lost, then additional protein should be provided and the subject reminded not to intentionally decrease their intake to speed weight loss (Lerman & Cave, 1989).

To date most of the reports of long-term weight maintenance are discouraging. Follow-up of individuals revealed many had regained their lost weight within 36 months. One study included data on 6000 subjects: 55 percent quit before completing the program, the 45 percent remaining lost 84 percent of their excess weight but had regained 59–82 percent of their initial weight by 30 months (Lerman & Cave, 1987; *Obesity and Health*, 1989, May). Another significant finding is that only 24 percent of the dieters were successful in their second attempt to lose weight as opposed to an 80 percent success rate the first time. The spectacular weight loss seems to occur only once (Lerman & Cave, 1989).

The poor long-term success emphasizes the need for a strong weight maintenance program which is continued after the patient is off the VLCD. Medically supervised VLCDs include education and teach behavior change; however, VLCDs provide no opportunity to practice the new behaviors while on the diet. Behaviors such as selecting and buying appropriate foods and learning new cooking techniques, portion control, stimulus control, and diminishing habits such as rapidity of eating and doing other things while eating are crucial to maintaining the weight loss and are best taught and reinforced during a maintenance phase. A lack of a strong maintenance phase appears to be the weakness of many programs, however, since it provides little profit (Pi-Sunyer, 1992).

EXERCISE

Exercise is thought to preserve lean body mass and maintain RMR during caloric restriction in mildly obese individuals (Class I and perhaps Class II), (Barrows & Snook, 1987a). This effect is particularly strong when the amount of protein consumed during diet restriction is less than 1.2 g/kg ideal body weight (Phinney, 1992). Additionally, exercise improves one's sense of well being and body image. However, the direct energy cost of exercise is surprisingly minimal; therefore, the greatest effects are cumulative, accomplished slowly with regular exercise over a long period of time. A single intense bout of exercise has little effect on energy balance and for the morbidly obese, intense and/or prolonged exercise is considered unrealistic and potentially dangerous. Ideally, the increase in exercise should not be offset by an increase in energy intake (Calles-Escandon & Horton, 1992). A surprising exception is observed with VLCDs. Exercise combined with very low calorie diets does not seem to consistently preserve the RMR or increase the rate of weight loss. We would anticipate that women following a VLCD and exercising would lose more weight than women following a VLCD without added exercise. However, more rapid weight loss or more positive nitrogen balance was not observed in the exercising group. The benefits of exercise may not be as obvious in this case but the exercising groups did learn skills which will be critical for long-term maintenance (Phinney, 1992). In fact, regular exercise is one of the best predictors for long-term successful weight loss (Kayman, Bruvold, & Stern, 1990).

Exercise cannot contribute significantly to a negative energy deficit unless there is a cumulative effect which is not offset by an increase in energy intake. Thermogenically there appears to be little difference between obese and nonobese individuals, i.e., no significant increase in efficiency which could explain the weight gain in the obese. The direct energy cost of exercise is surprisingly minimal, therefore, observed difference in thermic effect of food perhaps 25 percent would be eventually offset by increase in RMR due to increase in lean mass with weight gain (Calles-Escandon & Horton, 1992).

DRUGS

Drugs, as a treatment for obesity, have not received enthusiastic support by professionals. Theoretically, drugs ought to be the treatment of choice, no surgery and post operative complications; no severely restrictive diet which results in rebound weight gain for many; instead a pill promotes excess weight loss. Unfortunately, several problems regarding the use of drugs to treat obesity now interfere with the acceptance of drugs as a serious treatment option. First amphetamine, a strong appetite suppressant was used for the treatment of obesity before its potential for abuse was recognized. While this group of drugs is no longer approved for obesity treatment, the concern for potential drug abuse lingers and is still reflected in the Food and Drug Administration's restrictions regarding these drugs. Second, licensing agencies have restricted the use of drugs in the treatment for obesity as a "short term adjunct." Furthermore, "short term" has been interpreted as a couple of weeks. This assumes either that drugs are of limited value except as an initial stimulus when one begins a diet, or that the abuse potential precludes the use of drugs for a longer period of time. Since drugs have been demonstrated to be effective for as long as they are used, the first assumption is incorrect. Current drugs used for the treatment of obesity range from simple over-the-counter appetite suppressants to prescription drugs, and have little or no abuse potential and minimal side effects which eliminates the second assumption (Bray, 1992b).

The most problematic aspect of "short term" is that realistically it is not the first two weeks of a diet which are the hardest! And, if dieting stops after a two-week attempt, little of the tissue lost was fat. If an individual is 60 pounds over her desired weight and loses 2 pounds/week (a satisfactory rate of weight loss); 30 weeks of treatment are required to lose the excess weight. For many individuals to be successfully treated a minimum of 30–50 weeks may be required. However, physicians have received disciplinary action for treating obese individuals for more than a few weeks with drugs. This fact alone would discourage many professionals from prescribing drugs to facilitate appropriate weight loss.

Critics of the drug approach to treatment point to the long-term failures, that is, once the individual achieves the desired weight loss and discontinues the drug, the weight is rapidly regained. This is the third problem, the expectation that drugs should cure obesity. This view is unrealistic; drugs should be used in this case as a treatment similar to any chronic disease. Health professionals don't expect insulin to cure diabetes or antihypertensives to cure hypertension, and yet some physicians do expect a drug cure for obesity. The attitude that obesity is not a disease but rather a condition associated with a lack of willpower and gluttony undoubtedly is a factor in this expectation. Many professionals think obesity persists due to psychological factors and that once the weight is lost the problems are gone. However, research indicates that the obese population does not have more psychological problems than the nonobese population.

The pharmacology of obesity treatment today includes: appetite suppressants; inhibitors which limit the digestion of food (such as tetrahydrolipstatin); synthetic foods which offer the taste and satisfaction of rich foods without all the calories (for example, Olestra and Simplesse); and thermogenic drugs which increase the calories we burn without necessarily affecting the calories we consume. This last category of experimental drugs demonstrates some particularly interesting effects, an increase in muscle and reduction in fat stores similar to what is achieved with physical exercise.

Drugs may offer dramatic possibilities in the future. An injection of isoproterenol (a beta-adrenergic agonist) into one thigh of a women on a diet effectively increased fat mobilization from the injected thigh. Also, a cream containing aminophylline and yohimbine increased fat mobilization in the treated thigh. This suggests that there may be a way to spot reduce and treat regional fat deposits by a topical means. However, further clinical trials and testing must be completed and with the prevailing attitudes of professionals, the limitations posed by regulating agencies, and the inadequate funding we may have a long wait (Bray, 1992b).

SURGERY

"Most obese persons will not participate in outpatient treatment; of those who do, most will not lose a significant amount of weight, and of those who do lose weight, most will regain it" (Stunkard, Foster & Grossman, 1986). If we assume an average weight loss is 1.5 pounds per week, an individual who is 100 pounds overweight will have to faithfully follow a weight loss program for 67 weeks (1 year and 15 weeks) to achieve their ideal weight. Accomplishing this feat would appear to be highly unlikely. Additionally, binge eating is a major problem of the morbidly obese; these individuals report significantly greater psychological distress than do obese nonbingers including depression, anxiety, and obsessive-like behavior during dieting. Consequently, they demonstrate an increased risk for terminating treatment prematurely and rapidly regaining lost weight when treated by a conventional low calorie diet (Stunkard & Wadden, 1992).

Physicians considered the lack of success in treating obesity due to "the patient's lack of ability to control gluttonous dietary habits over a prolonged period of time." The attitude that "patients can't or won't lose weight on their own" led to the idea of a surgical approach which would "make them lose weight regardless of their intake" (Scott & Law, 1969). During the last 20 years there has been a truly alarming development of surgical procedures designed to induce weight loss. This era has been described by one surgeon as the "dark ages of surgery" (Kral, 1987). Procedures were developed and performed on hundreds of people without sufficient study to determine long-term problems. The supreme goal was achieving maximal weight loss. Although surgical approaches will result in weight loss, permanent weight loss in most cases, there are consequences which must be carefully evaluated and monitored. We have again learned some painful lessons this time from the early surgical procedures which we must consider to keep this form of treatment in perspective.

Surgical approaches to weight loss should be reserved for individuals with very high risk due to their obesity, or individuals with high risk and comorbid conditions. Clearly the risk of obesity must outweigh the risk of the procedure and possible long term complications (Bray, 1992a). Individuals who are 100 pounds above ideal standards or have a BMI > 40 require surgery. For these individuals the risk of obesity necessitates a permanent solution since weight loss with diet is < 5 percent of body weight with follow-up 1 year (Kral, 1992).

Most surgical procedures either induce malabsorption (intestinal modifications), reduce consumption (gastric modifications), a combination of both, or mechanically remove fat, i.e., lipectomy. There are approximately 30 surgical techniques which have been reported. The list of current procedures includes: jejunoileal bypass, biliointestinal bypass, duodenoileal bypass, ileogastrostomy, jaw wiring, gastric balloons, gastric bands, total gastric wrapping, gastroplasty and gastric bypass (Kral, 1987). The discussion here is limited to: (1) jejunoileal bypass (which taught us lessons we must not forget); (2) gastric bypass and vertical banded gastroplasty (because these are the most popular surgical procedures used today); (3) lipectomy (because of new developments); and (4) biliopancreatic diversion bypass (because it is scary).

Jejunoileal bypass (JIB):   In the early 1960s, Payne introduced the jejunocolic shunt (JCS) in which 36 cm of ileum was attached to the transverse colon as a surgical solution to the problem of obesity. Weight loss was described as profound, but severe electrolyte imbalances and diarrhea occurred. Most of his patients had their intestinal continuity reestablished and gained weight back to or above their presurgery weight (O'Leary, 1992). Modifications to reduce the severity of side effects of the JCS led to the development of the jejunoileal bypass (JIB). Many variations of this procedure have been reported but in general approximately 14" of proximal jejunum was attached to the distal 4" of terminal ileum. The continuous segment of small intestine was reduced from the normal 20–22 feet to approximately 2–2½ feet. A consequence of the surgery was the creation of a long blind loop of intestine which was not removed in the event of the need to reverse the surgery. This procedure drastically reduced the length of functional small intestine. The transit of food was so rapid, digestion was incomplete; and the surface area for absorption was so radically reduced that most of the food eaten passed through the gastrointestinal tract unabsorbed. It was anticipated that weight loss would occur regardless of what the patient continued to eat due to induced maldigestion and malabsorption (Deitel, 1989; Payne, DeWind, Commons, 1963; Payne & DeWind, 1969).

Results of the JIB: A number of conclusions are drawn from the literature: (1) weight loss was considered excellent (ranging from 59–235 pounds, average weight loss 112 pounds); (2) patients were generally satisfied (94% indicated they would make the decision to have surgery again); (3) improvements in physical mobility and health benefits were observed (blood lipid levels decreased, cardiac and pulmonary disease lessened); (4) early postoperative complications were minimal; (5) psychosocial responses were satisfactory to dramatic; (6) all patients developed diarrhea; (7) electrolyte imbalances could be managed; and (8) approximately 50 percent of the patients developed serious complications, such as liver failure, renal failure, kidney stones, gallstones, enteritis, decreased bone density, and even death. Complications could develop as late as 10 years following the surgery (Deitel, 1989; O'Leary, 1992; Olson, 1974).

Liver failure was the most severe complication which occurred in 40 percent of the cases (O'Leary, 1981). The cause was not originally understood but eventually several contributing factors were recognized: (1) hepatotoxic substances produced by bacteria in the bypassed portion of the bowel; (2) choline deficiency due to bacteria converting choline to trimethylamine; and (3) malnutrition, especially protein malnutrition which resulted in a reduced ability to synthesize lipoproteins (O'Leary, 1981).

Unexpected results revealed that with these patients malabsorption accounted for only a portion of the weight loss; most patients ate significantly less food after surgery and modified their intake to reduce fats and concentrated sweets. The diet modification was largely to avoid the adverse symptoms of diarrhea and steatorrhea associated with concentrated sugars or fats. Fried foods, nondiet pop, and gas producing vegetables and beans were frequently reported as troublesome. Some patients experienced 10–20 semiliquid stools per day and reported that they often had to get up in the middle of a meal to go to the bathroom, food transit was so rapid. Food records revealed a substantial reduction in the total number of calories consumed after surgery. Certainly part of this observation is due to adversive conditioning, but my patients also reported that following surgery they no longer craved sweets and that controlling their intake was much easier (Olson, 1974). The JIB is now discontinued in the United States in its original form due to problems associated with bacterial overgrowth in the blind loop and high rate of liver failure.

Gastric procedures: The recognition of the long-term complications of JIB persuaded many surgeons to turn to the stomach as the target for surgical treatment for obesity. Gastric procedures are collectively less successful than JIB in terms of weight loss, but have the distinct advantage of fewer and less serious side effects (Kral, 1987). Gastric procedures reduce the size of the stomach or restrict (gastric wrapping or banding) the amount of food one can eat. There were 5178 gastric operations reported to National Bariatric Surgery Association in Iowa between 1986 and 1989 (Mason, Renquist, Jiang, 1992; Grace, 1992).

In the gastric bypass (GB) procedure, the top of the stomach is sectioned off by a horizontal row of staples forming a pouch with less than one ounce (30 mls) capacity; the normal capacity of the stomach is approximately 1 quart (1000 mls). A portion of the jejunum is attached to the side of the pouch and an opening (stoma) is made to allow the contents to flow from the stomach pouch into the jejunum. Most of the stomach and all of the duodenum are bypassed; consequently many of the digestive functions of the stomach are circumvented. For example, when we consume concentrated foods the stomach adjusts the concentration (osmolarity) so that food leaving the stomach is the same concentration as the blood (isotonic). With this procedure, concentrated (hyperosmolar) food enters the jejunum; this causes an osmotic effect or drawing of fluid into the intestinal track contributing to the syndrome known as dumping (nausea, vomiting, bloating, diarrhea, dizziness, and sweating). People eat less due to the reduction in the size of the stomach and avoid certain foods to minimize adverse symptoms.

The vertical banded gastroplasty (VBG) creates a vertical pouch which has less tendency to stretch over time. A hole is punched in the stomach and a non-stretch band is placed through the hole around the created stoma. A vertical row of staples defines the pouch which is smaller (10–15 mls) than in the gastric bypass. This procedure preserves the normal sequence for the passage of food and thus eliminates the maldigestion and symptoms of dumping associated with the GB. In both procedures weight loss is accomplished by reducing the amount of food the individual eats; everything eaten, however, is essentially digested and absorbed, an important difference from the JIB (Dietel, 1989).

Results revealed weight loss associated with gastric procedures ranging from 40–50 kg or 35–70 percent of the excess weight (Kral, 1989). Rand (1986) reported better than typical results, a loss of 81 percent of original weight maintained for three years and markedly improved psychosocial outcome in patients. Weight loss is greater with GB than VBG due to the aversive conditioning, some maldigestion induced by this procedure, and changes which occur in gut hormones following GB (Kral,1992). Women lose less weight than men, and blacks lose less than Caucasians and Hispanics independent of socioeconomic status. One-third appear to be non-responders, that is these individuals lose less than a satisfactory amount of weight.

A particularly important point is that weight loss following both of these surgical procedures can be sabotaged by the diet consumed. Individuals who consume sweets, especially liquids, will not lose much weight with the VBG; whereas, with the GB weight loss is greater (due to adverse side-effects when sweets are consumed). However, an individual who nibbles all day long on high fat snacks like potato chips will fail to lose weight with the GB. Insufficient weight loss can occur in individuals who develop a pattern of overconsuming soft, liquid, or melting calorically dense food. Consequently, there has been some attempt to choose the best procedure for a particular patient by determining patterns in the diet history (Sugarman, Kellum, Engle, Wolfe, Starkey, Birkenhauer, Fletcher & Sawyer, 1992).

The non-responding superobese population requires a more aggressive approach. A staged approach of multiple operations has been suggested as necessary for a more effective initial operation (with increased risks of complications) if the individual is considered at risk of weight loss failure or weight regain (Kral, 1992).

Complications of gastric procedures include: persistent vomiting which occurs in as many as one-third of the patients due to eating behavior or to an obstruction of the stoma; gastritis can occur with GB due to bile pooling; hair loss; dumping syndrome (with GB) (diarrhea, gas, cramps, followed by hypoglycemia); 50–70 percent of patients demonstrate B_{12} deficiency and 36–50 percent iron deficiency; protein, folate, thiamin, and calcium deficiencies occur. Gallstones occur at 6 times the rate of nonsurgically treated obese individuals for the first 1–2 years post surgery. Complications seem to be more severe in GB than VGB (except in rare cases with protracted vomiting), in part due to the maldigestion which can result from this procedure. Even birth defects have been reported in fetuses of post-GB women perhaps related to B-vitamin deficiencies, and peripheral neuropathy has also been observed which responds to thiamin therapy (Halverson, 1992). Both gastric surgeries require lifelong surveillance (Kral, 1992).

Lipectomy: Suction lipectomy patients are mostly female; 95 percent of 3511 patients reported by Dillerud (1990) were women. The risks associated with this procedure are relatively small; a complication rate of less than 10 percent is cited which includes results which were less than ideal. In 100,000 reviewed cases there were 11 documented deaths and 9 non-fatal cases of serious morbidity, including infection, hematoma, hypovolemic shock, pulmonary embolism, and fat embolism. Less serious undesirable results include: waviness of the skin due to uneven fat removal, pain, pigmentation, bagginess when skin cannot contract sufficiently after fat removal and edema (ASPRS report, 1987).

Traditionally lipectomy has been reserved for the nonobese individual as a means to correct figure faults or contour irregularities (saddle bags or a protuberant abdomen). Typically only small amounts of fat are removed, the equivalent of 1–2 kg, which is hardly a solution for someone who is obese. The removal of fat is accomplished by the introduction of a hollow cannula through a small incision and the rather brutal ramming of this cannula to suck tunnels of subcutaneous fat (Kral, 1992).

Recently, reports of serial lipectomy for moderately obese women have been presented. Severe complications have been observed when more than 4 L of fat were removed without adequate transfusion; consequently, 1–2 L are now removed during one session. In one case a woman who had lost 70 pounds after a jejunoileal bypass stabilized at a size 20. After five serial suctions for a total removal of 7750 cc of fat she was a size 8 (Ersek, Philips, & Schade, 1991). While these results were quite dramatic, this case is not typical and the numbers of individuals studied is still small.

The advantage of direct fat removal is that lean tissue is maintained, unlike dieting where both fat and lean tissue are lost. Since lean tissue is the major determinant of energy requirements, if only fat is removed there would be no reduction in RMR due to calorie restriction or ultimate increase in metabolic efficiency due to loss of lean tissue.

Would the removal of adipose tissue affect set point? Adipose tissue appears to be sensitive to changes in fat cell size rather than fat cell number. Set point theory suggests that when an individual loses weight the fat cells shrink and lipogenic activity is stimulated. These shrunk cells have a reduced rate of lipolysis, reduced rate of fatty acid triglyceride recycling and an increased metabolic efficiency. The mechanism appears to promote refilling of the fat cells. Modest surgical removal of fat cells allows loss of fat without the compensatory shrinking of fat cells. This theoretically avoids triggering the increase in LPL. When the metabolic response to localized fat removal was studied in nonobese women there was no compensatory increase in the size of the remaining fat cells, no increase in metabolic efficiency or changes in regional adipose distribution (Lambert, 1991). The follow-up study completed one year after serial suctioning, revealed that the women not only had not regained the weight but had lost additional weight, an average of 15 pounds (Ersek, Philips, & Schade, 1991). These results are only presented for a small number of women and one year follow-up is not a long time; however, it appears that the removal of fat cells may have facilitated the maintenance of weight loss.

The results of this research are thought provoking. However, it should be pointed out that the women studied either had previously lost significant amounts of weight via a surgical approach (intestinal or gastric surgery) or were nonobese. There are two points to emphasize, (1) the removal of fat tissue was localized and averaged less than a total of 4000cc of fat; and (2) the women were not consuming calories in excess of their energy needs or there might have been compensatory increases in fat cells.

Biliopancreatic diversion or bypass: This procedure incorporates both the restrictive elements of gastric surgery and malabsorptive intestinal modifications. A small gastric pouch is created by a subtotal gastrectomy, volume 100–400 mls. The small intestine is divided at its midpoint and the distal (ileal) end is attached to the stomach remnant. The proximal end of the small intestine (duodenum), which is now separated from the stomach, is closed. However the ducts from the pancreas and gallbladder remain intact. The restructuring of the small intestine results in a path for food which is almost completely separate from the digestive enzymes and bile. Mixing of food and enzymes does not occur until the last 50 cm of ileum, significantly limiting digestion, and without digestion there is no absorption.

The early reports of BPB results were considered positive; patients lost at least 50 percent of their initial excess weight. In one report, weight loss achieved was > 80 percent of excess weight at 2 years postoperative. The major complication was protein malnutrition (incidence approximately 10%) and liver failure was thought to be rare. The weight loss was described as substantial and predictable, and greater than the loss achieved with gastric bypass (O'Leary, 1992). However, later reports revealed serious problems in 40–50 percent of the population such as decreased bone density, stomal ulcerations, kidney stones and malnutrition severe enough to require hospitalization for parenteral nutrition. In one study 28 percent of patients experienced such severe malnutrition that reoperation was required. Since this procedure is not totally reversible and the complications can be potentially life threatening, it should be reserved for only the superobese who have failed gastric procedures, and this type of malabsorptive operation should only be performed in special cases in centers with meticulous life-time follow-up (Brolin, 1992; Halverson, 1992; Kral, 1992).

The scary part is that we seem to be repeating history and not learning from past mistakes. The JCS was the first surgical procedure introduced to treat obesity; many patients died as a result of JCS so the JIB was developed. This procedure (JIB) was performed on over 100,000 individuals before the long-term risks were so obvious they could no longer be ignored; this led to the abandonment of malabsorptive procedures (intestinal procedures) in favor of gastric restrictive procedures. The gastric bypass (GB) was designed to limit intake but the side effects of dumping were originally considered undesirable and the vertical banded gastroplasty (VBG) was developed. Weight loss results with VBG were disappointing and surgeons who originally performed VBG are now reoperating and converting the revision to a GP because of the perceived added benefit of dumping. The goal again seems to be maximal weight loss and not the well being of the individual. The surgeries being performed are again deliberately designed to cause sufficient side effects that patients are forced to radically change their eating habits or suffer.

The biliopancreatic bypass not only induces the malabsorptive effects similar to the JIB but also imposes the restrictive nature of a GB. When we consider how severely altered the gastrointestinal track becomes, we should expect severe symptoms; we should anticipate all the problems associated with the intestinal bypass and the gastric surgeries, if not today, then in a few years. With this procedure we cannot know with any certainty what an individual actually absorbs; are they getting adequate nutrients? Even if a good diet is provided and consumed, there is no guarantee that they will be adequately nourished. Consequently, no woman who *ever* wishes to have children can have this surgery since there would be no guarantees for the adequate nourishment of the fetus.

Who should get this surgery? That is a very good question. Is maximal weight loss necessary? What is the definition of "successful" weight loss? What is success, achieving ideal body weight or losing sufficient weight to experience health and psychological benefits? The percentages of morbidly obese and superobese individuals who achieve ideal body weight is virtually zero. The medical literature in fact defines success in three different ways: (1) a loss of > 25 percent of preoperative weight, (2) a loss of > 50 percent of excess weight, or (3) a loss to within 50 percent of the ideal body weight (Brolin, 1992). These definitions all yield different results in terms of "success."

Research literature frequently presents data indicating the failure to achieve "success" without focusing on whether or not the individual experienced any physical or psychological benefits. In many cases there is improvement or resolution of the obesity-associated medical problems with a relatively modest weight loss. In other words most individuals do not need to lose a significant amount of weight in order to experience significant relief of symptoms and/or conditions caused or exaggerated by obesity (Brolin, 1992). Does it make sense therefore, to strive to achieve maximal weight loss at all costs? There is no answer to this question since there are no data on life expectancy after weight reduction to help formulate appropriate goal weights after surgical treatment (Kral, 1992). However, resolution of obesity-related symptoms ought to be considered more important than the amount of weight lost.

Surgery is not a cure by itself but rather a means to enforce a reducing diet. The most important part of the surgical weight loss approach can be summarized briefly: follow-up. Serious, even life-threatening complications may not occur until 10 years after the surgery. Unfortunately, many patients get lost along the way; they move, they feel good so they no longer believe supervision is required. They don't have time; they are dissatisfied with their weight loss and express anger by missing appointments. They are embarrassed about poor weight loss; or the surgeon has performed so many surgeries that maintaining life-time contact with all of them is impossible. Minimally there should be annual clinic visits after the second year (more often during the first two years); weight, blood pressure, and necessary laboratory studies which are tailored to the individual and the surgical procedure, should be completed.

PSYCHOLOGICAL FACTORS

Patients often do not recognize the full extent of their suffering until after successful weight reduction! Individuals who had maintained a 100 pound weight loss for three years following a gastric surgery when interviewed reported (100%) they would rather be deaf, dyslexic, diabetic, or have heart disease than be obese. Ninety-two percent would rather have a leg amputated and 90 percent would rather be legally blind than be obese. This was an unexpected result since most research in the area of "liability of disability" indicates that 62–95 percent of respondents would select their own disability when given an option. Even given the choice to be a multimillionaire and severely obese or normal weight and poor, all chose normal weight. Clearly the pain of obesity is very severe (Rand & Macgregor, 1991).

After surgical treatment patients demonstrate improved self-esteem, eating behavior, and body image. Marital satisfaction increased if there was some satisfaction before surgery. An early study claimed that bypass surgery led to divorce, but with more careful assessment, it was discovered that the tension and discord was due to increased assertiveness and a wider assumption of social roles by the patient. Often when the woman becomes more physically attractive and active the men feel threatened. Many of the husbands in my study frequently tried to sabotage their wife's efforts at weight control and when the women in desperation sought surgery, their husbands were not supportive. Improved psychological functioning enables patients to leave unhappy marriages. In unconflicted marriages, patients reported increased sexual satisfaction and increased marital happiness. One of the unique benefits of surgery is that these patients lose weight without the psychological distress experienced when dieting (depression, anxiety, weakness and preoccupation with food) (Stunkard & Wadden, 1992; Olson, 1974; Kral, Sjostrom & Sullivan, 1992).

PREDICTORS OF SUCCESSFUL WEIGHT REDUCTION

A number of studies have examined the common characteristics in individuals who demonstrate successful weight loss. The following patterns have been reported: (1) individuals who were more overweight, lost more weight, (2) the more prior programs tried the less weight loss occurred, (3) men participating in groups sessions and women seen in individual sessions lost the most weight, (4) the more sessions attended the greater the weight loss, (5) attendance at subsequent programs resulted in greater weight loss, (6) programs which included behavior modification were associated with greater weight loss, (7) increasing age resulted in less weight loss, (8) individuals having less than two children, and (9) weight loss during the first month is indicative of total weight loss, the greater the first month's loss, the greater the total loss, (10) individuals who use a self-reinforcement style, and (11) individuals who engaged in regular exercise were most successful. Most women who lost weight did so on their own and maintained the loss with exercise, altered dietary patterns, and self-monitoring (Allen, 1989; Wadden, et al., 1992; Foreyt & Goodrick,1993; Kayman, Bruvold, & Stern, 1990).

CONCLUSIONS

Women should carefully determine whether or not they are at risk before engaging in weight loss. Consider not only weight but also fat distribution. Is weight loss necessary to achieve health benefits? If the answer is yes, then they should be prepared to make a long-term commitment for a permanent solution. Can the weight be kept off and the potential complications of weight cycling be prevented? Is diet and exercise the right approach? If so, have realistic expectations, lose weight gradually, and don't anticipate miracles with exercise. Five 45-minute walks each week achieved gradually over 6 months can demonstrate significant improvements in mood, self-esteem, and perceived energy; and, exercise is also associated with an increased preference for carbohydrates over fat which helps reduce caloric intake (Foreyt & Goodrick, 1993). Modest weight loss can produce significant improvements in health. If more aggressive treatment is needed women should seek diet programs or surgeons that offer long-term maintenance diet phases or life-time follow-up after surgery. Ask questions before selecting any surgical procedure, while there can be significant benefits, there are also significant risks. Weight regain increases health risks, increases the sense of failure and loss of self-esteem; the costs of relapse are greater than staying overweight. Women should recognize fat thighs as a blessing (in terms of health risks) rather than a curse; this change in attitude will take considerable rethinking for our culture. Whichever approach is chosen the best advice is: don't be in a hurry and make a change that you can live with.

REFERENCES

ADA Report. (1989). Timely statement of The American Dietetic Association: Very low calorie weight loss diets. *Journal of The American Dietetic Association, 89*(7), 975–976.

ADA Report. (1990). Position of the American Dietetic Association: Very low calorie weight loss diets. *Journal of The American Dietetic Association, 90*(5), 722–726.

ADA Report. (1992). Economic benefits of nutrition services, Executive summary. The American Dietetic Association, Chicago, Illinois.

Allen, J. D. (1989). Women who successfully manage their weight. *Western Journal of Nursing Research, 11,* 657–675.

Alpert, S. S. (1988). The energy density of weight loss in semistarvation. *International Journal of Obesity, 12,* 533–542.

ASPRS Ad-Hoc Committee on New Procedures. (1987). Five-year updated evaluation of suction-assisted lipectomy. *Plastic Surgical Nursing, 7,* 142–147.

Barrows, K., & Snook, J. T. (1987a). Effect of a high-protein, very low calorie diet on body composition and anthropometric parameters of obese middle-aged women. *American Journal of Clinical Nutrition, 45,* 381–390.

Barrows, K., & Snook, J. T. (1987b). Effect of high-protein, very low calorie diet on resting metabolism, thyroid hormones, and energy expenditure of obese middle-aged women. *American Journal of Clinical Nutrition, 45,* 391–398.

Berg, F. M. (1993). Health risks of obesity, special report. *Obesity and Health.* North Dakota: Healthy Living Institute.

Blackburn, G. L., Wilson, G. T., Kanders, B. S., Stein, L. J., Lavin, P. T., Adler, J., & Brownell, K. D. (1989). Weight cycling: the experience of human dieters. *American Journal of Clinical Nutrition, 49,* 1105–1109.

Bray, G. A. (1989). Classification and evaluation of the obesities. *Medical Clinics of North America, 73,* 161–184.

Bray, G. A. (1992a). Pathophysiology of obesity. *American Journal of Clinical Nutrition, 55,* 488S–494S.

Bray, G. A. (1992b). Drug treatment of obesity. *American Journal of Clinical Nutrition, 55,* 538S–544S.

Brolin, R. E. (1992). Critical analysis of results: Weight loss and quality of data. *American Journal of Clinical Nutrition, 55,* 577S–581S.

Calles-Escandon, J., & Horton, E. S. (1992). The thermogenic role of exercise in the treatment of morbid obesity: A critical evaluation. *American Journal of Clinical Nutrition, 55,* 533S–537S.

Colditz, G. A. (1992). Economic costs of obesity. *American Journal of Clinical Nutrition, 55,* 503S–507S.

de Boer, J. O., van Es, A. J. H., Rovers, L. A., van Raaij, J. M. A., & Hautvast, G. A. J. (1986). Adaptation of energy metabolism of overweight women to low-energy intake, studied with whole body calorimeters. *American Journal of Clinical Nutrition, 44,* 585–595.

Deitel, M. (1989). *Surgery for the morbidly obese patient.* Philadelphia: Lea & Febiger.

Dillerud, E. (1990). Suction lipoplasty: A report of complications, undesired results, and patient satisfaction based on 3511 procedures. *Plastic and Reconstructive Surgery, 88,* 239–249.

Ersek, R. A., Philips, C., & Schade, K. (1991). Obesity can be treated by suction lipoplasty when combined with other procedures. *Aesthetic Plastic Surgery, 15,* 67–71.

Fisler, J. S., & Drenick, E. J. (1987). Starvation and semistarvation diets in the management of obesity. *Annual Review of Nutrition, 7,* 465–484.

Fisler, J. S. (1992). Cardiac effects of starvation and semistarvation diets: safety and mechanisms of action. *American Journal of Clinical Nutrition, 56,* 230S–234S.

Foreyt, J. P., & Goodrick, G. K. (1993). A non-diet approach to obesity. *Nutrition and the MD, 19,* 1–3.

Frankle, R. T., Yang, M. (1988). *Obesity and weight control: The health professional's guide to understanding and treatment.* Rockville, MD: Aspen Publishers.

George, L. B., Wilson, G. T., Sanders, B. S., Stein, L. J., Lavin, P. T., Adler, J., & Brownell, K. D. (1989). Weight cycling: The experience of human dieters. *American Journal of Clinical Nutrition, 49,* 1105–1109.

Gelfand, R. A., & Hendler, R. (1989). Effect of nutrient composition on the metabolic response to very low calorie diets: Learning more and more about less and less. *Diabetes/Metabolism Reviews, 5*(1), 17–30.

Grace, D. M. (1992). Gastric restriction procedures for treating severe obesity. *American Journal of Clinical Nutrition, 55,* 556S–559S.

Halverson, J. D. (1992). Metabolic risk of obesity surgery and long-term follow-up. *American Journal of Clinical Nutrition, 55,* 602S–605S.

Kayman, S., Bruvold, W., & Stern, J. S. (1990). Maintenance and relapse after weight loss in women: Behavioral aspects. *American Journal of Clinical Nutrition, 52,* 800–807.

Kern, P. A., Ong, J. M., Saffari, B., & Carty, J. (1990). The effects of weight loss on the activity and expression of adipose tissue lipoprotein lipase in very obese humans. *New England Journal of Medicine, 322,* 1053–1059.

Kissebah, A. H., Freedman, D. S., & Peiris, A. N. (1989). Health risks of obesity. *Medical Clinics of North America, 73,* 111–138.

Kral, J. (1987). Malabsorptive procedures in surgical treatment of morbid obesity. *Gastroenterology Clinics of North America, 16*(2), 293–305.

Kral, J. (1989). Surgical treatment of obesity. *Medical Clinics of North America, 73*(1), 251–264.

Kral, J. G. (1992). Overview of surgical techniques for treating obesity. *American Journal of Clinical Nutrition, 55,* 552S–555S.

Kral, J. G., Sjostrom, L. V., & Sullivan, M. B. E. (1992). Assessment of quality of life before and after surgery for severe obesity. *American Journal of Clinical Nutrition, 55,* 611S–614S.

Kreitzman, S. N. (1992). Factors influencing body composition during very low calorie diets. *American Journal of Clinical Nutrition, 56,* 217S–223S.

Kuczmarski, R. J. (1992). Prevalence of overweight and weight gain in the United States. *American Journal of Clinical Nutrition, 55,* 495S–502S.

Lambert, E. V., Hudson, D. A., Block, C. E., & Koeslag, J. H. (1991). Metabolic response to localized surgical fat removal in nonobese women. *Aesthetic Plastic Surgery, 15,* 105–110.

Laporte, D. J., & Stunkard, A. J. (1990). Predicting attrition and adherence to a very low calorie diet: A prospective investigation of the eating inventory. *International Journal of Obesity, 14,* 197–206.

Lerman, R. H., & Cave, D. R. (1989). Medical and Surgical Management of Obesity. *Advances in Internal Medicine, 34,* 127–164.

Linner, J. H., (1987). Overview of surgical techniques for the treatment of morbid obesity. *Gastroenterology Clinics of North America, 16*(2), 253–272.

Markman, B. S. (1987). Anatomic and metabolic aspects of adipose tissue. *Perspectives in Plastic Surgery, 1*(2), 158–172.

Mason, E. E., Renquist, K. E., & Jiang, D. (1992). Perioperative risks and safety of surgery for severe obesity. *American Journal of Clinical Nutrition, 55,* 573S–576S.

O'Leary, J. P. (1981). Liver failure after jejunoileal bypass: an appraisal. *International Journal of Obesity, 5,* 531–535.

O'Leary, J. P. (1992). Gastrointestinal malabsorptive procedures. *American Journal of Clinical Nutrition, 55,* 567S–570S.

Olson, B. A. (1974). Dietary patterns of post jejunoileal bypass patients. Unpublished data.

Olson, B. A. (1993). Women, obesity, and the results of medical management. *Clinical Issues in Perinatal and Woman's Health Nursing, 4,* 220–226.

Payne, J. H., DeWind, L. T., & Commons, R. R. (1963). Metabolic observations in patients with jejunocolic shunts. *American Journal of Surgery, 108,* 273–288.

Payne, J. H., & DeWind, L. T. (1969). Surgical treatment of obesity. *The American Journal of Surgery, 118,* 141–147.

Phinney, S. D. (1992). Exercise during and after very low calorie dieting. *American Journal of Clinical Nutrition, 56,* 190S–194S.

Pi-Sunyer, F. X. (1992). The role of very low calorie diets in obesity. *American Journal of Clinical Nutrition, 56,* 240S–243S.

Prentice, A. M., Jebb, S. A., Goldber, G. R., Coward, W. A., Murgatroyd, P. R., Poppitt, S. D., & Cole, T. J. (1992). Effects of weight cycling on body composition. *American Journal of Clinical Nutrition, 56,* 209S–216S.

Rand, C. S. W., Macgregor, A., & Hankins, G. (1986). Gastric bypass surgery for obesity: Weight loss, psychosocial outcome, and morbidity one and three years later. *Southern Medical Journal, 79*(12), 1511–1514.

Rand, C. S. W., & Macgregor, A. M. (1991). Successful weight loss following obesity surgery and the perceived liability of morbid obesity. *International Journal of Obesity, 15,* 577–579.

Scott, H. W., & Law, D. H. (1969). Clinical appraisal of jejunoileal shunt in patients with morbid obesity. *American Journal of Surgery, 117,* 246–253.

Seidell, J. C., Deurenberg, P., & Hautvast, J. G. A. J. (1987). Obesity and fat distribution in relation to health—current insights and recommendations. *World Review of Nutrition and Dietetics, 50,* 57–91.

Sjostrom, L. V. (1992a). Morbidity of severely obese subjects. *American Journal of Clinical Nutrition, 55,* 508S–515S.

Sjostrom, L. V. (1992b). Mortality of severely obese subjects. *American Journal of Clinical Nutrition, 55,* 516S–523S.

Staff. (1985). Alterations in metabolic rate after weight loss in obese humans. *Nutrition Reviews, 43*(2), 41–42.

Staff. (1985). Male pattern obesity as a risk predictor for coronary heart disease, stroke and death. *Nutrition Reviews, 43*(2), 44–46.

Staff. (1989, May). VLCD and obesity surgery after 5 years. *Obesity and Health, 3,* 33.

Staff. (1989, October). Behavioral risk survey. *Obesity and Health, 3,* 73.

Staff. (1990, March). VLCD specialists warn against hazards. *Obesity and Health, 4,* 17–19.

Staff. (1992). Gastrointestinal surgery for severe obesity: National Institutes of Health Consensus Development Conference Statement. *American Journal of Clinical Nutrition, 55,* 615S–619S.

Stunkard, A. J., Foster, G. D., & Grossman, R. F. (1986). Surgical Treatment of Obesity. *Advanced Psychosomatic Medicine, 15,* 140–166.

Stunkard, A. J., Stinnett, J. L., & Smoller, J. W. (1986). Psychological and social aspects of the surgical treatment of obesity. *American Journal of Psychiatry, 143*(4), 417–429.

Stunkard, A. J., & Wadden, T. A. (1992). Psychological aspects of severe obesity. *American Journal of Clinical Nutrition, 55,* 524S–532S.

Sugarman, H. J., Kellum, J. M., Engle, K. M., Wolfe, L., Starkey, J. V., Birkenhauer, R., Fletcher, P., & Sawyer, M. (1992). Gastric bypass for treating severe obesity. *American Journal of Clinical Nutrition, 55,* 560S–566S.

Van Gaal, L. F., Vansant, G. A., & Leeuw, H. D. (1992). Factors determining energy expenditure during very low calorie diets. *American Journal of Clinical Nutrition, 56,* 224S–229S.

Van Itallie, T. B., & Yang, M. U. (1984). Cardiac dysfunction in obese dieters: A potentially lethal complication of rapid, massive weight loss. *American Journal of Clinical Nutrition, 39,* 695–702.

Wadden, T. A., Van Itallie, T. B., & Blackburn, G. L. (1990). Responsible and irresponsible use of very low calorie diets in the treatment of obesity. *Journal of the American Medical Association, 263,* 83–85.

Wadden, T. A., Foster, G. D., Wang, J., Pierson, R. N., Yang, M. U., Moreland, K., Stunkard, A. J., & VanItallie, T. B. (1992). Clinical correlates of short- and long-term weight loss. *American Journal of Clinical Nutrition, 56,* 271S–274S.

Weststrate, J. A., Dekker, J., Stoel, M., Begheijn, L., Deurenberg, P., & Hautvast, J. G. A. J. (1990). Resting energy expenditure in women: Impact of obesity and body-fat distribution. *Metabolism, 39*(1), 11–17.

—————⫸●⫷—————

BOOKS, ARTICLES, AND PAPERS

ADA Report. (1989). Timely statement of The American Dietetic Association: Very low calorie weight loss diets. *Journal of The American Dietetic Association, 89,* 975–976.

This position paper issued by the American Dietetic Association identifies the benefits and risks of very low calorie diets (VLCDs), the appropriate criteria for selecting program participants, and recommendations for careful monitoring and maintenance.

ADA Report. (1990). Position of the American Dietetic Association: very low calorie weight loss diets. *Journal of The American Dietetic Association, 90,* 722–726.

This position paper provides a critique of the very low calorie diet (VLCD) approach to weight control which would be useful for health professionals. This brief paper includes an historical overview, the benefits and risks of VLCDs, criteria for patient selection, appropriate diet protocol and the role of monitoring by the health care team. The position paper stresses the importance of the credentialed, registered dietitian (RD), as someone who has specialized education and professional experience in nutrition. The RD is a nutrition expert, whereas, the title nutritionist has no legal definition that can be used by anyone.

ASPRS Ad Hoc Committee Report. (1987). Five-year updated evaluation of suction-assisted lipectomy. *Plastic Surgical Nursing, 7,* 142–147.

This report concludes that suction lipectomy is a normally safe and effective means of surgically contouring localized fat deposits that do not respond to diet and exercise, when performed by a properly trained surgeon. However, increased peer review and the development of guidelines to govern who is permitted to perform the procedure are needed. Complication rate is less than 10 percent which includes less than ideal results. Variations from the ideal are: waviness, pain, pigmentation, bagginess, edema. In the review of 100,000 cases the committee documented 11 deaths, 9 non-fatal cases of serious morbidity, such as, hematoma, infection, hypovolemic shock, intraperitoneal perforation, and pulmonary embolism.

Barrows, K., & Snook, J. T. (1987). Effect of a high-protein, very low calorie diet on body composition and anthropometric parameters of obese middle-aged women. *American Journal of Clinical Nutrition, 45,* 381–390.

The results of a very low calorie diet (VLCD) (420 cal/day, providing 70 grams of protein), on weight loss and body composition of 15 obese women, aged 30–54 years, are presented. The mean weight loss was 20 kg with a rate of loss of 1.1 kg/week. The researchers found the composition of weight loss was 83 percent fat and 17 percent lean body mass for the study (mean 18 week duration). This is a higher percentage of fat and lower percentage of protein than reported by other researchers. The accuracy of different anthropometric measurement techniques are compared for the obese population. Due to the excessive buoyancy associated with obesity, hydrostatic weighing is difficult. Fat folds in the obese are large and cannot be easily measured by skin-fold calipers and the fat folds are difficult to separate from muscle further increasing errors in measurement. Since body fat tends to shift toward the trunk area with age, a change which is not reflected in skin-fold measurements; and, since the relationship between body density and skin fold thickness is curvilinear, that is, a large increase in skin fold in obese subjects is associated with only a small change in body density, circumference measurements provided the best estimate of body density.

Barrows, K., & Snook, J. T. (1987). Effect of high-protein, very low calorie diet on resting metabolism, thyroid hormones, and energy expenditure of obese middle-aged women. *American Journal of Clinical Nutrition, 45*, 391–398.

The detailed composition of a commercial high-protein, VLCD is provided for this study. The weight loss was greatest during the first 12 weeks. RMR decreased by 21 percent for this group of women, which represents a reduction 355 calories in their resting metabolic rate. A surprise result was that weight loss did not continue during the 5 weeks of refeeding at 800 calories/day as expected. This plateau in weight loss was explained as a combination of noncompliance or increased cheating, the reduced RMR, and the lower energy cost of weight bearing activity. A comparison of methods of energy expenditure revealed that activity records overestimate energy needs of the obese. Included in the article is an explanation of the role of thyroid hormones on protein status and weight loss.

Berg, F. (1993). Health risks of obesity, special report. *Obesity and Health.* North Dakota: Healthy Living Institute.

This timely publication should be of value for a wide audience, professionals and nonprofessionals. Part I reviews the health risks of obesity, the significance of fat distribution, and the effects of aging on risks of obesity. Part II examines the risks of losing weight, effectiveness of various programs, weight cycling, and a section which questions the wisdom of treating obesity when no treatment is effective. Included in this section is an overview of the diet industry; this perspective is particularly enlightening and the information presented is not easily obtained. The publication raises important questions which need to be considered in future research.

Blackburn, G. L., & Bray, G. A. (1985). *Management of obesity by severe caloric restriction.* Littleton, MA: PSG Publishing Company, Inc.

This book is written by the experts in the area of very low calorie diets (VLCDs). Included in the book are chapters which address the following: the composition and effects on metabolic rate and nitrogen balance of VLCDs; effects of weight loss on various clinical diseases such as diabetes mellitus or risks for surgical patients; and expected desirable outcomes of weight loss as well as how to safeguard against undesirable consequences. Extensive research data is provided to document the chapters. From today's perspective the one obvious section missing from this book is long term results. Weight regain and subsequent greater difficulty with repeat weight loss is now recognized as a serious problem associated with VLCDs. However, at the date of publication, the long-term data regarding the problem of weight regain was not available. Regardless of its date, I still recommend this book as a significant contribution to the information available about VLCDs.

Bray, G. A. (1992a). Pathophysiology of obesity. *American Journal of Clinical Nutrition, 55,* 488S–492S.

The author presents an argument for a classification system using BMI (Body Mass Index) to distinguish between varying degrees of obesity without the pejorative connotations of many of the currently used labels, such as, superobese, massive or malignant obesity. This class system would be used to identify those with the greatest health risks and consists of the following: Class 0, 20–25 kg/m^2 (not obese); Class I, 25–30 kg/m^2 (low risk); Class II, 30–35 kg/m^2 (moderate risk); Class III, 35–40 kg/m^2 (high risk); and Class IV, > 40 kg/m^2 (very high risk). He further addresses the importance of fat distribution and progressive obesity as determinants in predicting risk. The classification system could also be used to determine the most appropriate approaches to treatment, i.e., diet versus drug versus surgery.

Bray, G. A. (1992b). Drug treatment of obesity. *American Journal of Clinical Nutrition, 55,* 538S–544S.

This article presents a very interesting perspective regarding the use of drugs for the treatment of obesity. While there are several types of drugs demonstrated to be effective, this approach to obesity treatment has been hampered by professional attitudes and state licensing agencies. First, professionals assume that drug treatment for obesity should be temporary, that is, a cure. A more realistic view would consider obesity as a chronic condition like hypertension with treatment provided continuously. The Food and Drug Administration has labeled these drugs for the "management of obesity as a short term adjunct." Practically, "short term" would have to be 30–50 weeks to achieve significant weight loss in most cases. Consequently, disciplinary action has been taken against physicians who have treated obesity for "more than a few weeks" with appetite suppressant drugs. The drugs being used today do not demonstrate the abuse potential of the amphetamines, and in fact, the amphetamine type drugs are no longer approved for the treatment of obesity. The mechanisms of drug effects range from appetite suppressants, (such as serotonergic agonists like fenfluramine and noradrenergic drugs like phenlypropanolamine), to thermogenic drugs (which increase energy expenditure without necessarily a decrease in intake), digestive enzyme inhibitors, and synthetic foods which are not significantly digested. Regrettably, funding for obesity research seems to be severely limited relative to the need, and the clinical trials which are required in the development of new drugs are extremely expensive.

Brolin, R. E. (1992). Critical analysis of results: Weight loss and quality of data. *American Journal of Clinical Nutrition, 55,* 577S–581S.

This is an interesting article which addresses some of the confusion regarding the definition of successful treatment for the obese population. Obviously to compare the surgical and diet weight loss approaches, there must be a uniform definition of a successful weight loss. Several different definitions of success are used in the medical literature, (1) loss of 25 percent of preweight, (2) loss of 50 percent of the excess weight, (3) loss to within 50 percent of ideal weight. The seriousness of this diversity becomes apparent when morbidly obese groups are compared to superobese. If weight loss alone is the criteria of success the superobese typically lose more weight than the morbidly obese; however, achieving a goal weight within 50 percent of their ideal is accomplished only by a small percentage. However, a much higher percentage of individuals (95%) demonstrated improvement or resolution of medical problems even without a "successful" weight loss. This indicates another problem with the existing definitions for success, failure to assess whether or not an individual benefited from the weight loss. Brolin proposes a classification system for success which considers both weight loss and whether or not the individual demonstrated improvements in medical conditions. This is an extremely important distinction since virtually no superobese individuals achieve their ideal body weight, and yet with seemingly modest weight losses, considerable improvements in the comorbid conditions can occur.

Calles-Escandon, J., & Horton, E. S. (1992). The thermogenic role of exercise in the treatment of morbid obesity: A critical evaluation. *American Journal of Clinical Nutrition, 55,* 533S–537S.

The effects of exercise on energy balance are compared between obese and nonobese individuals. The tacit goal was to determine whether or not defects in thermogenesis exist for obese individuals which may contribute to the development of their obesity. The following are systematically compared between these two groups: resting metabolic rate (RMR); the thermic effect of food; and the thermic effect of exercise. The results of the comparisons between obese and nonobese for each component are dismissed as insignificant. The energy cost of exercise can theoretically range from 5–40 percent of the total energy expenditure. However, the actual number of calories burned during an acute bout of exercise is surprisingly small. The thermic effect of exercise is equated to the post-exercise increase in oxygen consumption (oxygen debt). The increase in intensity of the thermic effect after exercise is proportional to the intensity of the bout of exercise and lasts between 4–24 hours. The magnitude of the increase ranges from 2–15 percent of RMR with 3–5 percent being the most common observation. Since the effect is very short lived and since it is unrealistic and perhaps even dangerous for the obese individual to exercise at a significant intensity for a prolonged period, the thermic effect of exercise is not considered important clinically. Exercise associated with diet restrictions and weight loss has been demonstrated by some to preserve lean body mass and maintain RMR, except during severe caloric restriction such as the VLCDs where exercise was associated with a decrease RMR. The effect of exercise on energy intake seems to differ between obese and nonobese individuals. The nonobese increase their energy intake proportional to the increase in energy output induced by exercise while the obese did not increase their energy intake. The differences in the thermic effect of food was also considered to be quantitatively small, the authors indicated that the reduced thermogenesis eventually would be offset by the increase in RMR due to the increase in lean mass associated with the weight gain. While the authors did not identify any significant differences in thermogenesis between obese and nonobese individuals, they did recognize the health benefits of exercise, such as the increase in insulin sensitivity, and improvements in cardiovascular fitness and blood pressure control.

Deitel, M. (1989). *Surgery for the morbidly obese patient*. Philadelphia: Lea & Febiger.

Deitel presents a diverse and in-depth discussion of surgical approaches for the treatment of obesity. Everything from jejunocolic intestinal bypass surgery to jaw wiring is included. The author provides the rationale behind the evolution of modifications of intestinal surgeries and the logic behind the switch to gastric

procedures. The surgical procedures are thoroughly illustrated, and the results (positive) and consequences of each surgery are explained in detail. The last portion of the book addresses the required follow-up care that is essential and problems that surface after weight loss, such as the need for plastic surgery.

---

deBoer, J. O., van Es, A. J. H., Roovers, L. A., van Raaij, J. M. A., & Hautvast, J. G. A. J. (1986). Adaptation of energy metabolism of overweight women to low-energy intake, studied with whole-body calorimeters. *American Journal of Clinical Nutrition, 44*, 585–595.

This article has become a classic study of energy expenditure and the adaptation during energy restriction in overweight women. Whole-body indirect calorimeter measurements are made before, during and after weight reduction, and after refeeding. The decrease in 24-hour energy expenditure was greater than expected from the change in body weight and body composition which the authors ascribed to (1) reduced diet-induced thermogenesis, (2) loss of body weight and fat-free mass, (3) lower energy costs of physical activities because of this lower weight, and (4) an adaptation, probably metabolic, to low energy intake.

Ersek, R. A., Philips, C., & Schade, K. (1991). Obesity can be treated by suction lipoplasty when combined with other procedures. *Aesthetic Plastic Surgery, 15*, 67–71.

This article presents two dramatic case results and data from 31 women who underwent serial lipectomy for the removal of fat. In one case a 31-year-old woman lost 150 pounds after an intestinal bypass. Four serial suctions removed 4600 cc of subcutaneous fat; additionally, she underwent an abdominal lipectomy, a thigh lift, and the surgical removal of excess fat and skin from her arms and back. The dramatic results are revealed in before and after pictures. The 31 patients averaged 3 suction procedures (range 2–11) for an average total removal of 3869 cc of fat, and an average of 1312 cc per session. After 3 years of follow-up 30 of the original patients could be located. The group had lost additional weight, an average of 15 pounds, and clothing sizes were reduced by 3 or 4 sizes. Exact reasons for the additional weight loss were speculated as improved self-image and motivation to further improve their appearance. The authors strongly advise that less than 2 L of fat be removed per session to avoid potential complications; in their results no serious complications were noted.

Fisler, J. S., & Drenick, E. J. (1987). Starvation and semistarvation diets in the management of obesity. *Annual Review of Nutrition, 7,* 465–484.

This review provides a thorough explanation of the biochemistry of fasting. Nitrogen losses in the obese are approximately 10 g/day (representing 65 grams of protein) on day 1 and decrease to 4 g/day (25 grams of protein) during the third week of a fast. Women typically demonstrate less negative nitrogen balance and achieve balance faster than do men on a VLCD. The composition of the weight loss during the initial two weeks is mostly water, some protein, and approximately 30 percent fat; after one month of fasting, 70 percent of the weight loss is fat. The obese lose less nitrogen/kg than the nonobese, 10g/kg vs. 20g/kg respectively. Additionally, the quality and quantity of protein affect nitrogen status. Most VLCDs now provide 1g/kg high quality protein. Some individuals lose protein at a faster rate than anticipated or desired; unfortunately, plasma protein levels are generally insensitive to the body protein deficit in fasting and do not correlate with nitrogen balance (except perhaps for complement C3) necessitating a nitrogen balance study. Sodium losses during the first 2–6 days can range from 2000–5700 mg/day then falls to < 350 mg/day by day 10. Potassium excretion initially is 1400–1800 mg/day, rises to 2700 mg/day on day 5, then decreases to 400–700 mg/day by one month. The source of the potassium loss is primarily lean tissue. When potassium is supplemented ammoniagenesis is suppressed and nitrogen losses are reduced. Calcium excretion by comparison seems minimal, 350 mg/day at the end of two weeks; however, 1.5 percent of the body's calcium can be lost during a two-month fast. This loss is exaggerated with potassium supplementation, the reduced ammoniagenesis increases the acidosis associated with ketosis and increases the calcium mobilization from bone to buffer the blood. The clinical problems that can occur with fasting are discussed. The appropriate population for this method of weight loss are individuals in the moderate or high risk category, BMI > 30 kg/m^2.

Frankle, R. T., & Yang, M. (1988). *Obesity and weight control: the health professional's guide to understanding and treatment.* New York: Aspen Publishers.

This book is highly recommended for anyone working with obese individuals. Each chapter of the book is written by a recognized expert. Contents include: appetite regulation; etiology of obesity; thermogenesis; metabolic adaptation to starvation; assessment of the obese person; VLCDs; behavior modification; exercise; surgery for obesity; drugs to treat obesity; and chapters which address special issues. Two particularly useful chapters for practitioners deal with eating management and nutrition counseling.

Gelfand, R. A., & Hendler, R. (1989). Effect of nutrient composition on the metabolic response to very low calorie diets: learning more and more about less and less. *Diabetes/Metabolism Reviews, 5,* 17–30.

This is a truly excellent review article on protein status of obese individuals during starvation and while adhering to very low calorie diets. The factors which promote protein sparing or increase protein losses are addressed. The effects of various diet components, an explanation of the composition of energy expenditure and the effects of serum triiodothyronine on body composition are also included. The authors have a very readable writing style for such a complex subject.

Grace, D. M. (1992). Gastric restriction procedures for treating severe obesity. *American Journal of Clinical Nutrition, 55,* 556S–559S.

Criteria for patient selection for gastric surgeries is provided: age 18–50 years, > 45 kg above ideal weight, and have failed a supervised diet. Reversible medical problems increase the indication for surgery as well as abdominal distribution of obesity. The characteristic patient profile is 85 percent female, 15 percent male, and mean age 36. Men seeking treatment tend to be 25 kg heavier than the women. The vertical banded gastroplasty (VGB) resulted in loss of 30 percent of the initial weight at one year for women. Approximately 92 percent of the patients were successful in losing > 25 percent of initial body weight. Follow-up is difficult; at one year 16 percent of patients could not be located; at five years, 71 percent were available. At five years, 41 percent had maintained a loss of > 25 percent of initial weight, 78 percent had lost > 10 percent of body weight. Long-term success is largely determined by diet post surgery and patient motivation.

Halverson, J. D. (1992). Metabolic risk of obesity surgery and long-term follow-up. *American Journal of Clinical Nutrition, 55,* 602S–605S.

Gastric surgeries for the treatment of obesity are in general considered much safer than the intestinal malabsorptive surgeries. However, vitamin deficiencies (B12 and folate) and iron deficiencies occur in a significant percentage of individuals following gastric surgery. In cases where the individual postoperatively experiences protracted vomiting, the complications can be quite severe. The author addresses the complications of jejunoileal bypass surgery and warns of the serious problems associated with the biliopancreatic bypass which is now being performed. He stresses that follow-up be long term and that all weight reduction methods produce a metabolic cost which can lead to critical organ damage, which must be monitored.

Kern, P. A., Ong, J. M., Saffari, B., & Carty, J. (1990). The effects of weight loss on the activity and expression of adipose tissue lipoprotein lipase in very obese humans. *New England Journal of Medicine, 322,* 1053–1059.

This study reveals some interesting and perhaps distressing news regarding the enzymatic changes which occur at the fat cell with weight loss. The subjects in this study lost a mean of 100 pounds the levels of lipoprotein lipase (LPL), the enzyme responsible for fat deposition, were assayed from adipose biopsy samples before and after weight loss had stabilized. The results indicated that heparin-releasable lipoprotein lipase increased in all patients, the immunoreactive protein increased significantly, and the LPL messenger RNA increased. The greater the initial body mass, the greater the increase in LPL with weight loss; although, the increase in LPL was not correlated with the amount of weight lost. This observation suggests a role for LPL in preserving fat mass; theoretically, an increase in LPL would increase fat deposition and increase the difficulty in maintaining weight loss. An additional observation in rodents, but not yet demonstrated in humans, is that increases in LPL increase food consumption. If this is true also for humans, it would provide a mechanism for the so called "set point theory."

Kissebah, A. H., Freedman, D. S., & Peiris, A. N. (1989). Health risks of obesity. *Medical Clinics of North America, 73,* 111–138.

These authors provide an indepth discussion of health risks of obesity with particular emphasis on how body fat distribution is determined and the metabolic effect of upper versus lower body obesity. Another section of this paper critiques obesity research and attempts to explain why there is still so much confusion and lack of consistent results in this area. This section points out many of the flaws in experimental design of published research which a critical reader should consider before comparing research and/ or attempting to draw conclusions.

Kral, J. G. (1987). Malabsorptive procedures in surgical treatment of morbid obesity. *Gastroenterology Clinics of North America, 16,* 293–305.

A review of selected surgical procedures, jejunoileal bypass (JIB), biliointestinal bypass (BIB), ileogastrostomy, duodenoileal bypass (DIB) and gastric bypass (GBP). Major long-term complications for JIB are identified: hepatic and renal failure, enteritis, arthritis, and deficiencies of electrolytes, vitamins, protein, and trace elements. Treatment and/or preventative measures for post jejunoileal patients are: supplementation with a multivitamin, calcium, magnesium, electrolytes; a low carbohydrate, high protein, low oxalate, low fat diet; antianaerobe antibiotics, and antidiarrhea medications. The author warns that the abuse of surgical procedures has led to rampant experimentation without appropriate concerns for long-term complications. Operations for morbid obesity need to be studied for a sufficient length of time to recognize the risks and hazards before being placed in routine use.

Kral, J. G. (1989). Surgical treatment of obesity. *Medical Clinics of North America, 73,* 251–264.

The author describes antiobesity surgery as "behavioral surgery" and explains that surgical approaches incorporate the concept that aversion is easier to condition than reward, and more difficult to extinguish. Overeating after surgical treatment results in a range of symptoms from nausea and vomiting to severe diarrhea and cramps. He describes the rationale behind some of the new modifications of intestinal procedures. For example, the biliointestinal bypass procedure attaches the blind loop of the intestine to the gallbladder. This modification reduces many of the traditional complications caused by stasis in the blind loop and excess bile in the colon. Bile characteristically is reabsorbed in the ileum so that very little reaches the colon, but with typical intestinal procedures all but 4 inches of ileum are bypassed, radically reducing absorption. Kral provides a summary of the results of various procedures; weight loss averages one third of the preoperative weight, or 55–60 percent of the excess weight. Individuals with the intestinal procedures (malabsorptive) have better success achieving and maintaining weight loss. Gastric surgeries may achieve a 92 percent loss of excess weight after 18 months but this diminishes to 63 percent after 72 months. Hence the most significant complication of gastric surgeries is weight regain due to the "soft diet syndrome," ice cream, cake, alcohol, etc. There are many documented health and psychological benefits associated with weight loss experienced

by patients. Patients demonstrate extraordinary gratitude even with only moderate weight loss; however, the author cautions there is the potential for serious side effects even with gastric surgeries and patients must be carefully monitored and adequate supplementation provided.

Kral, J. G., Sjostrom, L. V., & Sullivan, M. B. E. (1992). Assessment of quality of life before and after surgery for severe obesity. *American Journal of Clinical Nutrition, 55,* 611S–614S.

Most of the in-depth information about the severely obese has been obtained from surgical populations. While this population may not be representative of the total severely obese, they have provided valuable information. Psychological disturbances in general are not more prevalent among the obese; many of these individuals have been overweight since childhood and have developed a remarkable ability to adapt to their obesity. The exception to this pattern is depression which is more prevalent. Psychosocial functioning prior to surgery was highly correlated with successful weight reduction post surgery. Weight loss is associated not only with psychological improvements but also with improved physiological functions (improved breathing, sleeping, ambulating, sexual functioning, etc.), and improved economic status.

Kral, J. G. (1992). Overview of surgical techniques for treating obesity. *American Journal of Clinical Nutrition, 55,* 552S–555S.

Kral is one of the established leaders in the area of obesity surgery. He has consistently been a voice of reason against rampant experimentation. This review article gives a brief historical perspective of the various approaches of surgical treatment for obesity. Surgery is justified by extraordinarily high failure rates of nonoperative management, < 5 percent of body weight is lost with diet after one year. Kral stresses the need for meticulous follow-up even for the gastric surgeries. One of the most disappointing complications of gastric surgery is weight regain. The author explains how an individual can sabotage the intent of the surgery by altering their diet toward more high caloric liquids and soft or melting foods.

Kreitzman, S. N. (1992). Factors influencing body composition during very low calorie diets. *American Journal of Clinical Nutrition, 56,* 217S–223S.

This is an excellent article which addresses the factors that can influence the rate and composition of weight loss. The author explains the early fuels used by the body during dieting and leads the reader through the metabolic changes and adaptations which occur as dieting continues. He concludes the VLCDs produce consistent weight loss that is safe and predictable but warns that other weight loss approaches (surgery, magazine diets, behavior modification, etc.) should be closely scrutinized and the composition of weight loss audited. He also discusses the concept of the personal fat ratio (fat to FFM in the excess weight above the core fat-free body). This ratio stays constant through a wide range of body weights and differs from person to person and should be accounted for in studies to prevent bias since it is highly correlated to the composition of weight loss.

Kuczmarski, R. J. (1992). Prevalence of overweight and weight gain in the United States. *American Journal of Clinical Nutrition, 55,* 495S–502S.

Data from the Second National Health and Nutrition Examination Survey (HANES II) and HANES I is presented. Approximately 34 million United States adults are overweight, 19 million women and 15 million men. The data is divided by age, education attainment, income, sex, and race so that distinct patterns emerge. The author provides very detailed statistics of the overweight population in this country.

Lambert, E. V., Hudson, D. A., Bloch, C. E., & Koeslag, J. H. (1991). Metabolic response to localized surgical fat removal in nonobese women. *Aesthetic Plastic Surgery, 15,* 105–110.

The results of localized fat removal were studied in a population of weight stable, non-

obese women to determine the metabolic consequences. The size of the remaining fat cells as determined by biopsy did not change during the 1–2 months postoperative period. The RMR did not change and anthropometric measurements did not change. While 2 months' postoperative is considered short-term follow-up, the results demonstrate that the surgical removal of fat did not result in compensatory changes in fat cell size, or in metabolic efficiency, or in the distribution of fat in weight stable women. The removal of fat from a localized area through lipectomy allowed fat loss without the lean tissue loss associated with dieting and the ultimate reduction in RMR. It should be stressed, however, that these women were weight stable.

Lerman, R. H., & Cave, D. R. (1989). Medical and surgical management of obesity. *Advances of Internal Medicine, 34,* 127–164.

If you are looking for one article to provide an overview of the current approaches to the treatment of obesity, this is it. This is a very informative and thought provoking article. The authors cover everything: definitions of obesity; complications associated with obesity; benefits of exercise; results of behavior modification approaches; effectiveness of drug therapy; VLCDs; results of jejunoileal bypass, gastric reduction procedures, jaw wiring, and gastric bubbles; benefits of weight loss; long-term complications of various methods; attrition rates; and the consequences of excessive weight loss, e.g., the need for plastic surgery to remove excess skin. The article is well organized and the major points thoroughly supported.

Linner, J. H. (1987). Overview of surgical techniques for the treatment of morbid obesity. *Gastroenterology Clinics of North America, 16*(2), 253–272.

This article is an excellent review (complete with diagrams) of surgical procedures performed to induce weight loss. These procedures create a negative energy balance by reducing calories available for fat deposition either through malabsorption by way of a shunt (bypass) or gastric restriction which reduces dietary intake. Procedures highlighted include: jaw wiring, gastric bubbles and balloons, gastric banding, total gastric wrap, small bowel shunts, biliopancreatic shunts incorporating partial gastrectomy, and stomach staplings of many varieties. The emphasis of this article is on gastric surgeries. The Roux-en-Y gastric bypass is identified as the superior weight loss inducing procedure. This particular procedure can: (1) produce dumping syndrome when sweets are consumed; (2) elicit a satiety effect by distention of the jejunum due to food rapidly leaving the stomach; and (3) cause malabsorption due to reduced stimulation and coordination of digestive enzymes and bile with food. Complications of this procedure are not common; however, when ulcers do occur this poses a diagnostic and therapeutic problem. The distal stomach cannot be viewed via fiberoptics and these ulcers do not respond to H2 blockers and ultimately require surgery. A historical and medical perspective is given as the procedures evolved.

Markman, B. S. (1987). Anatomic and metabolic aspects of adipose tissue. *Perspective in Plastic Surgery, 1,* 158–172.

This is a very interesting article which presents an in-depth analysis of adipose tissue. The types of fat (subcutaneous versus deep or intraabdominal) and sites of fat (depots) respond differently to hormones and nutrition. The specific metabolic characteristics are discussed and visual presentations illustrate the anatomic and structural differences in fat depots. Biochemical explanations are given for many of the classically observed phenomena such as the difficulty women have in reducing fat from their hips and thighs.

O'Leary, J. P. Gastrointestinal malabsorptive procedures. (1992). *American Journal of Clinical Nutrition, 55,* 567S–570S.

This article presents the history of surgical procedures for the treatment of obesity with clear diagrams and descriptions of the basic procedures. The first recorded surgical procedure was presented in 1954, which involved surgical resection of the intestinal tract. Surgeons had observed

that patients undergoing massive intestinal resections experienced weight loss which was followed by weight stabilization. The jejunoileal bypass was developed and although it is still being performed in some countries, its use has become restricted in the United States due to the associated long-term complications. Weight loss is accomplished by the severe malabsorption induced by the short circuiting of the small intestine. A later variation of the malabsorptive model is the biliopancreatic diversion in which the stomach is reduced to a small pouch and the intestine is diverted so that digestive enzymes and bile do not mix with the food until the last 50 cm of the small intestine. Thus virtually all of the absorptive area is bypassed. While weight loss is significant, the side effects also seem significant and long-term results are not yet available.

Olson, B. A. (1974). Dietary patterns of post jejunoileal bypass patients. Unpublished data.

Sixteen patients, 15 women and one man, were followed post jejunoileal bypass to determine what effect the surgery imposed on preexisting eating habits. The patient population profile follows: mean age 34; 10/16 were single; race, 10 white, 6 black; onset of obesity, 11 childhood, 5 adult; months post op, 3–33 months. The mean weight loss since surgery ranged from 59–235 pounds; the average weight loss was 112 pounds. The mean weight loss during the first 3 months was 13.7 pounds; 6 months, 7.3; 12 months, 5.3; and 18 months, 3.2 pounds/month. Two patients whose weight plateaued were in their third year post surgery. All patients reduced their intake following surgery. Average pre-surgery intake was estimated at 6000 calories; post surgery, diet records demonstrated an average intake of 2170 calories. Foods most frequently mentioned as problems or avoided included: a commercially available fried chicken, fried food and gravy, spicy foods (i.e., spaghetti and pizza), beans (pinto, navy, lima beans), acid fruits (tomatoes and oranges), and raw vegetables (cabbage, onions, radishes and cauliflower). Seven of the 16 reported that they no longer craved sweets and were satisfied with a "reasonable" serving. This may be due to relief from guilt and failure to lose weight, a conditioned response to severe diarrhea associated with over-indulgence of sweets or fats; or some physiological change in appetite related to the surgery. Other benefits observed included: increased independence, three women moved from their parents home into their own apartments; improved employment status, four who were formerly unemployed obtained jobs; improved health, significant decreases in serum cholesterol and triglycerides, improved joint functions, and increased work capacity and pulmonary function.

Payne, J. H., DeWind, L. T., & Commons, R. R. (1963). Metabolic observations in patients with jejunocolic shunts. *American Journal of Surgery, 108,* 273–289.

This is a classic article in the evolution of intestinal surgery for the treatment of obesity. The jejunocolic procedure was introduced as a temporary measure to induce weight loss; failure to reverse the procedure resulted in very life-threatening consequences and frequently death. Much of the original rationale for a surgical approach to obesity is presented which provides insight which would be missed by reading only current research. Actual case studies are presented which reveal the difficulties of obesity for both the patient and the physician. A before and after picture illustrates the dramatic results but the high failure rate (weight regain with reversal) is also presented.

Prentice, A. M., Jebb, S. A., Goldberg, G. R., Coward, W. A., Murgatroyd, P. R., Poppitt, S. D., & Cole, T. J. (1992). Effects of weight cycling on body composition. *American Journal of Clinical Nutrition, 56,* 209S–216S.

Results of experimental yo-yo dieting are introduced. Eleven moderately obese women (82 kg, BMI 31.4) engaged in three 2-week cycles of (VLCD) weight loss followed by four weeks of free diet. Each subsequent weight loss was less; weight loss was 4.4, 3.3 and 3.0 kg respectively, during each 2-week cycle. Weight regain between cycles was 0.9, 2.2, and 1.8 during the free diet periods. The authors attribute the decreasing weight loss to increased noncompliance

rather than an increased efficiency. Body composition measurements did not reveal a disproportionate loss of lean tissue; however, their estimates of fat loss ranged from 105 percent (which is a good trick) to 67 percent. This variability suggests that there is difficulty accurately measuring body fat in the obese individual and that some methods do not provide accurate information. The authors, however, do not seem concerned with this variability and conclude that there are no adverse effects in terms of body composition with weight cycling. They further support their view with data from a rural Gambian population who routinely go through periods of weight cycling which coincides with food shortages. While the Gambian population did not demonstrate age-related loss of lean mass with repeated cycles of weight gain or loss of 2–3 kgs over the course of a year, this group is not really comparable to an obese population losing significant amounts of weight in short periods of time.

Scott, H. W., Law, D. H., Sandstead, H. H., Lanier, V. C., & Younger, R. K. (1970). Jejunoileal shunt in surgical treatment of morbid obesity. *Annals of Surgery, 171,* 770–782.

The authors provide a definition for morbid obesity which becomes the standard. The Scott procedure utilizes an end-to-end anastomosis. This prevents reflux of food into the bypassed portion of the small intestine resulting in a greater loss of weight relative to the Payne procedure. It was believed that reflux accounted for increased digestion and absorption which reduced the expected weight loss. The authors present details of the patients studied and provide partial explanations for the observed complications associated with this procedure.

Seidell, J. C., Deurenberg, P., & Hautvast, J. G. (1987). Obesity and fat distribution in relation to health—Current insights and recommendations. *World Review of Nutrition and Dietetics, 50,* 57–91.

This review article includes: a discussion of the newest quantitative methods for the determination of body fat (e.g., computed tomography (CT) and nuclear magnetic resonance imaging); descriptions and prevalence of obesity, the risks associated with obesity, fat patterning and associated risks with the abdominal fat distribution (including an impressive CT scan which illustrates differences between subcutaneous and intra-abdominal fat stores). The explanation of the metabolic differences between fat depots (locations of fat) and the types of fat (subcutaneous versus intra-abdominal or deep) was particularly informative. The authors provide a biochemical explanation for the observed differences in risk associated with each type of fat.

Stunkard, A. J., Foster, G. D., & Grossman, R. F. (1986). Surgical treatment of obesity. *Advanced Psychosomatic Medicine, 15,* 140–166.

This is a comprehensive article which addresses the definition of obesity, rationale for surgical approaches, and the risks associated with obesity. A detailed overview of the jejunoileal bypass and patient outcomes with special reference to the psychological improvements with weight loss.

Stunkard, A. J., Stinnett, J., & Smoller, J. W. (1986). Psychological and social aspects of the surgical treatment of obesity. *American Journal of Psychiatry, 143,* 417–429.

This article provides an in-depth discussion of the psychosocial benefits of jejunoileal bypass and gastric surgeries, including a rationale to justify this approach in the treatment of obesity. These authors are particularly effective in revealing the emotional pain associated with being obese and the desperate desire these individuals have to lose weight at any price. The authors present convincing evidence to support the use of radical approaches to facilitate weight loss.

Stunkard, A. J., & Wadden, T. A. (1992). Psychological aspects of severe obesity. *American Journal of Clinical Nutrition, 55,* 524S–532S.

The pain of obesity appears to be as great in 1992 as in 1986; however, today there is more

research to document the extent of the discrimination and humiliation associated with obesity. Additionally, there is more research to document the psychological results of weight loss after surgery. Surprisingly, many obese individuals do not recognize the extent of their suffering until after successful weight loss. Post-obese individuals (47 individuals who lost 45 kg of weight and maintained the loss for at least three years) unanimously chose being deaf, dyslexic, diabetic, or having heart disease rather than being obese again. Ninety-two percent would rather have a leg amputated and 90 percent would rather be blind than return to the obese state. When offered the choice of being normal weight or being a severely obese multimillionaire, all post-obese individuals chose being normal weight. Surgery and successful weight loss result in increased self-esteem, improved marital satisfaction (assuming there were no serious conflicts before surgery), improved body image, and improved eating patterns. The improved psychological functioning after surgery enables patients to leave unhappy marriages which had erroneously been interpreted in an earlier work as surgery for obesity causes divorce.

Sugarman, H. J., Kellum, J. M., Engle, K. M., Wolfe, L., Starkey, J. V., Birkenhauer, R., Fletcher, P., & Sawyer, M. (1992). Gastric bypass for treating severe obesity. *American Journal of Clinical Nutrition, 55,* 560S–566S.

Gastric bypass (GB) reduces the functional stomach to a small pouch which is connected to the jejunum by a 1 cm diameter opening. The remaining portion of the stomach and the duodenum is bypassed. This procedure results in weight loss due to an early sensation of fullness and an aversion to sweets. The direct routing of sweets into the jejunum induces dumping syndrome (symptoms ranging from nausea, vomiting, diarrhea, flushing, dizziness). Of the gastric procedures designed to induce weight loss, the gastric bypass promotes the greatest weight loss, exceeding the vertical banded gastroplasty (VBG). Two years following GB surgery, the weight loss approaches 66 percent of the excess weight, by nine years the loss is approximately

50 percent, indicating some weight regain. Weight loss with the VBG is approximately 43 percent at one year following surgery with gradual weight regain thereafter. The complications of gastric bypass, B-12 deficiency and anemia, are preventable with oral supplementation. The authors conclude that this procedure (GB) is the appropriate surgical approach especially for the obese addicted to sweets. The risks are minimal and the success is acceptable. The more drastic malabsorptive approaches should not be used except in the superobese or obese individuals who have severe health problems complicated by their obesity.

Wadden, T. A., Bartlett, S., Letizia, K. A., Foster, G. D., Stunkard, A. J., & Conill, A. (1992). Relationship of dieting history to resting metabolic rate, body composition, eating behavior, and subsequent weight loss. *American Journal of Clinical Nutrition, 56,* 203S–208S.

This study examined weight loss histories in 50 obese women to determine whether or not there was evidence of increased metabolic efficiency due to repeated efforts to lose weight. These women could be considered yo-yo dieters, reporting a minimum of four major attempts to lose weight before this particular study and weight loss period began. The mean age of the women was 40 years (mean body weight, 102 kg). The data for four dieting periods was obtained from histories. The reported attempts were at the following mean ages: the first, at 20, (mean body weight 71 kg); second, at 24 (body weight, 76 kg); third, at 28, (body weight, 85 kg); and fourth, at 30, (body weight 87 kg). This reflects the typical yo-yo pattern; the women gained back their lost weight and more evidenced by the greater body weight at each successive period. Unfortunately, body composition data was not available to determine if there were shifts in body composition toward increases in the percentage of fat. The authors point out that these women were able to lose weight at an acceptable rate and that when high cyclers (frequent dieters) were compared with low cyclers, there were no significant differences in the weight lost. They do concede that weight cycling was associated with increased body weight and fat and with greater waist and hip circumferences, but question whether the increased weight cycling led to increased weight or increased weight led to increased dieting, weight loss and eventual regain. However, we cannot dismiss the possibility of an increased energy efficiency since two efforts at weight loss were not directly compared. Definitive evidence must include measurements of RMR and body composition in two successive weight loss attempts matched to a control group of noncyclers. Additionally, some consistency must be imposed regarding what constitutes a diet, i.e., the amount of weight lost and/or duration of weight loss period, since these variables undoubtedly have an effect on metabolism.

Chapter 8

Research on Alcohol and Drug Use Among Women: A Review and Update

Tonda L. Hughes

INTRODUCTION

One of the most distinguishing features of recent literature is the increased focus on special populations of women. An increasing number of sources discuss alcohol- and drug-related problems among older women, widows, black and Hispanic women, lesbians, and women who have been sexually or physically abused. In fact, the *Journal of Drug Issues* devoted an entire issue in 1989 to alcohol and drug use among older minority women. Also important are several studies demonstrating women's greater physiologic vulnerability to the effects of alcohol as well as a study of female twins that lends support to the theory of genetic susceptibility to alcoholism.

Although this increased attention is promising, it represents only a beginning of research efforts. Furthermore, the literature reflects a dearth of information on other topics and special populations such as women and HIV, homeless, and native American women.

The annotated sources included in this chapter represent literature reviews, research studies, and the clinical and theoretical perspectives of authors from a number of disciplines. The sources cited do not reflect an exhaustive review but are intended to provide a representative look at current work related to women's use of alcohol and other drugs (AODs). Because of the large number of articles that focus on the effects of women's AOD use on the developing fetus or other pregnancy-related concerns and because this material is often considered in reviews on reproductive health issues, these sources were omitted from this chapter. In addition, although it is recognized that cigarette smoking is a significant women's health concern, studies focusing on this form of substance use are also not included.

SPECIAL POPULATIONS

OLDER WOMEN

Relatively little is known about the patterns and extent of alcohol and other drug problems among older women. Epidemiologic research on AOD use in this population is problematic at best; surveys have tended to produce more reliable estimates for men than women (Rathbone-McCuan, Dyer, & Wartman, 1991).

Many of the indicators used to gauge AOD problems such as those related to work, driving, legal or financial areas are more relevant for younger than

Portions of this chapter were adapted for use in Sullivan, E. (Ed.), *Nursing Care of Substance Abusing Clients*, C. V. Mosby (to be published Fall 1994).

older persons and for men than women. Older persons, particularly women, tend to drink alone and almost exclusively at home, thus limiting problematic interactions with others that are often used as indicators of AOD problems.

In a comparison of their results with those of national surveys conducted between 1971 and 1979, Wilsnack, Wilsnack, and Klassen (1984) found that heavy drinking among women over 50-years-old ranged from 1 percent to 5 percent; however, among women over 65-years-old, most of the surveys reported heavy drinking rates of only 2 percent. More recently, Robbins (1991) analyzed data from the 1985 National Household Survey on Drug Abuse (NHSDA), and found that women 55-years-old and older report drinking to intoxication only one day a year on average compared with an average of seven days in the past year for women 18 to 25 years old.

In general, the literature on older women reflects less concern about alcohol and drug abuse than about drug misuse. Drug misuse among the elderly, while having many causes, is often attributed to noncompliance. However, this term often reflects the perspective of the physician or other health care professional, and not the perspective of the client. As Garrity and Lawson (1989) point out in their study on the patient-physician relationship as it affects compliance in older minority women, physicians who explain the effects of a medication and the reasons for prescribing it find that their patients are more "compliant." Older women, especially older minority women, are frequently hesitant to question physicians or other health care providers. This reluctance is often mistaken for indifference and may result in faulty communication and incorrect use of medications.

Inappropriate prescription of drugs to older women (Glantz & Backenheimer, 1988) for such conditions as anxiety and depression represents another form of drug misuse. An area related to this but in which no studies were found is inappropriate medication of the institutionalized elderly, most of whom are women who receive drugs to control their behavior in overcrowded, understaffed, convalescent homes. Certainly, more research is needed to ascertain the extent of this problem. Drug misuse does not always originate with the individual. "Compliant" women who take the tranquilizers and other drugs prescribed for them may be abusing substances unknowingly and are also at risk for the development of drug dependency.

Although the number of women over 65 years of age who intentionally use illicit drugs is small, abuse of other drugs, particularly alcohol, may become a more significant problem in this age group if AOD-use patterns among younger women do not change. Furthermore, a number of factors associated with aging may place older women at risk for the development of AOD problems. For example, loss of income, bereavement, and chronic illness are ubiquitous aspects of growing old. Isolation, loneliness, depression, and boredom also may contribute to self-medication that can lead to AOD dependency.

Many of the barriers to identification and treatment that exist for all women, such as stigma, associated with AOD problems are more pronounced in the case of the older woman. Therefore, in order to decrease or contain this potentially growing problem, prevention and intervention efforts must address both drug misuse and abuse as well as barriers to help-seeking among this population.

RACIAL AND ETHNIC MINORITIES IN THE UNITED STATES

Alcohol and other drug research has only recently begun to focus on racial and ethnic minorities. Because few longitudinal or national studies have collected data on these groups, estimates of prevalence, patterns, and problems are rough at best. Further research is needed to better understand ethnic and cultural differences in AOD use and abuse and to assist in developing culturally appropriate responses.

Current studies of minority women focus primarily on two groups: blacks and Hispanics. The studies reviewed in this chapter are devoted primarily to elderly women or those who had some other related problem, such as acquired immunodeficiency syndrome (AIDS). No articles were found on native American or Asian American women. The AOD-use patterns of each of these minority groups need further attention as they make up an increasingly larger portion of the female population in the United States.

African American Women Available data on alcohol and drug use patterns and related problems among minority women, like those on minorities in general, are ambiguous. For example, some studies have reported that although African American women are more likely to abstain from alcoholic beverages than are white women, they are more likely than white women to drink heavily when they drink (Clark & Midanik, 1982). However, other national surveys have not found higher rates of heavy drinkers among African American women (Herd, 1988; Wilsnack, Wilsnack, & Klassen, 1984). African American women do appear more likely than women from any other racial/ethnic group to use crack cocaine (1.5% as compared with 1.3% Hispanic women and less than 1% white women) (NIDA, 1990) and are more likely to experience greater alcohol- and drug-related problems. For example, African American women between 15- and 34-years-old have rates of cirrhosis of the liver six times higher than white women of that age group (Leland, 1984, p. 78) and appear to be at increased risk of acquired immunodeficiency syndrome (AIDS) (Lewis & Watters, 1989).

Hispanic Women Most sources report that the majority of Hispanic women abstain from alcohol. However, the rate of abstention varies among different Hispanic groups. For example, Caetano (1984) found that the number of Mexican American women who abstained (71%) was substantially greater than that found among Puerto Rican (45%) and Cuban women living in the United States (48%). Although recent Hispanic immigrant women report the lowest levels of drinking, there is a progressive decline in absten- tion and an increase in moderate drinking in each succeeding generation of women following immigration (Gilbert, 1987). Problems related to drinking among young Hispanic women (e.g., loss of control over consumption, bel- ligerence, health problems) are not substantially fewer than those of men in the same age group whose rate of heavy drinking is eight times higher (USDHHS, 1987). Marianismo, a term used to describe Hispanic women's feelings of responsibility and obligation to care for others, to please men, and to have children, serves as a barrier to help-seeking among Hispanic women.

Native American Women   Native American women are only 1.4 times more likely than white women to be heavy drinkers (Leland, 1984); however, alcohol-related problems (particularly cirrhosis), are proportionately higher than for whites and other ethnic groups. For example, 31 percent of native American female adolescents report alcohol problems compared with 25 per- cent of white female adolescent drinkers (USDHHS, 1988). In addition, na- tive American women have rates of cirrhosis more than 36 times the rate for white women (Leland, 1984).

Asian Women   Asian-Americans' image as a hard working, highly edu- cated, "model minority" contributes to shame and denial that act as barri- ers to the identification and treatment of AOD abuse in this population, making it difficult to estimate the prevalence of problems. This is particu- larly true for Asian-American women who are socialized to defer to men, elders, and others in positions of authority. Asian-American women of all ethnic groups (Japanese, Chinese, Korean, Filipino, and Vietnamese) ap- pear more likely than women from all other racial/ethnic groups to abstain from the use of alcohol (USDHHS, 1990). However, as with Hispanic women, the amount and frequency of drinking among this population of women may increase with acculturation.

Whether AOD-related problems are grounded in cultural attitudes or have a significant physiologic basis should be ascertained. Are some groups more susceptible than others to the effects of alcohol? Do ethnic and racial minor- ity women drink excessively to escape reality, depressed socioeconomic con- ditions, poor living conditions and discrimination? Such information must be gathered in order to better understand the factors that contribute to use and to plan more effective outreach, prevention and treatment programs.

LESBIANS

Another heretofore neglected population of women who are beginning to receive more attention from researchers are lesbians. Although studies on this population have been few and methodologically flawed (Glaus, 1989), most sources report that lesbians have a greater incidence of drug and alcohol use. This perception is perpetuated in part, perhaps, because lesbians are thought to rely on bars more than their heterosexual counterparts for socialization.

In a study of homosexuals in Chicago that included 748 lesbians, McKirnan and Peterson (1989) found that gay women and men, although less likely than women and men in the general population to abstain from AODs, were also less likely to be heavy users of these substances. However, like other minority groups, gay men and women who do drink or use other drugs reported higher levels of problems associated with that use than members of the general population.

An additional finding of interest was that the gay women and men in this study were psychologically healthy and socially well-integrated. This finding was also reported by Deevey (1990) who studied older lesbians. This finding is particularly important considering that gay women and men often experience high levels of harassment and discrimination, factors thought to contribute to both AOD use and mental health problems.

According to Weathers (cited in Schilit, Lie, & Montagne, 1990) the unresponsiveness of alcohol service agencies to lesbian clients is one possible reason for the higher rate of alcohol abuse among lesbians. Weathers reports that most agencies responding to a survey reported judgmental and restrictive attitudes toward lesbians and regarded lesbianism as pathological. She describes three major types of negative interactions characterizing the lesbian alcoholic's experience with alcoholism agencies: (1) refusal of services if the women's sexual identity is known or suspected; (2) provision of services on a limited basis or with attitudes not conducive to support, growth, self-disclosure, or the maintenance of sobriety; and (3) provision of services directed toward isolating and "curing" lesbianism as the primary problem, with relatively little or no attention given to the alcoholism.

As with other areas of research on homosexuals and with other minority groups, funding is limited. Furthermore, with regard to research or clinical work with homosexuals, the researcher or clinician risks being labeled "gay" if interested in this population. Considering that homosexuals account for at least 10 percent of the United States population and that lesbians make up roughly half of this group, it behooves researchers and clinicians to pay more attention to this special population (Lewis & Jordon, 1989).

ADOLESCENT AND YOUNG WOMEN

Although national surveys of high school seniors report a decline in overall use of illicit drugs, it is estimated that American teens have the highest levels of illicit drug use among their age peers in any developed country in the world (Johnson, O'Malley, & Bachman, 1989).

In a report of 1990 findings, Johnson, O'Malley, and Bachman (1991) report the following prevalence rates for the most commonly used drugs among high school students: marijuana 27 percent, stimulants 9 percent, cocaine 5 percent, and tranquilizers 3.5 percent. Rates of use for each of these drugs has declined from the peak levels reached in the 1970s. Consumption of alcohol among most age groups has also declined; however, significant numbers of young women and men continue to drink, and many drink heavily. For example, 32 percent of high school students and 41 percent of college students report drinking 5 or more drinks in a row on at least one occasion in the two-week period prior to the survey (Johnson, O'Malley, & Bachman, 1991).

Young men report higher prevalence rates and levels of use for alcohol and almost all other drugs. Exceptions are stimulants, sedatives and tranquilizers, which young women use at the same, or higher, levels. There is some evidence to indicate that gender differences in alcohol use, particularly among the youngest age groups, may be narrowing (Grant, Harford, Chou, Pickering, Dawson, Stinson, & Noble, 1991; Windle, 1991). In addition, young women in high school and college are more likely than their male counterparts to be daily smokers.

Most of the studies reviewed in this chapter that focus on alcohol or drug use among adolescent and young women examined either the relationship of AOD use and sexual abuse or the relationship between AOD use and eating disorders. The limited attention to this population is surprising given all the national attention being paid to illicit drug use among the young. The highly visible "war on drugs" and "just say no" movements should be studied for their differential effectiveness in preventing drug abuse among young women and men. In particular, effectiveness of these and other prevention efforts on curtailing smoking and amphetamine use among young women should be explored. Perhaps different strategies, including those aimed at teaching healthier methods of weight control would be more effective for adolescent and young women.

HOMELESS WOMEN

Despite the fact that an increasing proportion of the homeless are women and children few studies have focused on this population. AOD abuse is the most common health problem of homeless adults (Weinreb & Bassuk, 1990). Whereas homeless mothers were previously thought to be less likely to abuse AODs than women without children, anecdotal reports from service providers suggest that an increasing number of women with children are abusing AODs, particularly alcohol and crack cocaine. A recent study conducted in Baltimore found that 67 percent of homeless women have an AOD-abuse problem (Breakey, Fischer, Kramer, et al., 1989). It was not clear how many of these women had children. Abuse of AODs can not only precipitate or prolong homelessness but can contribute to its adverse course and consequences. Homeless women who drink heavily are especially susceptible to certain health problems such as trauma (including physical and sexual abuse), thermoregulatory disorders (e.g., frostbite, gangrene), peripheral vascular disorders, and tuberculosis.

PROBLEMS RELATED TO ALCOHOL AND DRUG USE

PHYSICAL/SEXUAL ABUSE AND DRUG/ALCOHOL

Anecdotal and clinical reports, as well as research literature are increasingly documenting the relationships between AOD use and interpersonal violence. Three major relationships have been identified: (1) men who abuse AODs perpetuate violence against women and children; (2) women who have histories of current or past sexual or physical abuse are at higher risk for AOD abuse and addiction; and (3) women who abuse or are addicted to AODs are more vulnerable to physical abuse and sexual assault.

A recent editorial in the Journal of the American Medical Association cautions, however, that care should be taken when describing the relationship between interpersonal violence and AOD abuse (Randall, 1991) to avoid perpetuating the belief that alcohol causes violent behavior. Randall (1991) states that "each [problem] stems from different underlying factors and although many families are dually affected by both behaviors, the strength of a correlation between the two is still debated" (p. 461).

Miller, Downs, and Gondoli (1989) point out that most studies exploring the relationship between violence and AOD abuse have focused on male perpetrators' use of alcohol or other drugs. However, as a number of studies reviewed in this chapter illustrate, the relationship between violence and AOD abuse is complex and multifaceted.

Researchers studying AOD abuse among women must be aware of the high incidence of violence in these women's histories just as clinicians who work with abused women must consider the possibility of co-existing AOD-related problems.

AIDS AND AOD ABUSE

AOD abuse and AIDS are linked directly or indirectly in several important ways. The most widely recognized link has to do with HIV transmission through exchange of infected blood or blood products, most frequently among intravenous drug users. A second link has to do with the fact that

AODs can impair normal immune responses that protect the body from disease. Researchers believe that drugs, particularly morphine, cocaine, and heroin act as "cofactors" that can trigger the development of AIDS (NIDA Notes, 1992, p. 9). This hypothesis would help to explain why it takes less time for a drug abuser than a nondrug abuser to develop AIDS after becoming HIV positive. Finally, use of AODs is associated with other high-risk behaviors. For example, use of AODs reduces sexual inhibition and increases the likelihood of unprotected sexual acitivity. High-risk sexual activity includes vaginal or anal intercourse without a condom as well as other sexual behaviors that allow exchange of blood, semen, or other body fluids. Female addicts often trade sex for drugs or for the money to buy drugs. Both the number of sexual partners and the frequency of engaging in the above sexual behaviors increase the risk of exposure to HIV. Although there is some indication that HIV infection levels are becoming more stable, high rates of risk behaviors are still being reported in many areas across the country (Greenhouse, 1992).

Current research indicates that minorities are disproportionately affected by HIV and AIDS. Although African Americans make up only 12 percent of the total United States population, they account for 27 percent-to-28 percent of AIDS cases. Hispanics, who are 8 percent of the population, represent 16 percent of the people who have AIDS in the United States. Among Asian Americans, who are not overrepresented in total AIDS cases, rates of new AIDS cases increased by 150 percent between 1985 and 1988 (Sobel, 1991).

Most women who are HIV-positive or have AIDS acquire the infection through intravenous drug use or sexual contact with men who are intravenous drug users. The racial distribution of seropositive female IV drug users also reflects the disproportionate number of minority women who are affected by HIV. A study done by Schoenbaum, et al. (cited in Cohen, Hauer & Wofsy, 1989) of methadone clients in New York found that almost 75 percent of the female clients were African American or Hispanic and that nonwhite men and women had a higher antibody prevalence rate than white men and women. Further, Mondanaro (1989) cites a Centers for Disease Control (CDC) spokesperson as stating that the cumulative incidence of AIDS in African American and Hispanic women is more than ten times that found in white women (p. 78).

USE OF COCAINE

Although treatment providers report an increase in the number of women who are addicted to cocaine, this clinical impression has not been validated in recent epidemiologic studies. Like alcohol use, cocaine use has always been lower among women than men. The use of cocaine increased in the late 1970s and early 1980s but leveled off in the mid 1980s and began to decline in 1987. Among younger adults the decline was sharper for men than for women. However, for young adults 23 to 26 years old, the decline for men and women was approximately equal. In 1987, 19 percent of men and 13 percent of women who had been out of high school for one-to-ten years reported using cocaine in the previous year. Older men and women reported lower rates of use (USDHHS, 1988). Women who do use cocaine appear less likely than men to progress to regular use (Kandel, Murphey, & Karus, 1985). Apart from studies that focus on the effects of cocaine on the fetus or neonate, little attention has been given to women's use of cocaine. In a book on chemically dependent women, Mondanaro (1989) provides a brief overview of the little information we have on cocaine and women.

PHYSIOLOGIC CONSEQUENCES

Also noteworthy in recent years is the increasing number of studies demonstrating that women are more susceptible to the physiologic effects of alcohol than are men. Current explanations of women's greater physiologic vulnerability relate to the following: (1) lower total body water content; (2) diminished activity of gastric alcohol dehydrogenase (the primary enzyme involved in the metabolism of alcohol); and (3) fluctuations in gonadal hormone levels during the menstrual cycle.

Frezza et al. (1990) were among the first to demonstrate conclusively that under certain conditions women do not metabolize alcohol as efficiently as men and that this ability is almost completely impaired in alcoholic women. When moderate amounts of alcohol are ingested following a standard meal, women metabolize significantly less of the alcohol in the stomach than do men. Thus, more alcohol reaches the circulatory system and must be filtered through the hepatic portal system. This highly significant study has profound implications for prevention and treatment of alcoholism among women.

Mishra, Sharma, Potter and Mezey (1989) also attempted to shed light on the problem of women's greater vulnerability to alcohol. They studied nine pairs of male/female siblings to compare rates of ethanol elimination. They did find that women had higher mean rates of ethanol elimination but failed to demonstrate higher plasma acetate (an ethanol metabolite) levels in women.

In a third study exploring physiologic differences, Rabinovitz, Van Theil, Dindzans, & Gavaler (1989), studied men and women with advanced liver disease to determine whether the prevalence of gastrointestinal disorders was associated with gender. The only difference found was a higher incidence of gastric ulcer in women, which the authors attributed to women's greater proportion of body fat. That is, because alcohol does not distribute to fat, women who consume alcohol have higher systemic blood ethanol levels. This increased blood level may induce gastric acid hypersecretion, with the resultant development of gastric ulcer.

Exactly how these findings are related is not clear. Much more research is needed before the puzzle of women's greater vulnerability to alcohol is fully understood.

IMPLICATIONS FOR RESEARCH AND TREATMENT

A number of authors have criticized treatment programs for their lack of responsiveness to women's special needs (Mandel, Schulman, & Monterio, 1979; Marsh & Miller, 1985). This lack of responsiveness can, at least in part, be attributed to the relative dearth of research on chemically dependent women (Hughes, 1990).

According to data cited in a recent issue of *Alcohol Alert* (Alcohol and Women, 1990), the proportion of female alcoholics to male alcoholics in treatment is similar to the proportion of female alcoholics to male alcoholics generally (30% women to 70% men). These data are used to explain the considerably lower numbers of women in treatment, a fact frequently noted in the literature. An additional factor used to explain this difference is the fact that women more commonly seek treatment from other than traditional alcohol programs—including sources such as psychiatric or mental health counseling and personal physicians.

The review also summarizes some of the gender differences in barriers and motivators to seeking treatment. For example, whereas women are more likely to seek treatment because of family problems, men more often enter treatment via the criminal justice system or through employee assistance programs. Lack of child care is one of the most frequently reported barriers to treatment for alcoholic women.

More research that explores the differences in treatment needs of women and men as well as those of various ethnic, racial, and other minority groups of women is needed. As Caetano (1984) points out, drug and alcohol treatment must be culturally appropriate to be effective. Research focusing on factors that influence help seeking, treatment entry, and treatment outcome is greatly needed. Determining how and under what circumstances women seek help for alcohol and other drug problems, as well as which treatment models and program services are most beneficial for specific populations of women remains a critically important area of study.

REFERENCES

ADAMHA News (1992). Morphine, cocaine, heroin speed HIV growth. *ADAMHA News, Alcohol, Drug Abuse, and Mental Health Administration, 18*(2), 9, 19.

Alcohol and women (1990). *Alcohol Alert*. National Institute on Alcohol Abuse and Alcoholism. No. 10, USDHHS, Rockville, MD: Alcohol, Drug Abuse and Mental Health Administration.

Breakey, W., Fischer, P., Kramer, M., Nestadt, G., Romanoski, A., Ross, A., Royall, R., & Stine, O. (1989). Health and mental health problems of homeless men and women in Baltimore. *Journal of the American Medical Association, 262*, 1352–1357.

Caetano, R. (1984). Drinking patterns and alcohol problems in a national sample of U.S. Hispanics. In *Alcohol use among U.S. ethnic minorities.* National Institute on Drug Abuse. Research Monograph No. 18. DHHS Pub. No. (ADM)87-1435.

Cohen, J. B., Hauer, L. B., & Wofsy, C. B. (1989). Women and IV drugs: Parenteral and heterosexual transmission of human immunodeficiency virus. *Journal of Drug Issues, 19*(1), 39–56.

Deevey, S. (1990). Older lesbian women: An invisible minority. *Journal of Gerontological Nursing, 16*(5), 35–39.

Fillmore, K. M. (1985). When angels fall: Women's drinking as a cultural preoccupation and as reality. In S. C. Wilsnack & L. J. Beckman (Eds.) *Alcohol problems in women: Antecedents, consequences, and interventions.* New York: Guilford Press.

Frezza, M., DiPadova, C., Pozzato, G., Terpin, M., Baraona, E., & Lieber, C. S. (1990). High blood alcohol levels in women: The role of decreased gastric alcohol dehydrogenase activity and first-pass metabolism. *The New England Journal of Medicine, 322*(2), 95–100.

Garrity, T. F., & Lawson, E. J. (1989). Patient-physician communication as a determinant of medication misuse in older minority women. *Journal of Drug Issues, 19*(2), 245–259.

Gilbert, M. J. (1987). Alcohol consumption patterns of immigrant and later generation Mexican American women. *Hispanic Journal of Behavioral Sciences, 9*(3), 299–313.

Glantz, M. D., & Backenheimer, M. S. (1988). Substance abuse among elderly women. *Clinical Gerontologist, 8*(1), 3–26.

Glaus, K. O. (1989). Alcoholism, chemical dependency, and the lesbian client. *Women and Therapy, 8*(1/2), 131–145.

Grant, B. R., Harford, T. C., Chou, P., Pickering, R., Dawson, D., Stinson, F., & Noble, J. (1991). Epidemologic Bulletin No. 27. Prevalence of DSM-III-R alcohol abuse and dependence: United States, 1988. *Alcohol Health and Research World, 15*(1), 91–96.

Greenhouse, C. M. (1992). IV drug users may stop risky behavior when AIDS hits home. *NIDA Notes, National Institute on Drug Abuse, 7*(1), 18–19.

Harrison, P. A. (1989). Women in treatment: Changing over time. *International Journal of the Addictions, 24*(7), 655–673.

Herd, D. (1988). Drinking by black and white women: Results from a national survey. *Social Problems, 35*(5), 493–505.

Hughes, T. L. (1990). Evaluating research on chemical dependency among women: A women's health perspective. *Family & Community Health, 13*(3), 35–46.

Johnson, L. D., O'Malley, P. M., & Bachman, J. G. (1991). *Drug use among American high school seniors, college students and young adults, 1975–1990.* DHHS Pub. No. (ADM)91-1813, Rockville, MD: ADAMHA.

Johnson, L. D., O'Malley, P. M., & Bachman, J. G. (1988). *Illicit drug use, smoking and drinking by America's high school students, college students, and young adults: 1975–1987.* DHHS Pub. No. (ADM)89-1602, Rockville, MD: ADAMHA.

Kandel, D. B., Murphey, D., & Karus, D. (1985). Cocaine use in America: Epidemiologic and clinical perspectives. National Institute on Drug Abuse. Research Monograph No. 61. Pub. No. (ADM)87-1414.

Leland, J. (1984). Alcohol use and abuse in ethnic minority women. In S. C. Wilsnack & L. J. Beckman (Eds.), *Alcohol problems in women.* New York: The Guilford Press.

Lewis, G. R., & Jordon, S. M. (1989). Treatment of the gay or lesbian alcoholic. In G. Lawson & A. W. Lawson (Eds.), *Alcoholism and substance abuse in special populations.* Rockville, MD: Aspen.

Lewis, D. K., & Watters, J. K., (1989). Human immunodeficiency virus seroprevalence in female intravenous drug users: The puzzle of black women's risk. *Social Science Medicine, 29*(9), 1071–1076.

Mandel, L., Schulman, J., & Monteiro, R. (1979). A feminist approach to the treatment of drug-abusing women in a coed therapeutic community. *International Journal of the Addictions, 14*, 589–597.

Marsh, J. C., & Miller, N. A. (1985). Female clients in substance abuse treatment. *The International Journal of the Addictions, 20*, 995–1019.

McKirnan, D. J., & Peterson, P. L. (1989). Psychosocial and cultural factors in alcohol and drug abuse: An analysis of a homosexual community. *Addictive Behaviors, 14*, 555–563.

Miller, B. A., Downs, W. R., & Gondoli, D. M. (1989). Spousal violence among alcoholic women as compared to a random household sample of women. *Journal of Studies on Alcohol, 50*(6), 533–540.

Mishra, L., Sharma, S., Potter, J. J., & Mezey, E. (1989). More rapid elimination of alcohol in women as compared to their male siblings. *Alcoholism: Clinical and Experimental Research, 13*(6):752–754.

Mondanaro, J. (1989). *Chemically dependent women: Assessment and treatment.* Lexington, Massachusetts: Lexington Books.

National Institute on Drug Abuse (NIDA). (1990). *National Household Survey on Drug Abuse: Main Findings* (DHHS Publication No. ADM 90-1682). Rockville, MD: NIDA.

Sobel, K. H. (1991). NIDA Conferences convey information about AIDS prevention to minorities. *NIDA Notes, National Institute on Drug Abuse, 6*(3), 5–7.

Rabinovitz, M., Van Thiel, D. H., Dindzans, V., & Gavaler, J. S. (1989). Endoscopic findings in alcoholic liver disease: Does gender make a difference? *Alcohol, 6,* 465–468.

Randall, T. (1991). (Editorial). Domestic violence: The role of alcohol (reply). *Journal of the American Medical Association, 265*(4), 460–461.

Rathbone-McCuan, E., Dyer, L., & Wartman, J. (1991). Double jeopardy: Chemical dependence in older women. In N. Van Den Bergh (Ed.) *Feminist perspectives on addictions,* New York: Springer Publishing Company.

Robbins, C. (1991). Social roles and alcohol abuse among older men and women. *Family & Community Health, 13*(4), 49–62.

Schilit, R. Lie, G., & Montagne, M. (1990). Substance abuse as a correlate of violence in intimate lesbian relationships. *Journal of Homosexuality, 19*(3), 51–65.

U.S. Department of Health and Human Services (1990). *Alcohol and health* (National Institute on Alcohol Abuse and Alcoholism Publication No. ADM 281-88-0002). Washington, DC: United States Government Printing Office.

U.S. Department of Health and Human Services (1988). *National Institute on Drug Abuse, National Household Survey on Drug Abuse: Main findings 1985.* National Institute on Drug Abuse. Pub. No. (ADM)88-1586.

U.S. Department of Health and Human Services (1987). *Alcohol and health.* National Institute on Alcohol Abuse and Alcoholism. Pub. No. (ADM)87-1519.

Weinreb, L. F., & Bassuk, E. L. (1990). Substance abuse: A growing problem among homeless families. *Family & Community Health, 13*(1), 55–64.

Wilsnack, S. C., Wilsnack, R. W., & Klassen, A. D. (1985). Drinking and drinking problems among women in a U.S. national survey. *Alcohol Health and Research World, 9,* 3–13.

Windle, M. (1991). Alcohol use and abuse: Some findings from the National Adolescent Student Health Survey. *Alcohol Health and Research World, 15*(1), 5–10.

—————————⟫●⟪—————————

BOOKS AND ARTICLES

Alcohol and women (1990). *Alcohol Alert.* National Institute on Alcohol Abuse and Alcoholism. No. 10, USDHHS, Rockville, MD: Alcohol, Drug Abuse and Mental Health Administration.

This issue of *Alcohol Alert,* a series published to update alcohol research and treatment professionals on important issues related to alcohol abuse and alcoholism, focuses on the topic of alcohol and women. Recent research findings are reviewed to describe women's drinking patterns including those related to marital status and ethnic and racial group status. Women's greater physiologic vulnerability is explained by three possible mechanisms: (1) lower total body water content; (2) diminished activity of gastric alcohol dehydrogenase (the primary enzyme involved in the metabolism of alcohol); and (3) fluctuations in gonadal hormone levels during the menstrual cycle. The potential association between drinking and breast cancer risk is also discussed. Although findings are contradictory, some evidence exists to suggest that the consumption of one or more ounces of absolute alcohol daily can increase the risk of developing breast cancer.

Some of the salient treatment issues for female alcoholics are described. According to data cited in the review, the proportion of female alcoholics to male alcoholics in treatment (25% women to 75% men) is similar to the proportion of female alcoholics to male alcoholics generally (30% women to 70% men). These data are used to explain the considerably lower numbers of women in treatment, a fact frequently noted in the literature. An additional factor used to explain this difference is the fact that women more commonly seek treatment from other than traditional alcohol programs—including sources such as psychiatric or mental health counseling and personal physicians.

Similarly, women are believed to experience motivators and barriers to seeking treatment that are different than mens'. Whereas women are more likely to seek treatment because of family problems, men more often enter treatment via the criminal justice system or through employee assistance programs. Lack of child care is one of the most frequently reported barriers to treatment for alcoholic women.

The issue ends with a brief review of findings related to treatment outcomes. In one study of clients who completed treatment, for example, women had slightly higher rates of abstinence than men. Women had higher rates of abstinence if treated in a medically oriented facility, whereas men did better in a peer-group oriented facility. Treatment outcome was better for women treated in a facility with a smaller proportion of female clients and better for men in a facility with a larger proportion of female clients. The point is made that whether or not women should have separate treatment is an important one; however, supporting evidence is as yet insufficient to conclude what works better.

———————————————————

Allen, K. (1992). Establishing reliability of the Community Oriented Program Environment Scale on Chemically Dependent black females. *The International Journal of the Addictions, 27*(1), 93–106.

Just as instruments developed for and tested with men cannot be assumed to be valid and reliable indicators of women's experiences, neither can instruments tested with one ethnic or racial group be expected to provide valid and reliable outcomes for other racial/ethnic groups. This article reports the outcomes of a study to assess the reliability of the Community Oriented Program Environment Scale (COPES) when used with black women.

A nonprobability sample of 30 black women from three inpatient programs was selected to respond to the questionnaires. Although reliability of the overall COPES was .64, alpha scores for the subscales were generally lower—ranging from .38 to .64.

The author concludes that although the COPES is a widely used instrument, its usefulness with all subsamples of chemically dependent clients cannot be assumed.

Bepko, C. (Ed.), (1991). *Feminism and addiction.* New York: The Haworth Press, Inc.

This book, whose editor is a social worker in family practice, includes a collection of twelve chapters focusing on current work in the area of family therapy and addictions. A number of the authors' works are based on constructivist theory, which according to the editor, provide a philosophical framework for treatment that allows for the interactive recreation of experience that is collaborative and internal rather than external, hierarchical, and imposed (p. 2).

The book is divided into three parts. Part One: Theory, Research and Social Issues: Exploring Addictions in Context includes chapters on cocaine-using mothers and their babies, gender socialization and women's addictions, codependency, and feminist critique of the twelve steps. Part Two: Feminist Approaches to Training and Treatment of the Addictions includes chapters on couples therapy and treatment of lesbians and their families as well as the application of feminist principles in training clinicians to work in the field of substance abuse. Part Three: Special Issues in Treatment and Recovery: Reflections and Interventions focuses primarily on the concept of shame (viewed by the author as an important cause and result of addiction), and on the concept of codependency from both a male and female perspective.

The editor states that feminist analysis examines problems within the context of power and that addiction is "a disordered power arrangement embedded in gender" (p. 1). This statement appears representative of the overall perspective of the volume, i.e., the view of the etiology of addiction as being largely sociocultural. In this sense it is intended to stimulate further examination of conceptions of both gender and addiction.

Bergman, B., Larsson, G., Brismar, B., & Klang, M. (1989). Battered wives and female alcoholics: A comparative social and psychiatric study. *Journal of Advanced Nursing, 14,* 727–734.

Domestic violence is one of the most pervasive and serious of women's health problems. It is estimated that roughly one-third of all married women are battered by their spouses at some time during marriage. High levels of violence between dating, engaged, and cohabiting couples have also been reported. Furthermore, some investigators have found that women who drink heavily or are alcohol dependent are at increased risk of physical abuse.

These authors sought to explore the relationship between family violence and alcoholism. Forty-nine women seeking hospital treatment for injuries sustained during battering by spouses or male partners were compared with 49 alcoholic women and a control group consisting of 49 women hospitalized for injuries sustained in accidents. The control group was matched with the alcoholic and battered women on the basis of age and nationality. Women in each of the groups were interviewed using a structured questionnaire. Responses to questions concerning childhood experiences, current social circumstances, and experiences with battering were elicited. Symptoms of alcoholism and level of alcohol consumption were assessed using questions from CAGE and the Ten Question Drinking History. CAGE is a four-question instrument used to assess drinking problems. The acronym is derived from the four questions: (1) Have you ever tried to Cut down on your drinking?; (2) Have you ever become Angry or Annoyed when questioned about your drinking?; (3) Have you ever felt Guilty about your drinking?; (4) Have you ever needed an Eye opener in the morning (a drink when you first get up in the morning)? Psychiatric symptoms, including depression, were also assessed.

Two-thirds of the alcoholic women reported battering and the majority demonstrated patterns of severe, prolonged physical abuse very similar to those of the women seeking treatment for battering injuries. The two groups of battered women were also similar in that many of them had experienced more violence during their childhoods, cohabited with more men, and demonstrated a higher frequency of depressive symptoms than the control group. Battered women in each of the three groups had similar childhood environments and had cohabited with approximately the same number of men. What differentiated the battered women in the accident group from the other two groups of battered women in this study was the absence of depression and other psychiatric symptoms as well as the absence of serious alcohol or drug abuse problems. The authors conclude that being mentally healthy is of crucial importance if women are to break away from abusive relationships.

Blankfield, A. (1989). Grief, alcohol dependence and women. *Drug and Alcohol Dependence, 24,* 45–49.

This article was based on a pilot survey of 37 widows who had not remarried. These women formed part of a population of 221 Australian-born women admitted to an alcohol treatment unit. The widowed population was compared with their single, married, divorced, or never-married counterparts ($n = 85$) to determine whether differences existed in terms of when they became alcohol-dependent.

The results of this survey are unclear. The widows reported less excessive drinking in close relatives and more excessive drinking in their deceased spouses compared with the nonwidowed women. Alcohol dependence may exist before or develop after widowhood, but this study suggests that social isolation may be an important factor in both alcoholic and nonalcoholic widows who adapt less well. In addition, the authors suggest that the death of an alcoholic spouse could be more important than family history in triggering alcohol dependency in some widows or social isolation in others. They acknowledge that the relationship among the factors of loneliness, grief, and alcohol is still unclear. The potential for widows of alcoholics to develop abnormal grief reactions because of ambivalent feelings toward their spouses requires further exploration through prospective studies.

Blankfield, A. (1989). Female alcoholics. 1. Alcohol dependence and problems associated with prescribed psychotropic drug use. *Acta Psychiatr Scand, 79,* 355–362.

Blankfield reports the results of a study exploring the use of psychotropic drugs among a group of Australian alcohol-dependent women. Information about both licit and illicit drugs was collected from clients admitted to a particular treatment center over a 12-year period. The findings support previous reports of psychotropic drug use among alcoholic women. That is, significantly more alcoholic women (70%) than alcoholic men (40%) reported use of psychotropic drugs. Furthermore, women who reported psychotropic drug use were more likely to have attempted suicide (26% versus 18%), particularly when the attempt involved overdose (23% versus 12%). These findings reinforce the need for physicians to use increased caution when prescribing psychotropic drugs, particularly for women.

Blume, S. B. (1990). Chemical dependency in women: Important issues. *American Journal of Drug and Alcohol Abuse, 16,* 297–307.

This overview begins with an historical perspective on societal attitudes toward women's drinking. In a discussion of why women are underrepresented in treatment, Blume emphasizes the role of inadequate or male-biased methods of case-finding as social and cultural barriers. Blume reviews some of the recent findings concerning gender differences in the consequences of drinking and discusses psychological conditions that commonly co-exist with substance abuse. As have many other authors, Blume concludes that the stigma associated with problem drinking among women serves as a potent barrier to help seeking and contributes to the intense shame and guilt experienced by most alcoholic women. Blume concludes with a discussion of the influence of social and cultural values on the development and treatment of alcohol problems in women.

Bollerud, K. (1990). A model for the treatment of trauma-related syndromes among chemically dependent inpatient women. *Journal of Substance Abuse Treatment, 7,* 83–87.

This paper describes a protocol that has been developed and implemented in a 140-bed addiction treatment facility to identify and plan specialized adjunctive treatment for patients who have been victimized. The program consists of patient education regarding violence against women and its psychologic impact, brief individual psychotherapy, group psychotherapy, attendance at alcoholics anonymous (AA), and a 12-week outpatient after-care group. The author describes each of these components and provides clinical examples to illustrate their effectiveness.

Cohen, J. B., Hauer, L. B., & Wofsy, C. B. (1989). Women and IV drugs: Parenteral and heterosexual transmission of human immunodeficiency virus. *Journal of Drug Issues, 19*(1), 39–56.

The authors discuss the characteristics of women with HIV infection, ARC, and AIDS who are also intravenous drug users (IVDUs) The article also examines the characteristics of female sexual partners of male IVDUs with HIV infection or AIDS. The specific subgroups of female IVDUs have often been ignored because most studies examine IVDUs without regard to gender. The authors contend that this approach ignores the fact that female IVDUs may have little in common epidemiologically with their male counterparts. The same is true for studies of women with AIDS that include subjects who are IVDUs, sexual partners of IVDUs, or bisexual men, or who acquired the disease through a blood transfusion. Because female IVDUs make up a significant portion of both IVDUs and women with AIDS, it is necessary to investigate them as a discrete group.

Although it is difficult to estimate the number of female IVDUs in the United States, the authors, relying on data from the National Institute of Drug Abuse, believe the number to be approximately 500,000. Female IVDUs make up more than 50 percent of the women with AIDS. By the time they present with AIDS, they are often ill with drug-related infections, pregnant, and suffer from complications from their pregnancy. As many as 65 percent of babies born to women with AIDS will have HIV infection at birth. Most of these babies are born to IV-drug using women.

Psychological problems of female IVDUs with AIDs stem from coming to grips with the possibility of death from a chronic, debilitating disease, whether or not to tell their sexual partners they are infected, and the dilemma of what will happen to their children after they die.

Unlike their male counterparts, most female IVDUs are either married to or in a relationship with an IVDU. Because women in this group assume all the caretaking roles assumed by women in general and because they often assume the financial burden of caring for the family as well, these women may resort to prostitution for money and/or drugs. Female IVDUs also report more illness than their male counterparts. Such disorders as anorexia, bulimia, infections, including venereal disease, and psychological stress are prevalent.

Drug treatment programs often ignore or are intolerant of the special needs of female IVDUs. There are only four programs, in Chicago, San Francisco, Philadelphia, and Los Angeles specifically designed for pregnant women. Most programs require fees for service which many of these women cannot afford. Few programs concern themselves with specific issues such as job retraining, childcare, and prison sentences.

Despite the grim scenario sketched out above, the authors believe this problem can be combatted. They offer four broad policy recommendations as follows: (1) HIV education and prevention programs; (2) prevention and treatment programs for female IV drug users; (3) services targeted specifically for HIV-infected women and their families; and (4) research and surveillance activities. For each of their recommendations, the authors outline specific plans or make suggestions for implementation that are tailored to the needs of women. However, educating policymakers in state and federal governments is necessary if such programs and research are to be funded. The rate of HIV infection and AIDS-related deaths among gay men has begun to drop precisely because the gay male community organized prevention and treatment programs targeted specifically for their group. This must be done for female IVDUs and female partners of IVDUs with HIV infection and AIDS.

Corrigan, E., & Butler, S. (1991). Irish alcoholic women in treatment: Early findings. *The International Journal of the Addictions, 26*(3), 281–292.

In this study, a representative sample of women were interviewed based on consecutive admission to treatment centers in Ireland. Questions were asked related to drinking patterns, use of other drugs, parental drinking, and troubles associated with drinking.

Both the rationale and methodology of the study borrow heavily from an earlier study conducted in 1980 by Corrigan in the United States. In this study, a total of seven treatment centers participated, each contributing between 10 and 26 patients. The investigators attempted to control for selection bias and to create a representative sample. About half the women were from Dublin and the remainder from other towns and rural areas. Patterns and amounts of alcohol consumed varied, but 75 percent of the women reported that they drank at home alone.

For a majority of the women, both their fathers (87%) and mothers (54%) also drank. The married women had drinking husbands and they often drank together. A relatively high percentage, 30 percent, reported previous suicide attempts. A majority of the women reported use of drugs in addition to alcohol and a substantial number reported binge drinking.

Dahlgren, L., & Willander, A. (1989). Are special treatment facilities for female alcoholics needed? A controlled 2-year follow-up study

from a specialized unit (EWA) versus a mixed male/female treatment facility. *Alcoholism: Clinical and Experimental Research, 13*(4), 499–504.

A number of authors have emphasized the need for special provisions in the treatment of alcoholic women. In this study the investigators compared women treated in a specially-designed women-only program (n = 100) with those treated in traditional mixed-sex alcoholism treatment programs (n = 100).

The experimental treatment facility for women with early alcohol problems, the EWA-project, was opened in 1981 in Stockholm, Sweden. This facility is part of a broader-based project to reach women in the early stages of addiction. Treatment at the EWA facility includes thorough medical, psychiatric, social, and psychological assessments. Particular attention is given to employment and family concerns. Mothers and children receive help and support from a child psychiatrist. Treatment programs are individualized and include close contact with staff and involvement of families. Special problems of women are addressed and opportunities for exchanging experiences with other women are provided.

Baseline data for this study were collected following detoxification. The two groups were found to be comparable on the majority of 200 medical, social, and psychological variables. The women ranged from 18 to 67 years of age. About 90 percent in both groups were gainfully employed; most were white collar or worked in service production. About 20 percent reported reduced work capacity related to drinking. The median number of sick days reported was 30 (compared with a median of 22 days for women in the general population). The majority of women lived with a permanent male partner, one-half of whom were problem drinkers or alcoholic; about one-third of the women had children. A total of 60 percent of the women had been treated for psychiatric symptoms before admission for alcoholism; 20 percent of these had received inpatient treatment mostly because of depressive or anxiety reactions. One-fourth of the women had attempted suicide at least once. The median age of problem drinking for both groups was 35; all women described an increase in tolerance and impaired ability to control consumption. The majority (70%) consumed table wine only. Regular psychotropic use was reported by 15 percent; 40 percent used these drugs only periodically. Preferred drugs were benzodiazapines. Because of the exclusion criteria, none of the women used narcotics. Most of the women were self-referred (85%); only 15 percent were referred by physicians.

Treatment lasted an average of eight months for women in the EWA program and five months for the control group. The EWA group appeared to be more successful than the controls in several respects. For example, they needed less hospital care for alcoholism and showed a lower mortality. They had fewer relapses and a more positive social development (e.g., improvement in relationships with partner and with children). Work capacity improved in EWA but deteriorated in controls. The authors note that both the treatment and control groups were initially attracted by the existence of the EWA program; women who were randomly selected out of the EWA and into the control group stopped treatment sooner than women in the EWA program. They conclude that specialized treatment services such as those provided by the EWA program are important in attracting women to treatment at earlier stages of addiction and encouraging women to stay in treatment.

An additional finding of interest is that a significant number of the EWA women managed to return to social drinking. This finding is controversial and presents a dilemma for practitioners working with this population. Experts disagree on whether there should be a rigid requirement for total abstinence or a willingness to consider the possibility of returning to social drinking following a period of sobriety.

Davis, S. (1990). Chemical dependency in women: A description of its efforts and outcome on adequate parenting. *Journal of Substance Abuse Treatment,* 7(4), 225–232.

In this article, Davis defines chemical dependency as a maladaptive response to an inadequate upbringing. Although she begins by citing Alexander's work, which maintains that environment and genetic predisposition are causally related in producing chemical dependency, Davis focuses on the environmental affects of poor parenting on chemical dependency and discusses how they, in turn can lead to poor parenting by chemically dependent women. In fact, children who are abused, abandoned, or otherwise harmed psychologically, all too often repeat their victimization on their own children. The chemically dependent woman who becomes pregnant is typically from a dysfunctional family, is depressed, anxious, and has low self-esteem. She is often unemployed and socially isolated. This combination of attributes has disastrous effects on her children. They are frequently born addicted, may be abandoned or neglected, and become socially and psychologically maladapted.

Davis suggests that effective treatment programs must assist these women to resolve their own unmet childhood needs through teaching them reparenting skills.

Dritschel, B. H., Pettinati, H. M. (1989). The role of female occupations in severity of alcohol-related problems. *American Journal of Drug and Alcohol Abuse,* 15(1), 61–72.

It has been hypothesized that the stress arising from work may contribute to the development of alcoholism among women. This is thought to be true for both women employed outside the home because of role overload, and women who are homemakers because of role deprivation, boredom, loneliness, and feelings of incompetence and devaluation.

This study investigated whether occupational class is associated with alcohol abuse in women. Women who were admitted to two adult inpatient addiction treatment programs were invited to participate following the third week of treatment. Of the 66 women who gave consent to participate, 31 worked outside the home, 17 were homemakers, and 18 were unemployed workers. The unemployed workers were women who were unemployed at the time of admission but who had been employed outside the home for at least 20 hours per week for more than half of their adult lives.

The study participants were interviewed using the Addiction Severity Index and an occupational interview instrument developed by the authors. The three groups did not differ with respect to age, years of education, alcohol use in the month prior to admission, or years of alcohol use. In contrast to previously reported findings, substance abuse problems did not differ between the three occupation groups.

Differences were found, however, in employment problem severity ratings: the unemployed workers reported more severe employment problems than did the workers or homemakers. The employment severity rating reflects factors such as number of days worked and amount of money earned in past month as well as subjective ratings of the degree to which the women felt troubled by not finding a job, by problems arising in their current job, and by the perceived need for job counseling.

In addition, analysis of the ASI revealed a trend for workers to have family and psychological problems in addition to alcoholism. Not surprisingly, more unemployed workers than workers wanted a job change. However, although there were no occupation-related differences in the *intensity* of stress experienced, significantly more homemakers wanted a job change and felt that such a change would result in an improved outcome in recovery.

Because of the small sample size, the results of this study are not definitive. The finding that unemployed women had more severe employment problems could have been a consequence of excessive drinking, or drinking to excess may have occurred in response to an increase in job-related problems, or other unexplained variables may have influenced this finding. Studies using larger sample sizes and more sophisticated methodology are needed to disentangle this complex web of relationships and variables.

Fellios, P. G. (1989). Alcoholism in women: Causes, treatment, and prevention. In G. W. Lawson & A. W. Lawson (Eds.), *Alcoholism and*

Substance Abuse in Special Populations (pp. 11–29). Rockville, Maryland: Aspen.

This chapter, one of 16 written about various subgroups designated as "special populations," focuses on women and alcohol. The author provides a general overview of research related to the causes and treatment of alcoholism in women. One concern with the review is the date of many of the sources cited; almost one-half of the citations are for references written in the 50s, 60s, or 70s, and relatively few are from the past five years.

Perhaps related to the lack of more recent references are a number of statements that must be questioned. For example, Fellios includes in his discussion of causative factors the now largely abandoned theory of the empty nest. He states ". . . This family crisis may be a serious illness in the family, divorce, or children leaving the home. As a result, the center of their (the alcoholic women) life—their home—is suddenly empty. As they search for outside help they find few resources: no job, few close friends, and no interests outside the family. The result is anxiety, panic, profound loneliness, and nothing to cling to but drinking" (p. 18).

Fellios also comments several times that women have a high degree of denial of drinking problems. Perhaps more accurate is the tendency of family members, physicians, and other health care providers to ignore or deny signs and symptoms of alcohol problems among women.

Further, Fellios cites findings from two studies published in 1966 and 1968 that suggest unsatisfied dependency needs may be one of the causes of women's abuse of alcohol. Dependency theory as an explanation for the development of chemical dependency is based on assumptions concerning traditionally defined appropriate "male" and "female" behaviors and currently has little support or interest.

Finally, statements such as "Therapy begins with an initial interview which, in the case of female patients, should be handled with great delicacy" (p. 22); "social pressure affects women severely" (p. 17); The therapist must keep in mind that ". . . she [the alcoholic woman] may be confused about her social roles" (p. 22); and

". . . heavy drinking often began as a response to obstetrical stress and disappointment" (p. 13), clearly reflect a stereotypic view of alcoholic women as weaker, sicker, and more difficult to treat than alcoholic men.

Although numerous other examples can be presented, it is hoped that these suffice to convince the reader that the material in this chapter must be read cautiously and the author's conclusions questioned closely.

Frezza, M., DiPadova, C., Pozzato, G., Terpin, M., Baraona, E., & Lieber, C. S. (1990). High blood alcohol levels in women: The role of decreased gastric alcohol dehydrogenase activity and first-pass metabolism. *The New England Journal of Medicine, 322*(2), 95–100.

This article reports three significant findings: (1) the enzyme alcohol dehydrogenase, heretofore thought to act principally in the liver to metabolize alcohol, also acts in the gastric mucosa; (2) this activity varies with gender; and (3) it is diminished in both male and female alcoholics.

These findings are based on a study done on 17 nonalcoholic women 22 to 48 years old, 14 nonalcoholic men 26 to 53 years old, 6 alcoholic women 17 to 52 years old, and 6 alcoholic men 45 to 61 years old.

Each of these groups was administered doses of ethanol (0.3 g per kilogram of body weight) orally and intravenously in a randomized sequence one hour after eating breakfast. In both the alcoholic and nonalcoholic groups, blood ethanol concentrations were higher in women than in men after oral ingestion of alcohol. In contrast, there were no significant differences after intravenous administration. Furthermore, in the alcoholic subjects, first-pass metabolism (in effect, the amount of alcohol metabolized in the stomach) was lower for both men and women than in the nonalcoholic subjects. Most significant, and most disturbing, was the finding that in alcoholic women, almost no first-pass metabolism occurred, as evidenced by the fact that blood alcohol levels were almost identical after oral and intravenous administration. Because first-pass metabolism is a protective mechanism, in that it decreases the amount of alcohol that enters the liver

and systemic circulation, the fact that it is less in women than in men generally, and almost non-existent in alcoholic women, provides another, cogent explanation for women's increased vulnerability to liver damage and other adverse effects of alcohol consumption.

Although these findings are important in thinking about prevention and intervention strategies, some caveats are in order. The findings of Frezza et al. also demonstrated that the first-pass effect is offset when the amount of alcohol consumed at one time is high. Fasting also was demonstrated to eliminate the first-pass effect. Thus, before firm conclusions are drawn, additional studies must be performed, both to replicate these findings and to explore some of the possible causes for the unexplained findings in the study.

Garrity, T. F., & Lawson, E. J. (1989). Patient-Physician communication as a determinant of medication misuse in older minority women. *Journal of Drug Issues, 19*(2), 245–259.

This article reviews the literature on the patient-physician relationship as it affects compliance in taking prescription drugs and following other recommended regimens. Four factors are examined as they relate to the physician-patient encounter: teaching efforts of physicians; expectations of physicians and patients; relative activity and passivity of physician and patient; and affective tone. The article also looks specifically at the literature describing the physician-patient relationship in which the patients are older, minority women.

With regard to the general review, the authors conclude the following: patients are more likely to follow physicians' recommendations when the latter have explained the reasons for the regimen. But it is not known whether it is the explanation or the increased interest shown by the practitioner and increased satisfaction by the patient that explains the reason for following the medication protocol. With regard to expectations, several studies have shown that when expectations differed between patient and physician, a barrier to compliance occurred. With regard to the third aspect of the relationship, the degree to which both patients and physicians actively participated in the plan to manage the illness, studies have shown that more active patients who take responsibility for and negotiate with the physician about their care, are much more likely to take recommended medications. The final aspect of the patient-physician relationship has to do with the affective tone of the physician; in the studies cited by the author, there was a positive correlation between compliance and the friendliness of the physician.

Although the few studies that exist point to the fact that what is true for the population at large is also true for the older minority female patient, the barriers to compliance that exist with the general population are even greater with older female minority patients. These barriers include language, cultural, and gender differences: most physicians are white affluent men who often assume that their elderly female patients, especially those who cannot communicate to the contrary, are uninterested in the details of the medication regimen prescribed. Patients' silence or diffidence is sometimes mistaken for indifference to treatment. Interestingly, both women and men were more likely to ask questions of female physicians.

The conclusions of this study may seem self-evident to those readers well schooled in the dynamics of discrimination and stereotyping, but the article is valuable to any practitioner who cares for minority female patients because it points to the difficulty this group has in establishing a healthy rapport with practitioners.

Glantz, M. D., & Backenheimer, M. S. (1988). Substance abuse among elderly women. *Clinical Gerontologist*, 8(1), 3–26.

This article provides a thorough review of the literature on inappropriate drug and alcohol use among the elderly in general and among older women specifically. Unfortunately, as the authors note, little research has been done in this area on older adults and even less on women. Existing research, however, does point to the following: abuse of alcohol and illicit drugs does not seem to be a widespread problem among elderly women;

the risk is greater for drug misuse, either self-perpetrated or from inappropriate physician prescriptions. Adverse drug interactions are part of this problem. Elderly women are at greater risk than any other age-by-gender group for inappropriate physician-prescribed psychotropics. Some highlights of the discussions are as follows:

(1) Evidence supports the belief that older women either abstain from or use alcohol in moderation and are less likely to suffer the ill effects of this drug than are their male counterparts. As baby boomers age, however, this trend may not continue, as this age group of women tend to drink and use other drugs more than women in the generations before them.

(2) Older women use significantly more over-the-counter and prescription medication than do their male counterparts. Consequently, they experience a greater number of adverse reactions, the most serious problems being with psychotropic drugs prescribed by physicians. Long-term users of anxiolytics are likely to be older women who visit physicians specifically to obtain prescriptions for these drugs.

This article contains no startling revelations but does summarize the literature and provide a good overview of what may become an increasing problem in the future.

Glaus, K. O. (1989). Alcoholism, chemical dependency and the lesbian client. *Women and Therapy*, 8(1/2), 131–144.

This review article, written in a special issue of *Women and Therapy* entitled *Lesbianism: Affirming Nontraditional Roles*, focuses on alcohol and other drug dependency among lesbians.

The prevalence of alcohol and other dependencies among lesbians is unknown but reported to be high. Of the few studies that focus on lesbians, most have been plagued by methodologic flaws, including small and nonrepresentative samples. Nevertheless, some findings have occurred consistently enough across these studies to inspire some confidence in their reliability. For example, lesbians generally may be at greater risk for alcoholism because of a greater reliance on bars or other drinking situations as a way to socialize and "be out." Glaus reviews assessment and treatment issues unique to lesbian clients and makes recommendations for therapists.

Although the information reported in this article is not new, it emphasizes the great need for methodologically sound research that examines drinking and drug use practices in large and representative samples of lesbians. Such research is essential to avoid speculation and combat erroneous assumptions and to develop more effective methods of prevention, identification, and treatment of alcohol and drug problems among lesbians.

Gomberg, E. S. L. (1989). *Alcohol and women.* (Pamphlet series). New Brunswick, New Jersey: Rutgers University Center of Alcohol Studies.

This 28-page pamphlet, written by a well-known researcher and author in the field, provides state-of-the-art information about women and alcohol. Women's past and current drinking practices and society's attitudes and views of those practices are reviewed. Also reviewed are the antecedents, manifestations, and consequences of alcohol abuse.

Gomberg draws from her own and other's research to arrive at categories of women at high risk for alcohol abuse. These include (1) women with a family history of alcoholism, (2) women who are cohabitating, (3) women who are on their own: unmarried, divorced, separated, (4) women whose spouses, lovers, closest friends, or siblings are heavy or frequent drinkers, and (5) women who are unemployed or looking for work. In the section on consequences, Gomberg discusses women's greater physiologic vulnerability to the effects of alcohol as well as the unique social and job-related consequences that accrue to women who abuse alcohol.

Gomberg concludes with a brief section on treatment and prevention. She notes that, contrary to many reports, data *do not* support that alcoholic women have poorer prognoses than alcoholic men. Important factors to consider in developing or implementing treatment for women are outlined.

Gomberg, E. S. L. (1989). Alcoholic women in treatment: Early histories and early problem

behaviors. *Advances in Alcohol and Substance Abuse,* 8(2), 133–147.

In this report of a study of alcoholic women in treatment, Gomberg enters the debate about whether the behaviors found in adult alcoholics are a cause or consequence of heavy and prolonged drinking. She argues that it is logically impossible to attribute broken families, unhappy childhoods, and early deviant behavior to adult-onset alcoholism.

To determine whether differences exist in early life experiences, data obtained from interviews with 301 alcoholic women and 137 nonalcoholic women, matched on age and social class, were compared. The women were divided into three groups: those in their twenties, thirties, and forties. Findings indicate that the alcoholic and nonalcoholic women did not differ significantly in reports of experience of painful early life events, but did differ in reports of behavioral *response* to these events and in their *affective reactions* during their early years. The two groups also differed in reports of impulsive and adolescent behaviors, suggesting that childhood and adolescent impulse-control problems may be associated with earlier onset of alcoholism.

Gomberg acknowledges the limitations of retrospective and self-report data. However, she makes the point that there is no evidence to suggest that alcoholic women introduce more memory distortions than nonalcoholic women in reporting perceptions of early life experiences. She concludes that, this being the case, the consistent finding is that early life emotional/behavioral problems are reported to a significantly greater extent by alcoholic women than by nonalcoholic women.

Gomberg, E. S. L. (1989). Suicide risk among women with alcohol problems. *American Journal of Public Health,* 79(10), 1363–1365.

In this report Gomberg presents data focusing on suicide attempts of alcoholic women from a larger study of alcoholic women in treatment. Data collected from alcoholic women (*n* = 301) and nonalcoholic controls (*n* = 137) indicate that significantly more alcoholic women (40%) than nonalcoholic women (8.8%) report having made suicide attempts. Among alcoholic women, suicide attempts were twice as common at ages 20 to 29 than at ages 40 to 49; this age difference was not found among nonalcoholic women. Alcoholic women were more likely to smoke cigarettes and to use other drugs in combination with alcohol than nonalcoholic women; those who had attempted suicide were more likely than alcoholic women who had not attempted suicide to have used every drug asked about in the interview (i.e., nicotine, tranquilizers, stimulants, sedatives, marijuana, psychedelics, cocaine, and heroin). The number of nonalcoholic women who had attempted suicide ($n = 12$) was too small to make meaningful comparisons. Among alcoholic women there was a clear difference in reported psychiatric symptoms of suicide attempters and nonattempters. Those who had attempted suicide reported significantly more tension, indecisiveness, anxiety, and nervousness.

Gomberg concludes that the combination of youthfulness and alcohol and drug abuse is critical in predicting high suicide risk. She recommends that professionals in emergency rooms and in chemical dependency treatment programs become aware of the suicide potential among this high risk group.

Gorney, B. (1989). Domestic violence and chemical dependency: Dual problems, dual interventions. *Journal of Psychoactive Drugs, 21*(2), 229–238.

Domestic violence, like chemical dependency, has only recently begun to be recognized as a serious women's health problem. The authors review prevalence data related to domestic violence and discuss the role of alcohol and other drugs in violent family interactions. Gorney challenges the popular notion that men become violent only when intoxicated. She argues that the prevalence of violence between partners cannot be adequately explained simply as the consequence of alcohol or other drug abuse, nor can it be understood outside the context within which it occurs. The implications of failure to identify violence in chemically dependent relationships, as well as the importance of intervening with every family member is discussed. The author also describes factors that act as barriers to identifying and treating this complex problem. The importance of providing training and supervision for all mental health professionals in their assessment and treatment of both chemical dependency and domestic violence is emphasized.

Hammer, T., & Vaglum, P. (1989). The increase in alcohol consumption among women: A phenomenon related to accessibility or stress? A general population study. *British Journal of Addiction, 84*, 767–775.

This article is based on a survey of Norwegian women and their husbands and explores the factors of accessibility and stress to explain the increase in alcohol consumption among Norwegian women. As the authors note, because there is a clear relationship between increased consumption and increased rates of alcohol-related problems, it is important for prevention and treatment programs to discover which groups of women are increasing their consumption and what factors are associated with their doing so.

Two major hypotheses have been put forth to explain women's increasing alcohol consumption: stress and easier access, both physically and socially. The stress hypotheses is based on the assumption that as divorce becomes more prevalent and/or as women enter the work force in increasing numbers and experience role conflicts and multiple-role demands, they will be more likely to use alcohol to relieve stress. Studies have not been consistent in supporting this supposition, however, with several documenting that divorced, separated or unmarried women consume more alcohol than their married counterparts, while another found that employed women with small children drank less. The most important factor related to accessibility seems to be employment status: several studies have found that occupational status more than family dynamics, marital status, income, or urban residence was associated with the variance in alcohol consumption by women.

These authors examined alcohol consumption and working culture; alcohol and stress;

and alcohol in the family by analyzing data collected in a national health survey conducted in 1985. The main finding is that for the factor of accessibility, population density and the husband's drinking level were more associated with women's drinking level than were employment, personal income, or occupational type. For the factor of stress, population density and the husband's drinking level were more related than were marital status, stress at work, or "nervous" problems. As the authors note, their findings are contradicted by other studies that found that occupational status was the most important factor associated with women's alcohol consumption. These inconsistencies point up the difficulty in trying to account for a complex interaction of variables in a retrospective study. Prospective studies, designed to increase control of extraneous variables, are needed if these relationships are to be better understood.

Harrison, P. A. (1989). Women in treatment: Changing over time. *International Journal of the Addictions, 24*(7), 655–673.

The goal of this study was to examine the hypothesis that shifts in behavioral norms concerning drinking and drug use, combined with changing roles and expectations for women in American society, may have altered the profiles of women entering treatment for chemical dependency.

The study sample consisted of 572 women in treatment between 1986 and 1987 at 21 treatment centers in 11 states. The sample was divided into women 35 years and older (*n* = 260) and those under 35 years old (*n* = 312). The majority of the women were white, heterosexual, and well educated. Although the women over 35 years were 2.5 times as likely as the under 35 group to drink daily, the younger women were more likely to use marijuana, cocaine, stimulants, opiates, and hallucinogens on a regular basis.

One of the most striking differences between the two age groups was age of initiation of substance use. Four times as many younger women began drinking before age 16 (56% versus 14%). The difference for other drug use was even more dramatic: 47 percent of the younger

women began using drugs by age 15 compared with only 3 percent of older women. As a group, the younger women exhibited a much more complex array of childhood and recent problems than did the older women. For example, the younger women reported more frequent suicide attempts, treatment for depression or other emotional problems, childhood antisocial behaviors, symptoms of eating disorders, and physical and sexual abuse. Younger women also demonstrated more social dysfunction, greater dependence on welfare, higher rates of unemployment, and higher rates of alcohol and drug abuse by their spouses.

The authors acknowledge that a clear generational distinction cannot be made. Older women with more severe histories may be underrepresented in this sample. Furthermore, a response bias may exist, with younger women being more willing to acknowledge past events. Nevertheless, as the authors point out, chemical dependency treatment programs face a difficult challenge with respect to younger women now entering treatment.

Harrison, P. A., Hoffmann, N. G., & Edwall, G. E. (1989). Differential drug use patterns among sexually abused adolescent girls in treatment for chemical dependency. *International Journal of the Addictions, 24*(6), 499–514.

Both anecdotal reports and empirical studies report a high rate of sexual abuse among populations of women in treatment for chemical dependency.

These investigators sought to determine whether differences in drug-use patterns existed in four groups of sexually abused adolescent girls admitted for chemical dependency treatment. The four groups consisted of those who had experienced intrafamilial, extrafamilial, both intrafamilial and extrafamilial, or no sexual abuse. Of the 597 girls included in the study, 21 (3.5%) reported past sexual abuse; 43 (7.2%) reported both intrafamilial and extrafamilial sexual abuse, 47 (7.9%) reported intrafamilial sexual abuse only, and 120 (20.1%) reported extrafamilial sexual abuse only. Sexual abuse victims began substance use at earlier ages than nonvictims and more commonly used stimulants, sedatives, minor tranquilizers, and hallucinogens. Intrafamilial abuse victims, in particular, began to drink earlier than nonvictims: well over one-third began drinking before age 11. All sexual abuse victims were more likely to use substances "to get away from family problems," a finding that supports the self-medication hypothesis offered by the authors. The authors acknowledge the limitations of the study (e.g., lack of information about relationship of the perpetrator to the victim, frequency and duration of occurrence of abuse, use of coercion, intimidation or violence, and responses of others to disclosure of abuse). This study provides additional support for the argument that chemically dependent women have unique treatment needs.

Jackson, B. B., & Taylor, J. (1990). Evaluation of factors affecting alcohol consumption in African American women. *Perspectives on Addictions Nursing, 1*(3), 3–7.

This investigation explored the influence of four factors—psychological stress, social support, socioeconomic status, and religious orientation on alcohol consumption in African American women. Data were from a longitudinal study of women 25 to 75 years old (*n* = 599) who resided in a large city in the Eastern United States. Analysis of data revealed several interesting findings. For example, women with high numbers of stressful life events were found to consume more alcohol—both overall consumption as well as consumption of wine, beer, and hard liquor. Women of lower socioeconomic status were found to drink more beer than those from higher socioeconomic groups; however, socioeconomic status did not differentiate overall consumption; wine or hard liquor consumption did not differ according to socioeconomic status. Univariate relationships between religious orientation and social support and consumption were not statistically significant. However, more sophisticated analysis revealed a negative relationship between religious orientation and consumption of hard liquor.

The authors provide several interesting and plausible explanations for the findings. First, because almost 45 percent of the women in the study

had incomes of less than $7,000 per year, many may engage in "escape drinking" as a means of coping with economic and psychologic stress. Second, the inverse relationship between socioeconomic status and alcohol consumption was supported only for beer, indicating that the risk of drinking beer, the most affordable alcoholic beverage, increases as socioeconomic status decreases. The authors raise the question of whether socioeconomic status is a better predictor of beer consumption, and life events the better predictor of wine and hard liquor consumption. Certainly the possibility of different factors influencing alcohol consumption patterns differently is worthy of further investigation.

Jaffee, L., & Ahuja, S. (1989). Women and the role of physical activity in chemical dependency treatment. *Melpomene Journal, 9*(1), 20–28.

The treatment of chemical dependency has historically had as its sole focus withdrawal and abstinence from chemical substances. Only recently have the benefits of exercise and diet begun to be explored. As is true with most research on chemical dependency generally, the few studies that have explored the influence of physical fitness on recovery have been limited to men. This study focused on the effects of structured physical activity in the treatment of chemically dependent women. Specifically, the investigators explored women's experience or perceptions of the benefits of physical activity as a part of their treatment for chemical dependency. Findings from the study included the following: (1) the benefits of a structured physical activity program were not obvious for women currently in treatment; (2) for women in recovery (defined as abstinence from alcohol or other drugs for at least two months), 69 percent reported stress reduction as a primary benefit of a structured physical activity program; (3) women in recovery who had been exposed to a structured physical activity program were more likely (80% versus 58%) to view physical activity as a factor in recovery than those who did not have this exposure.

Although this research is limited by a number of methodologic weaknesses, e.g., use of convenience sample and wide variation in amount and type of physical activity reported, the positive effects reported by the women support the usefulness of including structured exercise as part of the treatment for chemically dependent women. Further research is needed to document what sorts of activities for what periods of time are most useful.

Kail, B. L. (1989). Drugs, gender, and ethnicity: Is the older minority woman at risk? *Journal of Drug Issues, 19*(2), 171–189.

In this introductory article to a special issue in the *Journal of Drug Issues* called "Drug Use and Minority Older Women," the author provides an overview of the topics to be covered in this issue, as well as discusses whether or not older minority women are at special risk for drug misuse. Drug misuse is broadly defined as taking incorrect amounts of a drug (too little or too much); discontinuing use prematurely; using out-of-date medications; sharing medications; or using medications that have been prescribed for another illness. The problem of over-medication of the institutionalized elderly is not discussed. The article focuses on four ethnic groups in the United States: blacks, Hispanics, native Americans, and Asian-Americans. These four groups of older women seem to experience more problems with medications than does the older white population, men or women. The reasons for these problems vary by ethnic group, although the underlying cause has directly to do with the fact that the health care system in the United States is still run by the white majority and operates with assumptions based on this dominant culture.

Specifically, older black women have problems purchasing medicine because they are generally poorer than older women in the other ethnic groups. Older Hispanic women are at risk for medication misuse because of language barriers and sometimes cultural values at odds with "white medicine." Native American women have difficulty accessing the health care system because of their physical distance from it.

The author discusses the policy implications of these findings, the overriding one being financing. Medicaid prescription costs must be reduced in order to enable some older minority women to afford medications. Another issue is access and finding ways to help those who need care to visit a physician. Such ethnic institutions as the church in the black community, and other similar social or religious organizations could monitor, assist, and support the medication regimen of their older female community members. Another issue is the education of physicians in the health care system. Knowing more about minority cultures, their language, beliefs, and dietary habits, would go a long way toward helping physicians understand the lived experience of the women they treat.

This article provides a valuable overview to this special issue, in that it thoroughly reviews the literature and summarizes the other articles in the special issue.

Kendler, K. S., Heath, A. C., Neale, M. C., Kessler, R. C., & Eaves, L. J. (1992). A population-based twin study of alcoholism in women. *Journal of the American Medical Association, 268*(14), 1977–1982.

These researchers sought to clarify the role played by genetic factors in causing alcoholism in women. The data analyzed came from a study of genetic and environmental risk factors for common psychiatric disorders in white female-female twin pairs from the Virginia Twin Registry. Subjects from this registry were interviewed if they were born between 1934 and 1971 and if both members had previously responded to a mailed questionnaire. The interviews were conducted by researchers who were unaware of the status of the co-twin; 1030 twin pairs were interviewed and the sample contained both monozygotic and dizygotic pairs.

Unlike previous studies of alcoholism in twins, this study took its subjects from the general population rather than from treatment facilities or medical records. In the latter case, at least one of the twins is also affected and proband concordance reflects only the degree to which the twins resemble each other for the chances of having had alcoholism. In the authors' study, the sample contains twin pairs in which neither twin is affected.

Of the 2,060 subjects, 128 (6.2%) were classified as alcoholic with dependence-tolerance;

57 (2.8%) as alcoholic without dependence-tolerance, and 172 (8.3%) as problem drinkers. For all levels of use concordance between twins was consistently higher in monozygotic than in dizygotic twins. Multifactorial threshold models suggested that the heritability of liability to alcoholism in women is in the range of 50 percent to 60 percent.

The researchers acknowledge three limitations in the study: (1) the final study sample was not completely representative because some twins moved out of the state and not all responded to the initial survey; (2) in the face of the substantial heritability found for alcoholism familial or environmental influences would probably be undetectable; and (3) the assessments were performed at only one point in time. Correcting for the unreliability of measurement or conducting interviews at multiple occasions may have produced an even higher incidence.

The authors conclude that their study results show that women should be well represented in major efforts now underway to determine the molecular basis of the genetic susceptibility to alcoholism.

Klee, L., Schmidt, C., & Ames, G. (1991). Indicators of women's alcohol problems: What women themselves report. *The International Journal of the Addictions*, 26(8), 879–895.

The investigators who conducted this study believe that current etiological studies have produced contradictory and inconclusive findings concerning women's drinking behaviors. They therefore chose to focus on indicators rather than etiological factors. As defined in this article, an indicator is "evidence that a woman has or is developing a drinking problem, as identified by the woman herself or by others." An indicator does not refer to causes or to risk factors.

This article presents findings that are part of a larger study, the goal of which was to develop a taxonomy of indicators of women's alcohol problems. The specific findings from the small study were gathered from indepth interviews of 65 women of different ages and ethnic groups who were in treatment for alcohol problems.

The findings are presented from an "emic" perspective, i.e., from the point of view of the women themselves, not the interviewers. These 65 women reported 3,769 responses in the five categories listed above. The largest number, 58.4 percent, appeared in the individual category. Both psychological and behavioral effects were in this category. Common responses were centered around self-image, aggression, and preoccupation with alcohol. Denial of the problem and certain beliefs about alcohol were also cited.

Physiologic indicators accounted for 15.7 percent of the total and included sleep, nutritional, neurological, gynecological, and hepatic disorders. The social category, having to do with the way others respond to the female problem drinker, contained 12 percent of all indicators. This category was designed to elicit what the respondents thought about how others related to them, and the authors believe that its percentage was lower because many of these issues were subsumed under the "individual" category.

Although much of what was reported in this study is not surprising, the authors have reinforced what has been reported in other studies: women are different from men in their experience of alcoholism and that treatment-specific programs must be developed to meet their needs.

Kress, M. K. (1989). Alcoholism: A women's issue, a disability issue. *Journal of Applied Rehabilitation Counseling*, 20(2), 47–51.

This article, written for rehabilitation counselors, provides a general overview of the literature on women and alcohol. The author focuses primarily on characteristics of women alcoholics and gender differences in the physiologic and psychological consequences of alcoholism. Other issues of particular concern to women, such as past sexual abuse, are discussed briefly. Several parallels between women alcoholics and physically disabled persons are also described. For example, both hold second class status, often face discrimination, particularly in employment, and may experience rolelessness. The problems faced by women who are both alcoholic and disabled are mentioned only briefly.

Some of the material in the article must be viewed cautiously. For example, the author misuses the term codependency to describe polyaddiction, or dependence on more than one drug. In another section she states that "Sexual abuse experienced during childhood appears to be a major contributing factor to women's alcoholism" (p. 48). She substantiates this claim by citing reports that 60 percent to 70 percent of women alcoholics have a history of sexual abuse. Although alarming, similar estimates have been made about other groups of women. Although increasing evidence suggests that an association exists, currently there is insufficient research to document a causal relationship between past sexual abuse and the development of alcohol problems among women.

Nevertheless, as the author points out, there is a great need for treatment programs and practitioners to address the unique problems and concerns of physically challenged women. Although some important points are made in this article, it provides relatively pedestrian coverage of an important topic.

Ladwig, G. B., & Anderson, M. D. (1989). Substance abuse in women: Relationship between chemical dependency of women and past reports of physical and/or sexual abuse. *International Journal of the Addictions, 24*(8), 739–754.

Women who have been sexually or physically abused are believed to be at risk for the development of chemical dependency. This research explored the incidence of physical and sexual abuse among chemically dependent, incarcerated women. For the 118 women studied, 27 percent reported sexual or physical abuse prior to entrance into prison; 20 percent reported a history of sexual abuse. This study is limited by its convenience sample. Furthermore, because data were gathered during an initial assessment on entrance into prison, the investigators had no control over the data-gathering process and were unable to validate responses. The article includes a brief description of an intervention model that focuses on client-identified needs. Although such a model may in fact be useful in the treatment of chemically dependent women, it is not clear why it is included here. The authors make several important points including the need for a sexual assault history as a routine part of all initial assessments.

Lewis, G. R., & Jordan, S. M. (1989). Treatment of the gay or lesbian alcoholic. In G. W. Lawson & A. W. Lawson (Eds.), *Alcoholism and Substance Abuse in Special Populations* (pp. 165–190). Rockville, Maryland: Aspen.

This rather lengthy chapter is written for counselors and others who treat chemically dependent clients. The chapter is divided into four major sections: (1) a history of homosexuality and alcoholism, (2) issues in counseling the lesbian or gay alcoholic, (3) alcoholism treatment and gay men, and (4) alcoholism treatment and lesbian women. The first two sections are long and are likely to be ignored by many readers. However, for those interested in the evolution of thought about homosexuality and its link to alcoholism, the first section is particularly useful. In the relatively brief section devoted to the treatment of lesbians, the authors focus on some of the issues of particular concern to this population. These include lesbian relationships, isolation and loneliness, age and aging, alcoholics anonymous, and homophobia and prejudice. The authors conclude with a summary of specific treatment implications related to each of these issues.

Lewis, D. K, & Watters, J. K. (1989). Human immunodeficiency virus seroprevalence in female intravenous drug users: The puzzle of black women's risk. *Social Science Medicine, 29*(9), 1071–1076.

This article discusses findings that were part of a larger study conducted by the authors in 1987, which consisted of structured interviews followed by the collection of serum samples from intravenous drug users (IVDUs) in two treatment programs and in three different street settings in San Francisco.

The findings discussed here are based on 155 female heterosexual IVDUs. Of the total sample of women 85 were white and 70 were black. The two groups were similar in median age and marital status, but differed in education level, employment status, and treatment status, with whites being more educated, more likely to be employed, and more likely to be in treatment programs. As has been the case in other studies, black women were demonstrated to have a higher HIV seroprevalence than did white women (21% versus 7%).

The authors examined the ethnic distribution of known risk factors: needle sharing; high-risk sexual partners; multiple partners; receptive anal intercourse; and partners who never used condoms. What is somewhat surprising about the results is that with the exception of lack of condom use by sexual partners, which a greater number of black women than white women reported (70% versus 58%), white women reported significantly more risk-producing behavior for every factor than did black women.

According to the authors, this study is the first to compare risk behaviors of black and white IVDUs. That the authors do not explain the sample's increased susceptibility may be because of cultural and social differences between the two groups. One explanation put forth by the authors is that the term "needle sharing" has different meanings for the two groups. For whites it means any level of sharing; for blacks it means sharing only with relative strangers, not with lovers or friends. Another difference might be that black men are less likely to admit their bisexuality to their female partners; thus, the question concerning sex with bisexual partners would be answered in the negative by black women who might be ignorant of their partners' sexual behavior. The authors also posit that black women may be more reluctant than white women to admit high-risk sexual behavior or that the research questions were not phrased in a culturally appropriate manner, certainly the case in the past with intelligence, achievement, and aptitude tests.

Attempts should be made to replicate the findings in this study and also to do follow up studies of this population group, as their increased susceptibility to HIV infection and to AIDS is a significant concern.

Lex, B. (1991). Some gender differences in alcohol and polysubstance abusers. *Health Psychology, 10*(2), 121–132.

This broad-based review of the literature and of the investigator's own work touches on a number of issues familiar to researchers on substance abuse and its effects on women. Some of the many findings noted and discussed are as follows:

A review of the literature indicates that women drink less than men, suffer disproportionately greater effects, have more associated affective disorders, and suffer more from the stigma of alcoholism. The majority of women and men reported using alcohol during 1988, according to the NIDA Household Survey of 1988. Both marijuana and cocaine use had declined in men and women.

Both men and women manifest disruptions in the hypothalamic-pituitary-gonadal axis, but more studies are needed to identify specific mechanisms of actions.

Women are reported to drink alone more frequently than men, use more tranquilizers, and are less well known to the criminal justice system. They are also more likely to have a family history of alcohol problems and to have spouses with alcohol problems.

With regard to cocaine use, women were less likely than men to report decreased libido and intoxication effects. Both men and women reported depression, job stress, and the need to feel more sociable as reasons for cocaine use. With regard to marijuana, men smoked more and showed a progressive increase in frequency, which was not observed in the female subjects.

The author ends this review with a call for more research into physiological as well as environmental causes of substance abuse. Saying that there is no valid dispute between "nature and nurture," the author calls for ongoing epidemiological research as the only way to keep clinicians informed so that they can design effective treatment strategies.

Lex, B. W., Mello, N. K., Mendelson, J. H., & Babor, T. F. (1989). Reasons for alcohol use by female heavy, moderate, and occasional social drinkers. *Alcohol, 6,* 281–287.

This study attempts to examine in women what has already been investigated in men: the correlation of drinking patterns with self-reported reasons for drinking. Specifically, this study looks at women's self-reports of drinking beliefs and behaviors in both their community and on a clinical research unit.

Twenty-six women were asked various questions from the Alcohol Use Inventory and the Alcohol Stages Index about three separate 21-day drinking periods: the heaviest 3-week period in the last year; the period immediately preceding their 5-week stay on the alcohol research unit; and the stay itself, during which they had unlimited access to their alcoholic beverage of choice for a 21-day period.

Based on information gathered in the questionnaires, the women were divided into three groups of social drinkers: heavy; moderate; and occasional. Some of the findings are as follows. The heavy social drinkers (mean > 5 drinks per study day) reported strong beliefs that drinking would help them relax. They reported engaging in solitary drinking "frequently" during the study period. They also reported behaviors thought to be associated with drinking that is out of control: worrying about alcohol supply, drinking in the morning, occasional inability to stop drinking. One unexpected finding was that both occasional and heavy social drinkers responded to social cues to drink; moderate drinkers did not do so.

This study was carefully conducted, but small sample size and the confounding effect of reported rather than observed behavior make the findings less than incontrovertible.

Lundholm, J. K. (1989). Alcohol use among university females: Relationship to eating disordered behavior (Brief report). *Addictive Behaviors, 14*, 181–185.

This article reports the findings of a study that examined the relationship between alcohol abuse and disordered eating patterns in 135 women enrolled at Iowa State University. The authors cite numerous studies reporting alcohol abuse in anorexics and in bulimic anorexics and were attempting to see if the relationship existed among nonhospitalized women. University women were selected because women of college age frequently report disordered eating behavior.

Disordered eating was examined using the Eating Disorders Inventory, and alcohol abuse

was assessed with the Million Clinical Multi-axial Inventory. Disordered eating was measured by comparing the responses on the eight scales of the Eating Disorders Inventory of women who scored high on the Million Inventory (≥ 13) with women who scored low (≤ 6).

Women who reported both bulimic episodes and frequent use of alcohol were dissatisfied with their body size. Those who reported bulimia but not frequent alcohol abuse reported more dissatisfaction with others and were particularly unhappy with interpersonal relationships.

Women who scored high on alcohol abuse differed from low scorers in the following ways: they experienced episodes of bulimia, a sense of alienation, and few close relationships, as well as insecurity, worthlessness, and inability to identify sensations of hunger and satiety. This constellation of attitudes and behaviors is quite similar to that of bulimics. These findings support the belief that bulimics, anorexics, and alcoholics all have a substance abuse disorder and that food is just one of several substances abused.

This study is important in that it examines a nonhospitalized population. It would have been enhanced by some discussion of prevention and treatment implications. In addition, the relationship between disordered eating, alcohol abuse, and depression should also be explored in future studies.

Mayers, R. S. (1989). Use of folk medicine by elderly Mexican-American women. *Journal of Drug Issues, 19*(2), 283–295.

This article provides a thorough review of the considerable literature on the use of folk healers, or curanderas in the Hispanic communities in the United States. Curanderas are Mexican and Mexican-American folkhealers who practice "curanderismo." This folk medicine requires knowledge in the healing properties of herbs, teas, and other substances found in nature. These medicines are supplemented by rituals, prayers, and other techniques to effect a cure.

Anthropologists, sociologists, and others who have studied this phenomenon over the last thirty years differ on the implications of this practice for the general health and well being of Hispanics. Earlier studies tended to be critical of both the practice and the culture for engaging in it because it prevented those who needed "scientific" health care from receiving it. Later studies have found that curanderismo does not supplant but acts as a complement to health care provided by the dominant culture.

With regard to elderly Mexican-American women, it has been found that this group uses curanderismo more than any other Hispanic group. This finding is not surprising given the fact that in Hispanic cultures women are still viewed as the ones most interested in the health and illness of their families and communities.

Three concerns emerge from this fact: these women will use home remedies in lieu of medications prescribed by physicians; will not go to a physician if a curanderismo cure is available; and may experience adverse drug interactions if they rely on both forms of medication simultaneously. The first concern, however, seems to have been ruled out by previous studies, which point not to curanderismo but to poor communications and barriers to access as the causes of noncompliance. The second concern, choice of curanderismo over health services of the dominant culture, seems also to be unfounded. One study, for example, found that the two most important reasons for noncompliance were lack of money and lack of insurance. The third concern is particularly true for elderly Hispanic women, because they often do not tell their physician or family about concurrent drug use. Some folk medicines have adverse side effects and may cause adverse drug interactions. In this case, it behooves the physician who treats this population to inform her or himself about curanderismo so as to anticipate this situation and perhaps get information at history-taking about the use of folk medicine.

This article provides a thorough review of the literature and clarifies some of the confusion and contradiction that has existed about the importance of curanderismo in the Hispanic culture.

McKirnan, D. J., & Peterson, P. L. (1989). Alcohol and drug use among homosexual men and women: Epidemiology and population characteristics. *Addictive Behaviors, 14,* 545–553.

McKirnan, D. J., & Peterson, P. L. (1989). Psychosocial and cultural factors in alcohol and drug abuse: An analysis of a homosexual community. *Addictive Behaviors, 14,* 555–563.

Alcohol and drug use among gay men and women has been a subject of great speculation but relatively little research. Most reports include estimates of high rates of use. However, much of the speculation is based on anecdotal reports or biased studies. Research on homosexual populations has been plagued by small, nonrepresentative samples, most of which have been taken from bars, support groups, or psychiatric or other treatment settings.

These two papers report the findings of a survey of alcohol and drug use among gay men and lesbians. Although the sample was not random, respondents were solicited from a much wider range of settings than in previous studies. For example, surveys were distributed in newspapers, community organizations, clinics and health related organizations, and during community events; only 5 percent of the respondents obtained the survey in a bar or similar setting. The majority of respondents were men ($n = 2,652$); only 22 percent ($n = 748$) were women.

The first paper presents characteristics and patterns of alcohol and drug use. For example, only 13 percent of the men and 15 percent of the women reported abstinence from alcohol, as compared with 23 percent of the men and 34 percent of the women who abstain in the general population. The lower number of abstainers did not however, translate into a higher proportion of heavy drinkers; more gay men and women were moderate drinkers than men and women in the general population. A paradoxical finding was that the homosexual sample showed higher rates of alcohol *problems* as defined by shortened versions of the dependency and loss of control scales used in national studies of the general population. Similar trends were also found for drug use: 56 percent of the homosexual sample used marijuana in the year prior to the survey, in contrast to approximately 20 percent of the general population. The corresponding yearly figures for cocaine use were 23 percent among the homosexual sample versus 8.5 percent in the general population. As with alcohol, *heavy* use of other drugs was less common in the homosexual sample. Thus, significantly more gay men and women use alcohol or drugs than in the general population, although this does not translate into substantially higher rates of heavy use. The gay and lesbian sample demonstrated far less of a decline in both alcohol and drug use across age groups than does the general population, and less of a gender difference.

The central hypothesis in the second paper is that attitudinal and cultural sources of vulnerability are central to understanding the effects of stress and other variables on substance abuse. Attitudinal vulnerability represents learned expectations regarding the effects of alcohol or drugs, while a cultural emphasis on bar settings is more specific to urban homosexual communities. Both variables were strongly related to alcohol abuse, although correlations with drug use were less consistent. The authors conclude that further research is needed to determine whether these differences in findings for alcohol and drug abuse are a result of the vulnerability measures being alcohol-related, or whether they reflect a difference in the effect of these variables.

Finally, although the respondents reported discrimination and harassment because of their sexual orientation, rates of depression, alienation, and general stress were relatively low. This is an important finding and indicates that contrary to previous reports, gay men and women, at least those in this sample, are psychologically healthy and socially well-integrated. This research is also important in that it represents one of the broadest attempts to document more accurately alcohol and drug use, and factors related to use among gay men and lesbians.

Miller, B. A., Downs, W. R., & Gondoli, D. M. (1989). Spousal violence among alcoholic women as compared to a random household sample of women. *Journal of Studies on Alcohol, 50*(6), 533–540.

Most studies exploring the relationship between violence and substance abuse have focused on the perpetrator's (usually a man) use of chemical substances. Few studies have examined the victims' use of alcohol or drugs in the context of violence. In order to assess this relationship, the investigators compared 45 women selected from treatment agencies and alcoholics anonymous groups with 40 nonalcoholic women randomly selected from households. The authors describe in some detail data obtained from two-hour interviews with the two groups of women. Interview questions focused on early family relationships, including sexual and physical abuse and family history of alcoholism. The Michigan Alcoholism Screening Test (MAST) was used to measure alcohol intake and the Conflict Tactics Scale (CTS) was used to measure violence. The CTS includes indices of negative verbal abuse, moderate violence, and severe violence.

Several important differences were found between alcoholic and household women. Alcoholic women reported a greater number of childhood stressors including parent's divorce, separation, remarriage, or death. The alcoholic women were more likely to have had at least one alcoholic parent and to have had difficult or violent relationships with their fathers. Alcoholic women were likely to report higher levels of negative verbal abuse, moderate violence, and severe violence than the household women. For example, approximately 25 percent of the alcoholic women had been kicked, hit, or hit with a fist as compared with 5 percent of household women.

The authors acknowledge that although the findings suggest a strong link between spousal violence and women's alcoholism, generalizability of the results is limited. For example, women who seek treatment may differ from women who do not. A similar limitation, not noted by the authors, is the potential bias in the household women. Although selected from random households, only 26 percent of eligible respondents agreed to participate. Thus, the women who agreed to participate may differ from those who refused. Finally, the temporal ordering of spousal violence is unknown. Additional research is needed to determine whether the violence preceded or followed problem drinking.

Mitchell, J. E., Pyle, R., Eckert, E. D., & Hatsukami, D. (1990). The influence of prior alcohol and drug abuse problems on bulimia nervosa treatment outcome. *Addictive Behaviors, 15,* 169–173.

In this study, the authors used data from a two-to-five year follow-up study of 100 patients in an outpatient cognitive behavioral group psychotherapy treatment program for bulimia nervosa at the University of Minnesota. The authors attempted to determine the effects of a prior diagnosis of alcohol or other drug (AOD) abuse on the long-term outcome of patients who were diagnosed with bulimia. Their overall outcome was comparable to the outcome of the patients who had not had AOD abuse problems.

Because some researchers believe that bulimic eating behaviors and AOD abuse may be interchangeable behaviors for some, the authors wanted to find out if patients with co-morbidity would escalate their AOD use to compensate for loss of bulimic behavior. They did not find this to be the case. Their overall outcome was comparable to the outcome of these patients who had *not* had AOD abuse problems. Despite a small sample size, the fact that the patients studied had already gained some control over their AOD problem, and the fact that the treatment program used elements common to both kinds of problems, lends support to the premise that this co-morbid condition can be successfully managed.

Mishra, L., Sharma, S., Potter, J. J., & Mezey, E. (1989). More rapid elimination of alcohol in women as compared to their male siblings. *Alcoholism: Clinical and Experimental Research, 13*(6):752–754.

This study had a two-fold purpose: to compare men and women for their rates of ethanol elimination and to investigate any differences by sex in the accumulation of acetate, an ethanol metabolite. Nine pairs of natural siblings were studied to reduce genetic variability. Ethanol was infused intravenously in a dose of 0.6 g/kg of body weight over 45 to 60 minutes, and serial blood samples were obtained for 5 hours. The mean rate of ethanol elimination was higher in seven women, the same in one, and lower in one compared with their male siblings.

The significance to women of this study and others like it is that the rate of ethanol elimination is thought to be associated with susceptibility to liver injury caused by alcohol consumption. It is known that women develop alcoholic liver disease with a lower daily alcohol consumption than men, even after intake is corrected for body weight. This increased susceptibility may be caused by increased rate of ethanol metabolism, with increased formation of metabolites such as acetaldehyde or acetate, which are thought to mediate the toxic effects of ethanol.

Although this study clearly demonstrated that the women had a higher mean rate of ethanol elimination, it did not demonstrate higher plasma acetate levels. The investigators were unable to do more than speculate about this observation, assigning the cause to lower levels of testosterone or greater binding of acetaldehyde by hepatic proteins in women. (acetaldehyde is metabolized to acetate).

The researchers should be commended for their attempt to control for genetic variability and other confounding factors (all subjects had normal nutritional status and were free of hepatic, cardiac, or renal dysfunction). That its results do not point to a clear physiologic cause for the increased susceptibility of women to alcohol is disappointing but should not deter further investigators in this area.

Murray, J. B. (1989). Psychologists and alcoholic women. *Psychological Reports, 64,* 627–644.

Although the title of this paper suggests a focus on issues related to the treatment of alcoholic women of particular importance to psychologists, the scope of the article is much broader. Murray presents a comprehensive overview of research findings related to women and alcohol. Following the review the author summarizes the findings, suggesting gender differences in five broad areas: heredity, drinking patterns, physiologic responses, psychologic responses, and treatment and prevention. Because the article is very well referenced (123 sources), it serves as a valuable resource, particularly for educators and researchers interested in the topic of alcoholic women.

Neisen, J. H., & Sandall, H. (1990). Alcohol and other drug abuse in gay/lesbian populations: Related to victimization? *Journal of Psychology and Human Sexuality*, 3(1), 151–168.

The American Psychological Association (APA) dropped the definition of homosexuality as a disease in 1973; nevertheless, the stigma and general prejudice against homosexuals remain.

This article reports the findings from a study of inpatients at Pride Institute, a 28-day inpatient chemical dependency treatment program specifically for lesbians and gay clients. Using retrospective chart review, the study explored the prevalence of sexual abuse in recovering clients admitted between September 1986 and April 1987. The investigators defined sexual abuse as either one or more incidents of (1) rape involving intercourse or attempted penetration, or (2) oral or anal contact with the genitals of either the person being abused or the abuser. Nearly 50 percent of the 201 inpatients (50 women and 151 men) studied reported being sexually abused. Significantly more of the women reported a history of sexual abuse (70% versus 42%).

This study is important for several reasons. First, it uses a narrow definition of sexual abuse, which allows easier comparisons with findings from other studies. Second, it reports data from homosexuals—a significantly understudied population. Finally, unlike the majority of other studies in this area, rather than focusing on men only as perpetuators of abuse and violence it includes data on the victimization of men. The authors are careful to point out that the prevalence rates reported by both men and women in this study are similar to those reported by chemically dependent heterosexuals in other studies,

lest the conclusion be drawn that sexual abuse causes homosexuality.

These findings emphasize the need for additional research to more clearly understand the links between homosexuality and substance abuse as well as between sexual victimization and substance abuse.

Perodeau, G. M., & Kohn, P. M. (1989). Sex differences in the marital functioning of treated alcoholics. *Drug and Alcohol Dependence, 23,* 1–11.

Despite extensive data on the impact of alcoholism on the family unit, there has been limited research on alcoholic marriages, particularly when the wife is the alcoholic. Furthermore, data from studies in which the alcoholic is the husband cannot be extrapolated because of differences in roles, social status, and the stigma attached to drinking.

In this article, the authors report the findings from a study of 55 alcoholics in treatment (31 men and 24 women) compared with a matched control group of social drinkers. Spouses of both alcoholics and nonalcoholics were also sampled. Both respondents and spouses completed three questionnaires designed to evaluate marital functioning.

Significant findings are summarized as follows: (1) nonalcoholics reported better marital functioning than alcoholics; (2) female alcoholics reported more troubled marital relationships than did male alcoholics and felt more responsible for creating the problems because of their drinking; (3) spouses in both cases reported strained relationships; (4) alcoholic couples were not as congruent as their nonalcoholic counterparts in deciding whether or not to end an unhappy relationship; (5) alcoholic wives had been more active in ending their marriages than their husbands, just the opposite of alcoholic husbands with nonalcoholic wives.

Some important implications of these findings are as follows: therapy for married female alcoholics should attempt to encourage these women to externalize some of their guilt feelings and assertiveness training would be beneficial for these women by enabling them to express their needs rather than converting them into the self-destructive act of drinking. Alcoholic husbands, on the other hand, should be encouraged to accept more responsibility for the problems their drinking causes.

There are some limitations to the study's generalizability in that it did not compare alcoholic marriages with other clinical groups, it examined only treated, middle-class couples, and it examined only intact marriages. Nevertheless, these findings warrant further investigation, as they point to significant differences in attitudes of alcoholic men and women toward the influence of their drinking on marriage.

Rabinovitz, M., Van Thiel, D. H., Dindzans, V., & Gavaler, J. S. (1989). Endoscopic findings in alcoholic liver disease: Does gender make a difference? *Alcohol, 6,* 465–468.

Although it has been documented that women are more susceptible to the hepatotoxic effects of alcohol than are men, little data exist as to the extent of gastrointestinal involvement in advanced alcoholic liver disease. Furthermore, even less is known about whether or not this involvement is affected by gender.

The purposes of this study were (1) to ascertain the prevalence of various endoscopic findings in the gastrointestinal tract of persons with advanced alcoholic liver disease, and (2) determine if prevalence is affected by gender.

The study was retrospective; the subjects (49 men and 26 women) were all diagnosed with severe disease before the study began. The amount and duration of their drinking was neither controlled for nor monitored. The following upper gastrointestinal disorders were found: esophagitis; esophageal varices; gastritis, gastric varices; gastric ulcer; duodenitis; and duodenal ulcer. The only significant difference by gender was in the prevalence of gastric ulcer (23.1% for the women versus 6.1% for the men).

The authors speculate that this difference exists because of variations in body weight and composition. A higher proportion of female body weight is fat to which alcohol does not distribute, resulting in higher systemic blood levels in women than in men. These higher blood levels may induce gastric acid hypersecretion, with the resultant development of gastric ulcer.

Although the authors failed to support their hypotheses for any of the gastrointestinal findings except gastric ulcer, this failure may be more a function of study design than of physiologic fact.

Robbins, C., & Clayton, R. R. (1989). Gender-related differences in psychoactive drug use among older adults. *Journal of Drug Issues, 19*(2), 207–219.

This article is based on a study that analyzed descriptive data from the 1982 and 1985 National Household Studies on Drug Abuse (NHSDA). The analyses are of data on four kinds of psychoactive drugs: sedatives, tranquilizers, stimulants, and analgesics. Information about men and women of different ages and ethnic groups was examined.

The authors acknowledge that the analyses are limited in that the household surveys underrepresent the drug-using population in the United States because they did not survey persons in prisons, hospitals, dormitories, rest homes, motels, military institutions, or the homeless. All these groups are thought to misuse drugs at a higher rate than the population in general.

The results of the analyses indicate that analgesics are the most widely used and stimulants the least widely used of the four drugs. Women report greater use of prescribed drugs, particularly tranquilizers; more than one in ten women reported using tranquilizers in the past year. But in the 65 and older group, men report more use of sedatives, stimulants, and tranquilizers.

With regard to ethnic differences, Hispanic women report a high level of prescription analgesic use, and the ethnic minorities in the United States report less use of medically prescribed psychotropic drugs. Although the data do not indicate a severe problem in the use of these drugs among the populations examined, the authors note that the surveys' exclusion of institutionalized populations and the fact that people tend to underreport drug use generally may belie these results.

Schlesinger, S., Susman, M., & Koenigsberg, J. (1990). Self-esteem and purpose in life: A comparative study of women alcoholics. *Journal of Alcohol and Drug Education, 6*(1), 127–141.

In this questionnaire-study of 120 subjects, the investigators examined two issues affecting female alcoholics: self-esteem and purpose in life. The aim of the study was to determine the relationship between these two factors. The group of 120 women was divided into four subgroups: (1) female alcoholics; (2) male alcoholics; (3) non-alcoholic women; (4) non-alcoholic women in treatment for psychiatric disorders.

This study was designed to enable the researchers to determine whether gender or alcoholism itself is more significantly related to the lack of self-esteem and hopelessness that is well-documented in female alcoholics.

The results of the study indicate that female alcoholics can be distinguished from the other groups by a distinctive constellation of symptoms including a severe lack of self-esteem and meaninglessness. These symptoms were most pronounced in unmarried and minority women. The study results further support the belief that alcoholism cannot be reduced to chemical dependency but includes psychological and social factors, and for women the psychological toll is greater than for men.

Schilit, R., Lie, G., & Montagne, M. (1990). Substance abuse as a correlate of violence in intimate lesbian relationships. *Journal of Homosexuality, 19*(3), 51–65.

These authors, like many others reporting on the prevalence of alcohol abuse among lesbians, cite estimates that approximately one-third of gay women abuse alcohol. They are careful to point out, however, that these estimates are based on only a few studies of lesbians. Not noted by the authors is the fact that these studies are, almost without exception, based on nonrepresentative samples.

Although there is increasing evidence to support an association between substance abuse and violence in heterosexual relationships, this relationship in homosexual couples has, to date, been largely ignored. Apart from the fact that homosexuality remains a stigmatized lifestyle, other reasons exist that likely explain this lack of attention. Of primary importance is the effort within the lesbian community to maintain the appearance of a collective and cohesive unit.

The findings discussed are based on responses of 104 (29.7% response rate) self-identified lesbians who completed a mail survey. Of the women who responded, 39 percent reported abusive relationships; of those, 64 percent reported that their partners used alcohol or other drugs (AODs) prior to the battering episodes. In addition, 64 percent of the women reported that they, themselves had used AODs prior to the battering episodes. Frequency of partner drinking was related to the number of incidents of battering. Interestingly, 88 percent of the lesbians surveyed reported drinking moderately (fewer than two drinks on one occasion) or that they do not drink at all. However, 8 percent of the respondents and 6 percent of their partners use other drugs at least once a day. The most commonly used drugs are marijuana, hashish, antianxiety drugs, and cocaine. Whether the use of antianxiety drugs was nonmedical or prescribed was not clear.

The authors also note that fewer than one-half of the women who were battered sought help. This finding points to the need for more attention and more services devoted to the mental health needs of lesbians. Although limited by the low response rate and nonrepresentative sample, these findings do indicate that battering among lesbian couples exists. However, whether the pattern and relationships of substance abuse and battering are similar for homosexual and heterosexual couples needs further study.

Shore, E. R., & Batt, S. (1991). Contextual factors related to the drinking behaviors of American business and professional women. *British Journal of Addiction, 86,* 171–176.

In this survey of 453 professional or business women in the Wichita, Kansas area who agreed to answer the survey, questions were asked about alcohol use, attitudes and knowledge. Because there were no data on the group to establish population characteristics, a sampling method could not be developed and the results cannot be generalized to other groups.

The investigators' examination of the data indicate that contextual factors, specifically those directly related to drinking, are important in understanding women's drinking behaviors. Level of consumption and number of negative consequences were positively correlated with the level of drinking of spouses and best friends.

Two findings are particularly noteworthy: (1) increased age was predictive of increased consumption but had fewer negative consequences, the most frequent of which was driving under the influence; (2) multiple roles in these women were not correlated with increased consumption, i.e., job stress and other factors associated with working were not shown to contribute to increased consumption.

Turnbull, J. E. (1989). Treatment issues for alcoholic women. *Social Casework, 70*(6), 364–369.

Although there has been considerable interest in treatment outcome of alcoholics generally, the majority of published studies have focused on men, or have combined both men and women as though there were no differences between them. Turnbull provides a basic, though relatively thorough overview of gender differences in etiology and consequences of alcoholism. She focuses primarily on treatment including barriers to treatment and issues related to assessment and intervention. Turnbull concludes with a brief discussion of issues related to alcohol problems among ethnic minority women and lesbians.

Van Den Burgh, N. (Ed.) (1991). *Feminist perspectives on addiction.* New York: Springer Publishing Company.

This edited volume provides a refreshing and much-needed alternative perspective on the development, progression, and treatment of addiction. The feminist perspective values process as equally important to product and supports the belief that the personal is political. Other values consonant with a feminist approach include working collaboratively, valuing personal

experiences, encouraging growth and development, caring for others, building supportive relationships, and believing in the interconnectedness of people and events. The application of these principles is discussed in the context of research and treatment of various forms of addiction.

The book is divided into three parts. Part One: Gender roles, power, and addiction provides a feminist framework for understanding the etiology and treatment of addiction. Part Two: Substance Dependencies presents a feminist perspective on several specific forms of addiction including alcoholism and other drug addiction and eating disorders. Of particular importance (because of the dearth of related literature), are chapters on lesbian alcoholics in treatment and chemical dependency in older women. Part Three focuses on Process Dependencies and describes addictive behaviors related to gambling, relationships, sex, and work.

Contributors to the volume include a number of well-known researchers and clinicians representing a diverse range of experience. As noted by the editor, the chapters include both theoretical and practical information making the book useful for clinicians, academicians, and researchers in a variety of settings.

Waterson, J., & Ettorre, B. (1989). Providing services for women with difficulties with alcohol or other drugs: The current U.K. situation as seen by women practitioners, researchers and policy makers in the field. *Drug and Alcohol Dependence, 24,* 119–125.

This paper reports the findings of a survey focusing on services for chemically dependent women in the United Kingdom. Respondents were attendees of two conferences that addressed issues related to women's problems with alcohol and other drugs. Although surveys were completed by only 65 (54%) of the conference participants, respondents represented a wide range of researchers, policy makers, and service providers. Overall, the findings suggest that special services for women are limited in the United Kingdom. Women-only groups and female employees were the most commonly reported special services. The lack of facilities for child care and persistent stigmatization of chemically dependent women were the most commonly reported problems. The authors note that although these problems have long been identified, the gap between research and practice has not yet been bridged.

Weiner, H. D., Wallen, M. C., & Zankowski, G. L. (1990). Culture and social class as intervening variables in relapse prevention with chemically dependent women. *Journal of Psychoactive Drugs, 22*(2), 239–248.

Relapse, a complex, poorly understood phenomena continues to be one of the most frequent outcomes of chemical dependency treatment. These authors discuss the problem of relapse in lower-class, socially and economically deprived public-sector women and argue that it must be seen in the context of these women's lives.

The authors began by describing similarities and differences between the public sector and working, middle class populations of women, both of whom are treated at Eagleville Hospital. Similarities include low self-esteem, guilt, dependence on others, disruption in family and intimate relationships, family history of substance abuse, childcare responsibilities that act as a barrier for entry into treatment as well as a reason for premature departure, and a history of sexual abuse. Distinct differences also exist in that the working and middle-class women generally have some social supports and are likely to return home following treatment. They often possess educational skills and work experience suggesting that life-management coping skills have been developed and used in the recent past. In contrast, the women of lower-socioeconomic status are far less likely to have adequate life-management coping skills. They generally have minimal educational or vocational skills, little or no work experience, and limited social supports. Although they are often in need of long-term residential treatment, family responsibilities often require them to return to settings characterized by poverty, illiteracy, poor housing, unemployment, broken families, high crime rates, violence, drug dealing and use, inadequate schools, high infant mortality rates, poor health care, and inadequate public services.

The authors describe the gender-specific program developed in 1969 at Eagleville Hospital in Pennsylvania. A few of the noteworthy components of the program include adjunctive therapies such as art and horticulture therapy, assertiveness and relaxation training, social skills development, exercise, and adult basic education teaching and tutoring. Approaches to common treatment issues including low self-esteem, dependency, poor coping skills, and family concerns are discussed. Relapse and relapse prevention training focuses on five major areas: (1) emotional and spiritual well being; (2) family relationships; (3) intimate relationships; (4) the social environment; and (5) coping skills. Finally, relapse prevention with dually diagnosed patients is discussed and a case study is presented to illustrate the implementation of the program.

Weinstein, D. L. (Ed.). (1992). *Lesbians and gay men: Chemical dependency treatment issues.* Binghamton, NY: Haworth Press.

This collection of ten articles is from the annual conference, "Ten Percent of Those we Serve: Treatment of Alcoholism and other Addictions Among Gays and Lesbians." According to the editor, the articles included in the book are part of the conference goal of increasing health care providers' skills in working with lesbian and gay clients.

Although most of the articles are clinical rather than research based, they cover a wide range of issues and provide information useful to clinicians and researchers interested in the area of substance abuse prevention and treatment. Of particular interest is the lead article by Carter Heyward, a well-known feminist theologian who is openly lesbian and who is recovering from alcoholism and bulimia. Her paper provides a provocative look at homophobia and addiction within the social context of alienation and heterosexism.

Subsequent chapters address issues involved when heterosexual therapists treat homosexual clients and the challenges of working with clients who are HIV positive or have AIDS. Kus, a nurse-sociologist who specializes in gay men's studies and alcohol studies, explores spirituality in everyday life and makes recommendations for clinicians who work with gay men. Shifrin and Solis's article focuses on working with gay and lesbian adolescents and emphasizes the importance of substance abuse prevention, gay and lesbian youth in straight service settings, and the role of the family in treatment. They provide specific suggestions to school and social agency staff in promoting healthy homosexual identity formation. Rothberg and Kidder's article addresses issues important in working with lesbians who grew up in alcoholic families and the influence of that experience on adolescent development, maturation, and subsequent intimate relationships. McNally and Finnigan report findings from McNally's dissertation research focusing on stages of recovering the lesbian alcoholic's identity formation. They stress the importance for successful recovery of understanding these stages. The final three articles focus on dual diagnosis, the application of family therapy concepts in the treatment of lesbians and gay men, and the mechanics of planning an experiential weekend workshop for gays and lesbians.

As the editor notes, many additional areas related to the treatment of lesbian and gay male alcoholics need attention. However, this collection provides an important resource to clinicians and researchers who are interested in learning more about this understudied topic.

Weisner, C., & Schmidt, L. (1992). Gender disparities in treatment for alcohol problems. *Journal of the American Medical Association*, 268(14), 1872–1876.

Using structured, in-person interviews, these researchers compared men and women defined as problem drinkers, with regard to prevalence, characteristics, and treatment-seeking patterns. Problem drinkers were defined as those who met at least two of the following criteria: (1) in a one month period, consuming at least five drinks on at least one occasion; (2) experiencing one or more alcohol-related social consequences; and (3) having at least one or more alcohol dependence symptoms.

Specifically, the researchers examined women's access to treatment in a range of alcohol-specific and non-specialized health care systems. For most subjects, alcohol-treatment services were the most frequently used, but high percentages of subjects also reported using services found in the criminal justice system, mental health, and emergency service milieus. The wide range of services and settings used by problem drinkers demonstrates that the burden of dealing with this problem is shared by some agencies that are not designed to provide specialized care. The study found that, generally, women were more likely than men to have used mental health services, whereas men more often seek help through the criminal justice system *when* they used non-specialized services. The authors believe this pattern supports the supposition that women delay treatment until their problem is more severe.

The article concludes with the call for more cross-sectional research to clarify the effects of gender differences in help-seeking patterns. They believe the over representation of women in non-alcohol specific health care systems is cause for concern about the effectiveness of the care they receive.

Yandow, V. (1989). Alcoholism in women. *Psychiatric Annals*, 19(5), 243–247.

This brief overview covers an extensive range of topics including fetal alcohol syndrome, women's greater vulnerability to alcohol, the effects of drinking on sexuality, and the relationship between alcoholism and other psychopathology. Although most of the information presented is not new, the author does not support many debatable contentions with references. In addition, several statements are made that are unclear or questionable. For example, the author states (under the heading "Genetic Factors"), that "Cohabitation, especially in the lesbian population, is also a risk factor for women" (pp. 244–245). Whether the implication is that women who cohabit are more at risk than those who are married or live alone is unclear. Further, this distinction concerning lesbians is especially of concern because "cohabiting" is the only socially recognized living arrangement for lesbians whose relationships are not recognized legally. The author does make a number of important points including the fact that there are appallingly few treatment programs that offer child care and other special services for women. The statement that more money is spent on advertising one brand of beer than that allocated for the entire national research budget emphasizes the enormity of the task faced by researchers and health care professionals in trying to learn about and control alcohol abuse in cultures that promote drinking as an acceptable part of adult life.

Young, E. B. (1990). The role of incest issues in relapse. *Journal of Psychoactive Drugs, 22*(2), 249–258.

Recent studies have found that over 75 percent of chemically dependent women in inpatient settings report childhood sexual abuse. Women victimized by sexual abuse are at high risk for the development of a variety of problems including low self-esteem, depression, anxiety, alienation and the inability to sustain relationships, the repetition of abusive relationships, sexual dysfunction and dependence on alcohol and other drugs, as well as other addictions.

The author discusses at some length the following points: (1) the role of addictive behaviors in defending against memories of sexual abuse; (2) the risk that unidentified incest material may precipitate relapse or result from relapse; (3) the fact that relapse may indicate the presence of other addictions that must be identified in order for recovery to proceed; and (4) the often compounding problem of sex and love addiction. She emphasizes that these issues must be considered, and if present, included in the treatment/relapse prevention plan.

Chapter 9

Women's Cardiovascular Health

Karyn Holm
Sue M. Penckofer

INTRODUCTION

Preventing and treating heart disease in women is the challenge of the future. Approximately 485,000 women die of cardiovascular disease annually as compared to 233,000 who die from all forms of cancer with 42,800 of this number from breast cancer and 49,000 from lung cancer (American Heart Association, 1993). While these statistics are alarming, they support the urgency of the problem. Over the years, issues surrounding women and heart disease have evolved from initiatives designed to help women prevent heart disease in their spouses to contemporary initiatives designed to help women prevent heart disease in themselves. It was almost three decades ago, long before heart disease was considered a problem in women, that over 10,000 women came together to learn how to protect their husbands against heart disease (Oregon Heart Association: Husbands and Hearts, November, 1964). Since that time, statistics have steadily accumulated suggesting that heart disease is taking on increased importance as a women's health issue. In October, 1989 the first conference on heart disease in women was held in Washington, D.C. At this conference, sponsored by the American Heart Association, the most current information on the incidence, diagnosis and treatment of coronary heart disease (CHD) in women was presented. In addition, information regarding the impact of estrogen and the effect of the multiple roles women now assume on the development of CHD was also discussed.

Current understanding of risk factors for heart disease in women is that they are for the most part not entirely dissimilar from those in men. For both sexes there are those factors which are unchangeable and those which are amenable to risk factor modification. For example, age (being older), race (being black), gender (estrogen seems to be protective against heart disease) and family history (relatives with heart disease) are factors that we can do nothing about, except be cognizant that these factors are instrumental in the development of heart disease. However, the modifiable risk factors, for example smoking, high blood pressure, and elevated serum cholesterol are all responsive to programs of risk factor modification.

Regarding those risk factors for which intervention(s) have proven successful, there are a number of issues for women. First of all, it is clear that although there is increased momentum to study women and heart disease risk, our primary knowledge base has been male dominated. Furthermore, as we gather knowledge about heart disease in women, it will be important to compare these findings to those findings of the traditional male model.

Current indications are that there is bias in the diagnosis and treatment of women. For example, researchers have shown that physicians take a less aggressive approach to the management of coronary artery disease (CAD) in women than in men (Steingart et al., 1991); that women hospitalized for CAD undergo fewer major diagnostic and therapeutic procedures than men

(Ayanian & Epstein, 1991) and that more males than females undergo coronary artery bypass surgery (CABS) upon diagnosis of coronary artery obstruction (Becker, Corrao & Alpert, 1988; Krumholz, Douglas, Lauer & Pasternak, 1992). It has also been demonstrated that late referrals for surgical intervention may increase the operative mortality seen in women following bypass (Khan, Nessim, Gray, Czer, Chaux & Matloff, 1990).

The extent of disease rather than gender alone may be more important when examining in-hospital mortality rates for men and women. A recent study reported that women had more severe disease which accounted for their higher in-hospital mortality when compared to men undergoing percutaneous transluminal coronary angioplasty (Bell, Holmes, Berger, Garratt, Bailey & Gersh, 1993). In addition, there is evidence to indicate that women present with signs/symptoms of angina as compared to men who present with acute myocardial infarction (MI) or sudden death as their initial manifestation of CHD (Holm, Penckofer, Keresztes, Biordi & Chandler, 1993). A recent study demonstrated that if angina was the first clinical manifestation of heart disease, women had a longer survival and decreased risk of MI/death when compared to men. If MI or sudden death were the initial presentations for women, subsequent MI or cardiac death or survival was comparable to men of the same age and diagnosis (Orencia, Bailey, Yawn & Kottke, 1993). Therefore, the need to educate women on the clinical presentation and early diagnosis is crucial. What becomes problematic as noted by Orencia and colleagues (1993) is that although current assessment and diagnostic testing for women is problematic, aggressive measures should be sought to improve early diagnosis given the evidence that women have better survival outcomes if angina is identified early.

Finally, there are gender disparities in clinical decision-making (Council on Ethical and Judicial Affairs, American Medical Association, 1991) as well as gaps in clinical science due to the exclusion of women (Cotton, 1990). This is particularly true for elderly women (Gurwitz, Col & Azorn, 1992; Wenger, 1992) and women of color (Liao, Cooper, Ghali & Szocka, 1992). In this review, we summarize contemporary literature and highlight implications for women in improving CHD risk. Based upon an exhaustive literature search for the years 1986 to the present, the aim is to gain appreciation of heart disease in women in order to design successful interventions.

Over recent years, the literature concerning women and heart disease has increased dramatically. The expectation is that over ensuing years, we will come to better understand how women can decrease their cardiovascular risk and improve their lifestyles via primary prevention. With a large proportion of women living longer, factors associated with hormonal therapy will continue to be important. Knowing that heart disease risk in both genders increases in a linear fashion with age, with women experiencing greater risk in postmenopausal years, hormonal therapy will continue to be held by many as the sole answer to heart disease in postmenopausal women. As care providers and advocates for women in the health care system of today and tomorrow, it is our responsibility to insure that women not only understand cardiovascular risk factor modification aimed at smoking cessation, dietary modifications, and increased physical activity but also understand their family and personal health history in order to make informed decisions.

REFERENCES

American Heart Association. (1993). *The 1993 Heart and Stroke Facts Statistics.* American Heart Association, Dallas, Texas.

Becker, R. C., Corrao, J. M., & Alpert, J. S. (1988). Review: Coronary artery bypass surgery in women. *Clinical Cardiology, 11*, 443–448.

Bell, M., Holmes, D., Berger, P., Garratt, K., Bailey, K., & Gersch, B. (1993). The changing in-hospital mortality of women undergoing percutaneous transluminal coronary angioplasty. *JAMA, 296*(16), 2091–2095.

Cotton, P. (1990). Examples abound of gaps in medical knowledge because of groups excluded from scientific study. *JAMA, 263*(8), 1051–1056.

Council on Ethical and Judicial Affairs, American Medical Association. (1991). Gender disparities in clinical decision making. *JAMA, 266*(4), 559–562.

Gurwitz, J. H., Col, N. F., & Avorn, J. (1992). The exclusion of the elderly and women from clinical trials in acute myocardial infarction. *JAMA, 268*(11), 1417–1422.

Holm, K., Penckofer, S., Keresztes, P., Biordi, D., & Chandler, P. (1993). Coronary artery disease in women: Assessment, diagnosis, intervention, and strategies for life style change. *AWHONN's Clinical Issues, 4*(2), 272–285.

Krumholz, H., Douglas, P., Lauer, M., & Pasternak, R. (1992). Selection of patients for coronary angiography and coronary revascularization early after myocardial infarction: Is there evidence of referral bias? *Annals of Internal Medicine, 116*(10), 785–790.

Liao, Y., Cooper, R., Ghali, J., & Szocka, A. (1992). Survival rates with coronary artery disease for black women compared with black men. *JAMA, 268*(14), 1867–1871.

Oregon Affiliate of the American Heart Association. (1964). *Hearts and Husbands.* Paper from the Hearts and Husbands—First Women's Conference on Coronary Heart Disease by the Oregon Affiliate of the American Heart Association, Portland, November 6th.

Orencia, A., Bailey K., Yawn, B., & Kottke, T. (1993). Effect of gender on long-term outcome of angina pectoris and myocardial infarction/sudden unexpected death. *JAMA, 269*(18), 2392–2397.

Steingart, R. M., Packer, M., Hamm, P., Coglianese, M. E., Gersh, B., Geltman, E. M., Sollano, J., Katz, S., Moye, L., Basta, L. L., Lewis, S. J., Gottlieb, S. S., Bernstein, V., McEwan, P., Jacobson, K., Brown, E. J., Kukin, M. L., Kantrowitz, N. E., & Pfeffer, M. A. for the Survival and Ventricular Enlargement Investigators. (1991). Sex differences in the management of coronary artery disease. *The New England Journal of Medicine*, *325*(4), 226–230.

BOOKS AND ARTICLES

Austin, M. A., King, M. C., Bawol, R. D., Hulley, S. B., & Friedman, G. D. (1987). Risk factors for coronary heart disease in adult female twins. *American Journal of Epidemiology, 125,* 308-318.

A strong genetic component for levels of low density lipoprotein (LDL), high density lipoprotein (HDL) and relative weight but not for systolic and diastolic blood pressures was found in this study of risk factors for CHD. The sample consisted of 434 adult female twin pairs for whom estimates of heritability, adjusted for shared environmental and behavioral influences were examined for key risk factors. The findings may help explain why some women continue to have high levels of coronary risk factors despite following recommendations for risk factor modification. For these genetically heart disease prone women, we will need to develop and test more aggressive risk factor modification programs which may prove useful in overcoming inherent predisposition to CHD in women.

Beard, C. M., Kottke, T. E., Annegers, J. F., & Ballard, D. J. (1989). The Rochester coronary heart disease project: Effect of cigarette smoking, hypertension, diabetes, and steroidal estrogen use on coronary heart disease among 40- to 59-year-old-women, 1960 through 1982. *Mayo Clinic Proceedings, 64,* 1471–1480.

For the years 1960 to 1982 all new cases of CHD among mid-life Rochester, Minnesota women were identified and matched with community control subjects. Of all of the risk factors, cigarette smoking accounted for a greater percentage of myocardial infarctions and sudden unexpected deaths (64%) than hypertension (45%) or diabetes (13%). Furthermore, estrogen exposure reduced CHD by 14 percent, leading the investigators to conclude that steroidal estrogens should be prescribed for all women aged 40 to 59 years. Again, we have strong indications of the protective effect of estrogen against CHD. Because the evidence is rapidly accumulating for the health benefits of estrogen replacement therapy for perimenopausal, menopausal and postmenopausal women, it is time to carefully analyze the risks and benefits of estrogen replacement in this age group.

Castelli, W. P. (1988). Cardiovascular disease in women. *American Journal of Obstetrics and Gynecology, 158,* 1553–1560.

In this article, the major emphasis is on serum cholesterol and serum lipids as primary indicators of cardiovascular disease in women. Hypertension, elevated serum glucose levels, obesity, and smoking are also highlighted. The author stresses that the rates for MI are similar for women as they are for men, but that for women, symptoms of CHD will occur at an older age. As longevity increases for both sexes, we can expect that more woman than ever before will live for many years past menopause. Therefore, issues associated with estrogen replacement therapy will continue to surface until estrogen replacement therapy is shown to be safe and effective for the majority of women or until reasonable alternatives to estrogen replacement therapy are identified and tested.

Fiebach, N. H., Viscoli, C. M., & Horwitz, R. I. (1990). Differences between women and men in survival after myocardial infarction. *JAMA*, *263*(8), 1092–1096.

Gender is often cited as an independent risk factor for MI, the assumption being that men have greater mortality and morbidity following MI. In this study of survival differences between the sexes following MI, it was demonstrated that mortality rates were not significantly different between women and men for in-hospital deaths. Furthermore, observed mortality rates were more related to individual risk factors than to gender differences.

Holm, K., & Penckofer, S. (1992). Cardiovascular risk factors in women. *The Journal of Myocardial Ischemia*, *4*(1), 25–46.

In absolute terms, more women than men will die from CHD because for whatever reasons women live longer than men. Data from the Framingham study indicate that few women will die from CAD before menopause. Furthermore, national statistics indicate that ischemic heart disease (IHD) peaks in women 15 to 25 years following menopause. For both sexes, CHD rates increase with age. Therefore, when examining the relationship between menopause and IHD, the confounding influence of age must be considered.

Holm K., Penckofer, S., Keresztes, P., Biordi, D., & Chandler, P. (1993). Coronary artery disease in women: Assessment, diagnosis, intervention, and strategies for life style change. *AWHONN's Clinical Issues in Perinatal and Women's Health Nursing*, *4*(2), 272–285.

As a professional group composed almost entirely of women, nurses can assume a leadership role in promoting a healthy life style for women. For each of us, this translates into

insuring that we ourselves practice what we tell our patients, i.e., what we preach.

Penckofer, S., & Holm, K. (1993). What you should know about women and heart disease. *Nursing '93*, 42–46.

A case study approach is used to illustrate examples of women who may present with CHD. An overview of modifiable and nonmodifiable cardiac risk factors and their unique contribution to CHD in women is addressed. In addition, a risk questionnaire designed specifically for women (adapted from the Arizona Heart Institute) is included to assess your own cardiovascular risk.

Perlman, J. A., Wolf, P. H., Ray, R., & Lieberknecht, G. (1988). Cardiovascular risk factors, premature heart disease, and all-cause mortality in a cohort of Northern California women. *American Journal of Obstetrics and Gynecology*, *158*, 1568–1574.

There is a definitive need to screen women for risk of heart disease as our knowledge to date indicates that lifestyle modifications may significantly improve quality of life and risk of cardiovascular disease. These investigators identified that among premenopausal women, smoking, high blood pressure and diabetes were the strongest predictors of cardiovascular disease with associated risks of 2.8, 10.5, and 11.6 respectively. Of these factors, the one which can be directly altered is smoking with hypertension and diabetes benefitting from indirect interventions.

Smoking

Berman, A. M. (1989). Facts on women and smoking. *Journal of the American Medical Women's Association*, *44*(2), 55.

In this short article from Harvard University's Institute for the Study of Smoking Behavior and Policy, we are presented with the most current facts concerning women and smoking behavior. While smoking rates in men have declined to a greater extent than those in women, among women college graduates, only 17.1 percent are currently smokers compared to 31 percent of women whose education stopped at high school. This statistic alone has important implications for women's health. College graduates are responding to contemporary warnings about the health hazards associated with smoking, while their less educated sisters are ignoring the Surgeon General's pleas for a smoke-free society.

Khaw, K-T., Chir, M. B. B., Tazuke, S., & Barrett-Connor, E. (1988). Cigarette smoking and levels of adrenal androgens in postmenopausal women. *The New England Journal of Medicine, 318*(26), 1705–1709.

These researchers examined the relationship between cigarette smoking and adrenal androgens in a sample of 233 white, postmenopausal women 60- to 79-years of age. They found that in those women currently smoking cigarettes, the mean plasma levels of adrenal androgens were higher than in those who were nonsmokers. The differences in androgen levels remained after adjustments were made for age and body mass index (BMI). These findings suggest that the possible decreased risk of breast and endometrial cancer often associated with cigarette smoking is probably not as related to estrogen as it is to androgen levels. While this issue requires further study, women should realize that when weighing the benefits and risks associated with cigarette smoking, the risks continue to outweigh the benefits.

Krauss, R. M., Perlman, J. A., Ray, R., & Petitti, D. (1988). Effects of estrogen dose and smoking on lipid and lipoprotein levels in postmenopausal women. *American Journal of Obstetrical Gynecology, 158*, 1606–1611.

In a study of the combined effects of conjugated estrogen use, age, BMI, and smoking on plasma lipid and lipoprotein levels, these researchers found that estrogen was associated with reductions in low-density lipoproteins (LDLs) and increases in high density lipoproteins (HDLs). A maximum LDL cholesterol level reduction was

reached at a dose of 1.25 mg., after which point increasing the dose of estrogen had little effect. In smokers, the elevations of HDLs and the decreases in LDLs were not as dramatic. Therefore, the benefits associated with estrogen are not realized to the same extent in smokers.

Palmer, J. R., Rosenberg, L., & Shapiro, S. (1989). "Low yield" cigarettes and the risk of nonfatal myocardial infarction in women. *New England Journal of Medicine, 320*(4), 1569–1573.

Tobacco companies are currently promoting newer brands of cigarettes with reduced yields of nicotine and carbon monoxide. In this study, risk of MI was compared to current smokers by the nicotine and carbon monoxide yield of the cigarettes they smoked. The estimated relative risk of MI in those who smoked low yield cigarettes was similar to the relative risk in those who smoked high yield cigarettes. These findings suggest that women who switch to low yield brands are doing little or nothing to reduce their risk of MI.

Rigotti, N. A. (1990). Cigarette smoking and body weight. *New England Journal of Medicine, 320*(14), 931–933.

Smoking remains the single most important preventable cause of death in the United States today. Furthermore, the gender gap is narrowing and if it continues, women will outsmoke men by the mid-1990s. For many women, smoking is still perceived as an effective means of weight control and is a major deterrent to quitting. Research has indeed demonstrated that smokers weigh 5 to 10 pounds more than nonsmokers of comparable age and height. Until we are clear as to the underlying mechanisms, we must continue to counsel people to quit smoking. For the woman smoker, it is important to stress that any weight gain can be minimized by an exercise program and a balanced diet.

Rimm, E. B., Manson J. E., Stampfer, M. J., Colditz, G. A., Willett, W. C., Rosner, B., Hennekens, C. H., & Speizer, F. E. (1993). Cigarette smoking and risk of diabetes in women. *American Journal of Public Health, 83*(2), 211–214.

The association between smoking and the incidence of noninsulin-dependent diabetes (NIDDM) was examined in 114,247 nurses who in 1976 were free of diabetes, cardiovascular disease and cancer. Findings revealed that current smokers had an increased risk of diabetes with a dose-response trend for risk of diabetes among heavier smokers. The relative risk of diabetes, adjusted for obesity and other risk factors was 1.42 among women who smoked 25 or more cigarettes daily as compared to nonsmokers. Because both smoking and diabetes are important risk factors for CAD in women, this important link provides further evidence for the value of smoking cessation.

Rosenberg, L., Palmer, J. R., & Shapiro, S. (1990). Decline in the risk of myocardial infarction among women who stop smoking. *The New England Journal of Medicine, 322*(4), 213–217.

The importance of smoking cessation is reinforced by the findings of this study. Here the smoking habits of 910 patients who had suffered their first MI were compared to the smoking habits of 2,375 controls. The relative risk of MI among current smokers as compared with women who never smoked was 3.6. However, most of this increase in risk had dissipated after approximately 2 to 3 years. Because most smokers wonder how long it will take to be free of the risks associated with smoking, the findings of this study give important information.

Royce, J. M., Hymowitz, N., Corbett, K., Hartwell, T. D., & Orlandi, M. A., for the Commit Research Group. (1993). Smoking cessation factors among African Americans and whites. *American Journal of Public Health, 83*(2), 220–226.

A paradox is that African Americans tend to smoke fewer cigarettes per day and tend to begin smoking later in life than do whites, yet their smoking-related disease mortality is

higher. Smoking fewer cigarettes implies that cessation should be easier. However, prevalence of smoking in African Americans continues to exceed that of whites. Here smoking patterns and attitudes that influence smoking cessation and relapse among African Americans were explored. Primary results in this sample of $n = 3,418$ (54.7% women) were that compared with whites, African Americans who smoked less than 25 cigarettes per day were 1.6 times more likely to smoke within 10 minutes of awakening. However, African Americans reported a strong desire to quit smoking and reported serious quitting attempts over the past year. Thus, smoking cessation interventions might be effectively targeted for this large segment of our population.

Williamson, D. F., Madans, J., Anda, R. F., Kleinman, J. C., Giovino, G. A., & Byers, T. (1991). Smoking cessation and severity of weight gain in a national cohort. *New England Journal of Medicine, 324*(11), 739–745.

Change in smoking status was related to change in body weight in a cohort of continuing smokers ($n = 748$ Men; $n = 1,137$ Women) and quitters of at least one year ($n = 409$ M; $n = 359$ W) who comprised the National Health and Nutrition Examination Survey (NHANES I) sample. The mean weight gain with smoking cessation while adjusting for age, race, education, alcohol, illness, baseline weight and physical activity was 2.8 kilograms (kg) in men and 3.8 kg in women. Major weight gain (> 13 kg) was observed in 9.8 percent of the men and 13.4 percent of the women who had quit smoking. Further, the relative risk of major weight gain in those who quit smoking, as compared to those who continued smoking was 8.1 (95% confidence interval 4.4 to 14.9) in men and 5.8 (95% confidence interval 3.7 to 9.1) in women, remaining high regardless of the duration of cessation. For both men and women, predictors of weight gain were race (being black), age (under the age of 55 years), and smoking greater than 15 plus cigarettes per day. Major weight gain, therefore was demonstrated to occur in only a small portion of those who quit smoking. However, this does not negate the need for effective methods of smoking cessation which concentrate on maintenance of baseline weight.

Cholesterol

American Heart Association. (1993). *The 1993 Heart and Stroke Facts.* American Heart Association, Dallas, Texas.

Elevated cholesterol is one of the major risk factors for heart disease. The level of risk is dependent on the value of the serum cholesterol concentration in the blood (mg/dl = milligrams per deciliter). As the level of blood cholesterol increases, so does the risk for heart disease. Low risk is a level below 200 mg/dl, moderate risk includes values from 200 to 239 mg/dl and a level over 240 mg/dl is associated with increased risk. Studies have shown that cholesterol levels in women exceed those of men from age 20- to 24-years and from age 45 years on up. In 1989 an estimated 55 million adult women had serum cholesterol levels of 200 mg/dl or higher. More than 60 percent of white females and 54 percent of black females were included in this group.

Bush, T., Fried, L., & Barrett-Connor, E. (1988). Cholesterol, lipoproteins, and coronary heart disease in women. *Clinical Chemistry, 34,* (8B), 60–70.

The associations found between cholesterol and heart disease have been based on studies of men and cannot be assumed to hold true for women. Here: (a) the relationship between cholesterol, HDL and LDL to the incidence of CHD; (b) the determinants of cholesterol and lipoprotein values in women; and (c) the research suggesting that modification of lipid profiles in women is associated with a change in CHD risk are examined. The conclusions were: (a) the HDL cholesterol seems to be the most important lipid for women when examining risk potential for CHD and the LDL cholesterol particle is less dense in women than in men indicating perhaps less atherogenic potential; (b) determinants of the concentrations of cholesterol, HDL and LDL are genetic but are not sex-linked; (c) there is no data presently available to indicate whether changes in cholesterol or lipoprotein values will change coronary disease risk, but there is evidence to indicate that exogenous estrogen administration can reduce cardiovascular risk by increasing the levels of HDL.

Cohn, B., Brand, R., & Hulley, S. (1989). Correlates of high density lipoprotein cholesterol in women studied by the method of co-twin control. *American Journal of Epidemiology, 129,* 988–999.

There is evidence to indicate that genetic factors may explain a large amount of the variability of HDL cholesterol in women. This study examined those variables that are associated with HDL cholesterol even after adjustment for familial factors (genetic and nongenetic). Female twins (monozygous and dizygous) were used to adjust for the familial influences to study the relationship between HDL and the risk factors of smoking, postmenopausal estrogen use, alcohol use, leisure exercise and body mass. Results indicated that the association between smoking and HDL and body mass and HDL were negative while the association between estrogen use and HDL was positive. The relationship for all three of these risk factors was found to be independent of familial variables. The association between alcohol (one to two drinks per day) and HDL was positive but may not be independent of familial influence. Finally, the association between exercise and HDL was not evident in monozygous twins after adjustment for familial variables. It was concluded that perhaps exercise may be explained by factors shared by monozygous twins. It was suggested that those factors which are independent of familial influence (smoking, body mass and estrogen use) may be more amenable to intervention for women.

Johansson, S., Bondjers, G., Fager, G., Wedel, H., Tsipogianni, A., Olofsson, S., Vedin, A., Wiklund, O., & Wilhelmsson, C. (1988). Serum lipids and apoprotein levels in women with acute myocardial infarction. *Arteriosclerosis, 8*(6), 742–749.

It has recently been argued that the protein component of the lipoprotein called the "apoprotein" is the more sensitive indicator of CHD risk. The main apoproteins in HDL are Apo A-I and Apo A-II while Apo-B and Apo-E are the main apoproteins of LDL and VLDL (very low density lipoprotein). This study compared a sample of women less than 55 years of age (n = 59) who suffered their first acute MI with those from a random sample in the same population (n = 140). Those women with acute MI had higher mean values of cholesterol, triglycerides, Apo-B and Apo-E and lower levels of HDL and Apo A-I than controls. However, after adjustment for age, cholesterol level was not different between these two groups. In addition, smoking, high serum triglyceride, history of hypertension, age, low levels of Apo A-I and high levels of Apo-E were risk factors independently contributing to the first nonfatal MI in these women. Therefore, evidence indicating that certain apoproteins characterize young women with acute MI requires further study to examine the extent of their importance as indicators of CHD risk in women of all age groups.

Manolio, T., Ettinger, W., Tracy, R., Kuller, L., Borhani, N., Lynch, J., & Fried, L., for the CHS Collaborative Group. (1993). Epidemiology of lower cholesterol levels in older adults: The Cardiovascular Health Study. *Circulation, 87*(3), 728–737.

Although decreased cholesterol has been associated with improved levels of cardiovascular health, recent research questions if levels too low can also be detrimental to one's health. This study investigated a sample of men (n = 2,091) and women (n = 2,714) aged 65 to 100 who participated in a multicenter Cardiovascular Health Study. Cholesterol levels <160 mg/dl were evident in 11.6 percent (n = 242) of men and 3.7 percent (n = 101) of women. Low cholesterol levels were associated with a higher prevalence of diabetes and lower levels of HDL-C, LDL-C and factor VII in both men and women. In addition, for women, cancer in the past five years, low income and increased creatinine were also reported. The relationships identified in this study suggest that some poorer health outcomes have been observed in adults with cholesterol levels <160 mg/dl. Further investigations to examine the mortality

and morbidity of patients with low cholesterol is needed.

Meilahn, E., Kuller, L., Stein, E., Caggiula, A., & Matthews, K. (1988). Characteristics associated with apoprotein and lipoprotein lipid levels in middle-aged women. *Ateriosclerosis, 8*(5), 515–520.

Evidence indicates that perhaps measurements of apoprotein levels are more stable and reliable than lipid values which may be extremely variable. Therefore, this study identified how certain characteristics (age, obesity, alcohol, smoking and exercise) affected apoprotein (Apo A-I, Apo A-II, Apo-B) and lipoprotein (HDL, LDL) values in healthy, premenopausal women (n = 541). Results indicated that with increasing age, the apoproteins, particularly Apo-B increased while the lipoproteins did not (p < .05). In addition, although blacks had higher A apoproteins and lower B apoproteins and lipoproteins, when compared to whites, the difference was not significant. Obesity was associated with elevated LDL and Apo-B and markedly low HDL and a modest decrease in Apo A-I values. Alcohol intake was positively associated with increased HDL, Apo A-I and Apo A-II. Smokers had elevated LDL and Apo-B levels and lower HDL and A apoproteins. Activity was not an independent predictor of apoprotein and lipid concentration. Therefore, results indicate that individual characteristics affect not only lipoprotein but aproprotein values and with an improved understanding of apoproteins, perhaps better predictors of risk for CHD in women can be identified and interventions appropriately implemented.

Diet

Khaw, K., & Barrett-Connor, E. (1987). Dietary fiber and reduced ischemic heart disease mortality rates in men and women: A 12-year prospective study. *American Journal of Epidemiology, 126*(6), 1093–1102.

The relationship between intake of dietary fiber and risk of heart disease is in its infant stages of research although early studies suggest an inverse relationship between the two. As dietary fiber intake increases, the risk of CAD decreases. Because of the lack of prospective studies on dietary fiber and heart disease in women, this study investigated the relationship between intake of dietary fiber at baseline in 859 men and women and followed this cohort 12 years to assess IHD mortality. Results showed that dietary fiber intake was reduced in both men and women who subsequently died of IHD. There was a statistically significant increase in risk of heart disease in men compared to women when dietary fiber intake was less than 16 gm/24 hours. Dietary fiber intake also positively correlated with HDL cholesterol in men and negatively correlated with LDL and total cholesterol in women. Overall, the relative risk for IHD in both men and women are similar when associated with dietary fiber intake.

La Vecchia, C., Gentile, A., Negri, E., Parazzini, F., & Franceschi, S. (1989). Coffee consumption and myocardial infarction in women. *American Journal of Epidemiology, 130*(3), 481–485.

Conflicting results of various studies examining the relationship between coffee consumption and risk of heart disease have been found in the literature. This case-control study examined 262 women who suffered MI and 519 controls who were admitted to the hospital for nondigestive tract disorders. Results showed an increased risk of heart disease for heavy (four or more cups per day) caffeine-containing coffee consumers. The strongest risk factor found in this study was the combination of heavy coffee consumption and cigarette smoking. Increased risk was also found in hyperlipidemic women who were heavy coffee drinkers. The authors hypothesize that coffee causes an increase in total cholesterol and women can effectively decrease their serum cholesterol level by reducing their coffee consumption.

Mensink, R., & Katan, M. (1989). Effect of a diet enriched with monounsaturated or polyunsaturated fatty acids on levels of low-density and high-density lipoprotein cholesterol in healthy women and men. *The New England Journal of Medicine, 321*(7), 436–441.

The risk of heart disease increases with elevated levels of LDL. A diet which reduces the intake of saturated fat will lower these LDL levels. This study, unlike previous studies, focuses on the effect of two separate diets on serum lipoprotein levels in both men and women. One group received a diet high in monounsaturated fats and the other group received a diet high in polyunsaturated fats. Thirty-two women and 28 men were included in the study. Findings indicated that in women, lipid levels did not fluctuate with stage in the menstrual cycle. Both diets were found to decrease levels of LDL cholesterol. Levels of LDL cholesterol did not vary between men and women when saturated fat was removed from the diet, but the levels of HDL cholesterol decreased in men as compared to women. The effects of diet on HDL cholesterol in women needs to be further researched as evidenced by the results of this study.

Sharlin, J., Posner, B. M., Gershoff, S. N., Zeitlin, M. F., & Berger, P. D. (1992). Nutrition and behavioral characteristics and determinants of plasma cholesterol levels in men and women. *Journal of the American Dietetic Association, 92*(4), 434–440.

As part of a cholesterol screening project, the relationship of cholesterol levels to individual characteristics was examined. More than $1/3$ of men and $1/3$ of women had cholesterol levels falling in the moderate to high categories with 17 percent of women and 10 percent of men having extremely high levels. Further analysis revealed that the women with elevated cholesterol levels were older than those with low cholesterol levels, were less likely to follow a vegetarian diet, were overweight, were hypertensive and had significantly higher fat intake than those with lower cholesterol levels. When counseling women about cholesterol lowering strategies, it is wise to consider the interaction of all of these factors.

Stampfer, M., Colditz, G., Willett, W., Speizer, F., & Hennekens, C. (1988). A prospective study of moderate alcohol consumption and the risk of coronary disease and stroke in women. *The New England Journal of Medicine, 319*(5), 267–273.

Although studies in men reveal a relationship between moderate alcohol consumption and decreased risk of CAD, these studies have not been done with women. HDL levels found to be higher in women when compared to men, are thought to be further elevated following moderate alcohol consumption. This study prospectively examined a cohort of registered nurses and assessed their consumption of beer, wine, and liquor. It was found that among middle-aged women, moderate alcohol consumption decreased the risk of CHD and ischemic stroke, but increased the risk of subarachnoid hemorrhage. While these findings are similar to those found in men, previous research has shown that alcohol consumption has been associated with an increased risk of breast cancer and hypertension in women. Therefore, the benefits and risks of alcohol consumption in women needs further study.

Stampfer, M., Hennekens, C., Manson, J., Colditz, G., Rosner, B., & Willett, W. (1993). Vitamin E consumption and the risk of coronary disease in women. *New England Journal of Medicine, 328*(20), 1444–1449.

The role of antioxidants in the prevention of CHD has had widespread interest. This study examined the dietary questionnaires (which included an assessment of vitamin E) mailed in 1980 of women who participated in the Nurses' Health Study. For those women who took vitamin E supplements for more than 2 years, their risk of CHD was .59 (95% confidence interval, .38 to .91) after adjusting for other antioxidants (i.e., multivitamins), age and other cardiac risk factors. There is evidence that vitamin E use may be associated with decreased risk of CHD, however, before public recommendations are made regarding vitamin E use, more information

is needed preferably by results of randomized clinical trials.

van Beresteijn, E. C. H., Korevaar, J. C., Huijbregts, P. C. W., Schouten, E. G., Burema, J., & Kok, F. J. (1993). Perimenopausal increase in serum cholesterol: A 10-year longitudinal study. *American Journal of Epidemiology, 137*(4), 383–392.

Serum total cholesterol and dietary intake were measured annually (1979 to 1989) in 167 healthy perimenopausal women (initially 49 to 56 years) residing in the Netherlands. The intent was to observe the natural course of serum total cholesterol as well as the influence of dietary fat intake during and following cessation of ovulation. From 2 years prior to 6 years following menopause, serum total cholesterol concentration increased on the average by at least 1.1 mmol/liter (19%). Lowering of serum cholesterol was more responsive in women who had an increased intake of polyunsaturated fatty acids. The major implication is that increasing the intake of polyunsaturated fats may be an effective way to counteract the expected rise in total cholesterol as women age.

Obesity

Burkman, R. (1988). Obesity, stress and smoking: Their role as cardiovascular risk factors in women. *American Journal of Obstetrics and Gynecology, 158,* 1592–1597.

CHD is the leading cause of death in older women. Although a strong relationship between heart disease and obesity in men has been suggested, the relationship in women is not as clear. This review article cites studies documenting the association of obesity with CHD. It is noted that although obesity is positively correlated with other risk factors such as high cholesterol, diabetes and hypertension; the direct relationship of obesity and CHD is nonexistent or very weak in women. Nevertheless, because of its association with other risk factors, it is reported that maintenance of a "reasonable weight" is essential and approaches such as behavior modification programs, support groups and physical activity programs are recommended.

Despres, J-P., Moorjani, S., Ferland, M., Tremblay, A., Lupien, P., Nadeau, A., Pinault, S., Theriault, G., & Bouchard, C. (1989). Adipose tissue distribution and plasma lipoprotein levels in obese women: Importance of intra-abdominal fat. *Arteriosclerosis, 9,* 203–210.

Recent prospective studies have shown that "truncal obesity" which is characterized by excess abdominal fat is associated with increased morbidity and mortality from CHD. Although previous research studies have used the waist to hip ratio and subcutaneous skinfold as measures of abdominal fat, this study is unique in that computerized axial tomography (CAT) was used to measure intra-abdominal fat. Fifty-two premenopausal women aged 35.6 ± 5.5 years were measured for fat mass (percent of body fat x body weight), intra-abdominal fat by CAT scan, waist and hip circumferences, and plasma lipoprotein and apoproteins values. Results indicated that fat mass was not correlated with plasma lipoproteins, however "deep abdominal fat" measured by CAT scan (L4 to L5) was negatively correlated with HDL and ratios of HDL/LDL, Apo A-I/Apo B, HDL_2/HDL_3. Similar findings were noted when the waist to hip ratio was correlated with the plasma lipoproteins. Interestingly, however, the waist to hip ratio better explained the variance observed in the dependent variables of HDL, HDL_2 and HDL Apo A-I and deep abdominal fat explained more of the variance observed in the ratios of HDL/LDL, Apo A-I/Apo-B and HDL_2/HDL_3. Therefore, the authors argue that the waist to hip ratio may be the more cost-effective method of measuring abdominal fat and in epidemiologic studies, it may be the "best anthropometric measure." It is suggested that research continue to examine the association of obesity and lipoprotein alterations in women and reasons for the relationship (i.e., cause-effect) be further explored.

Folsom, A. R., Kaye, S. A., Sellers, T. A., Hong, C. P., Cerhan, J. R., Potter, J. D., & Prineas, R. J. (1993). Body fat distribution and 5-year risk of death in older women. *JAMA, 269*(4), 483–487.

BMI (ratio of weight in kilograms per height in meters squared) and waist to hip ratio were evaluated for their association with mortality risk in older women. A random sample of 41,837 women (55 to 69 years) with a total mortality of 1,504 deaths were studied. BMI was associated with mortality in a J-shaped fashion meaning that mortality was highest in the smallest as well as the most obese. Waist to hip ratio was associated, however, with mortality in a dose response fashion and was unrelated to weight loss prior to baseline. Waist to hip ratio was also associated with higher rates of early deaths among the leanest women. Therefore, a better indicator for risk of death in older women is the waist to hip ratio which should be routinely measured in older women.

Folsom, A., Prineas, R., Kaye, S., & Soler, J. (1989). Body fat distribution and self-reported prevalence of hypertension, heart attack, and other heart disease in older women. *International Journal of Epidemiology, 18*(2), 361–367.

This study examined the association between fat distribution and the prevalence of hypertension, heart attack and other heart diseases by method of self-report in Caucasian, postmenopausal women from Iowa (n = 40,000). Fat distribution was measured by the subject's self-report of current body weight and height as well as waist and hip circumferences (tape measures were sent to participants). BMI [weight (kg)/height (m²)] and waist to hip ratios (WHR) were calculated for the purposes of data analyses. Overall, subjects who reported hypertension, heart attack or other heart disease (i.e., arrhythmias, congestive heart failure) were older and had greater BMI and WHR ($p \le .0001$). The joint relationship of BMI and WHR was then examined for each disease category. There was a significant, positive relationship between both BMI and WHR and the prevalence of hypertension. Although a significant positive association existed between WHR and the prevalence of heart attack and other heart diseases, the relationship of these disorders with BMI was not significant. Therefore, these authors concluded that the relationship between body fat distribution and the incidence of cardiovascular disorders in women aged 55 to 69 needs further investigation, particularly since limitations in this study design (i.e., temporality) prevented identification of causal mechanisms.

Frank, A. (1993). Futility and avoidance: Medical professionals in the treatment of obesity. *JAMA, 269*(16), 2132–2133.

In this essay, two traditional arguments are said to be without any basis in fact. First, that there is absolutely nothing that can be done about obesity and second, that once weight loss occurs, recidivism rates are too high. Frank argues that women can sustain a comprehensive program, losing weight and even maintaining it. While obesity is not curable, it can be managed. Remember we do not abandon our diabetic patients or forsake our alcoholic patients who we cannot cure, but can manage with our best efforts.

Lichtman, S. W., Pisarska, K., Berman, E. R., Pestone, M., Dowling, H., Offenbacher, E., Weisel, H., Heshka, S., Matthews, D. E., & Heymsfield, S. B. (1992). Discrepancy between self-reported and actual caloric intake and exercise in obese subjects. *New England Journal of Medicine, 327*(27), 1893–1898.

Many obese people fail to lose weight even though they restrict their calorie intake to less than 1,200 kcal per day. Two explanations, either low energy expenditure or underreporting of caloric intake were studied in 224 people presenting for treatment. In group 1 (9 women and 1 man) total energy expenditure and actual energy intake were assessed for 14 days by indirect calorimetry and analysis of body composition. Individuals in group 2 (67 women and 13 men) who were without history of diet resistance, served as controls. There was no significant difference between groups 1 and 2 in terms of food and exercise. Thus, low energy expenditure was excluded as a mechanism of self-reported diet resistance. However, those in group 1 underreported their actual food intake and overreported their physical activity by 47 ± 16 percent and 51 ± 75 percent respectively. Further, those in group 1 perceived a genetic cause for their obesity, used thyroid medication at high frequency and perceived their eating as normal. These findings must be considered when working with obese women who are striving to correct a weight problem.

Manson, J., Colditz, G., Stampfer, M., Willett, W., Rosner, B. Monson, R., Speizer, F., & Hennekens, C. (1990). A prospective study of obesity and risk of coronary heart disease in women. *New England Journal of Medicine, 322*(13), 882–889.

Currently, one out of five Americans is obese (20% or more above their ideal body weight). Previous studies examining the relationship between obesity and CHD have included only men and have not controlled for factors such as smoking, diabetes or hypertension. This prospective study of female registered nurses aged 30 to 50 years examined the impact of the following on the risk of fatal and nonfatal CHD: weight at 18 years of age, weight gain from 18 years of age to present, and current obese status [measured by the Quetelet Index = Weight in Kilograms/(Height in Meters)^2]. Since obesity was noted to be inversely related to smoking and increased age, adjustment was made for these factors. Results indicated that those women who were in the heaviest Quetelet Index had a risk of fatal and nonfatal MI that was three times greater than the leanest group. Current obese status rather than obesity at the age of 18 years was a stronger determinant of CHD risk. In addition, gaining weight during adulthood increased coronary risk twofold. These researchers concluded that obesity was clearly a risk factor and a cause of mortality and morbidity observed in women with CHD.

VanItallie, T. (1990). The perils of obesity in middle-aged women. *New England Journal of Medicine, 322,* 928–929.

This editorial commentary discusses the tendency of previous epidemiologic studies to underestimate the serious consequences of obesity. It emphasizes that in order for a strong relationship to be demonstrated between obesity and CHD in women, prospective studies must have larger sample sizes and follow-up periods of significant duration. In addition, the problems in measuring body fat content must be examined. A criticism noted by this author is the failure of previous researchers to use waist to hip ratios when examining obesity since this has been reported to be a better predictor of CHD risk. Finally, it is concluded that although methods to treat obesity have not been extremely successful, efforts need to focus on a better understanding and evaluation of treatment modalities.

Diabetes and Hypertension

Fiebach, N., Hebert, P., Stampfer, M., Colditz, G., Willett, W., Rosner, B., Speizer, F., & Hennekens, C. (1989). A prospective study of high blood pressure and cardiovascular disorders in women. *American Journal of Epidemiology,* *130*(4), 646–654.

Hypertension has been identified as a risk factor for cardiovascular disease, however, few research studies have included women. This sample of 119,963 nurses aged 30 to 55 were followed for the development of CHD and stroke based on self-reports of high blood pressure and other risk factors noted six years earlier. Three hundred and eight cases of CHD (66 fatal) and 175 cases of stroke (50 fatal) were documented. Coronary and stroke events (fatal as well as nonfatal) occurred more often in participants who had reported high blood pressure. In addition, those reporting high blood pressure were noted to have higher levels of cholesterol ($p < .01$), more diabetes mellitus (DM) ($p < .01$) and a greater BMI ($p < .01$). After controlling for age and other risk factors, relative risk was 3.5 for CHD and 2.6 for stroke in the women who had reported high blood pressure. It was concluded that high blood pressure is an independent predictor for risk of CHD and stroke in women and that the relative risks calculated in this study

may even be underestimated since information on the severity as well as the treatment of the hypertension was not available.

Lobo, R. (1988). Lipids, clotting factors, and diabetes: Endogenous risk factors for cardiovascular disease. *American Journal of Obstetrics and Gynecology, 158*(6), 1584–1591.

This review article describes the impact of lipids, clotting factors and diabetes as risk factors for cardiovascular disease. Both Type I and Type II DM are identified as independent risk factors associated with the development of atherosclerosis, however the severity and duration of the diabetes do not seem to be related to this risk. It is noted that after adjustment for age, diabetic women have a 5:1 greater risk of CHD than nondiabetic women. In addition, glucose intolerance which is associated with increased coronary risk, seems to be greater in women than men. Finally, it is reported that diabetics have twice the risk of MI and a greater incidence of death following infarction than nondiabetics. It is concluded that women may have a coronary risk level that is equal to or greater than their male counterpart when there is the presence of diabetes.

Scheidt-Nave, C., Barrett-Connor, E., & Wingard, D. (1990). Resting electrographic abnormalities suggestive of asymptomatic ischemic heart disease associated with non-insulin-dependent diabetes mellitus in a defined population. *Circulation, 81*(3), 899–906.

A sample of 2,223 (1,236 women, 987 men) adults aged 50–89 were studied to examine the influence of NIDDM and impaired glucose tolerance (IGT) on resting electrocardiographic (ECG) abnormalities (Q or QS wave changes, complete left bundle branch block, ST segment depression, T wave changes). Asymptomatic IHD was defined as the absence of chest pain and one or more ECG changes while symptomatic IHD was defined as any history of MI or chest pain accompanied by ECG changes. Overall, IHD was more common in NIDDM women and men and women with IGT. In addition, there was a significant association between ECG changes and NIDDM in both men and women. Finally, the ECG changes associated with possible MI were more prevalent among women with NIDDM. The results indicate that asymptomatic patients with NIDDM can have significant resting ischemia on ECG which may have implications for future prognosis and treatment.

Sewardsen, M., Vythilingum, S., & Jialal, I. (1988). Abnormal glucose tolerance is the dominant risk factor in South African women with myocardial infarction. *Cardiology, 75,* 381–386.

Research studies addressing the impact of risk factors on the development of CHD in women have focused primarily on those persons living in the western countries. This research study is unique in that South African women of Indian (Asian) descent were studied. A sample of 90 women (26 to 60 years of age) who were at least three months post-MI were matched on age and sex to a control group and examined for the following risk factors: DM, impaired glucose tolerance (IGT), hypertension, hypercholesterolemia, hypertriglyceridemia, smoking, family history of MI and obesity. DM was the major risk factor reported in 78 percent of this study group and was observed six times more frequently than in the general South African Indian female population. Also of serious concern was that the prevalence of Type II diabetes in younger women (≤ 45 years; 79%) was consistent with older women (> 45 years; 77%). Hypertension, lipid abnormalities and family history of MI were noted to occur more frequently in older women. It is suggested that abnormal glucose may be the reason for the alteration in lipids noted in diabetics. The authors report that although smoking is an important risk factor in Westernized countries, there is a low prevalence of smoking among Indian women. Therefore, diabetes is the key risk factor with hypertension and lipid abnormalities having synergistic effects in older women of this population.

Wing, R., Bunker, C., Kuller, L., & Matthews, K. (1989). Insulin, body mass index, and cardiovascular risk factors in premenopausal women. *Arteriosclerosis, 9,* 479–484.

Menopause may be a time associated with changes in a woman's body weight, lipid levels and blood pressure. Therefore, to effectively evaluate the relationship between insulin, glucose, BMI and risk factors for the development of cardiovascular disease, a healthy sample ($n = 489$) of premenopausal women aged 42 to 52 who were nondiabetic and normotensive were examined. Results indicated that BMI and fasting insulin were correlated with the following cardiovascular risk factors: blood pressure (systolic and diastolic), triglycerides, HDL and its subfractions and apolipoprotein B (APO-B). To further isolate the relationships between BMI, insulin and these risk factors, subjects were split into tertiles. It was identified that for those subjects who were in the lowest BMI tertile, insulin had no effect on the cardiovascular risk factors of systolic blood pressure, triglycerides or APO-B. Similarly, there was no effect of BMI for subjects in the lowest insulin tertile on these risk factors. However, when subjects were in the middle and upper tertiles, there was a significant effect of body weight and insulin on coronary risk. The authors state that both BMI and insulin levels contribute to coronary risk level in healthy, premenopausal women and it is suggested that the unknown effect in menopausal women warrants further investigation.

Physical Activity

Blair, S. N., Kohl, H. W., Paffenbarger, R. S., Clark, D. G., Cooper, K. H., & Gibbons, L. W. (1989). Physical fitness and all-cause mortality: A prospective study of healthy men and women. *Journal of the American Medical Association, 262*(17), 2395–2401.

In this study of 10,344 men and 3,120 women over an average of eight years, there were 240 deaths in men and 43 deaths in women. When adjustments were made for age, death from all causes in both men and women declined with increased physical fitness. This was particularly true for cardiovascular disease. This study adds credibility to the importance of physical activity in the prevention of disease. For today's woman who is actively involved with career and family responsibilities, creating opportunities to be physically active should be emphasized in both work and leisure.

Fletcher, G. F., Blair, S. N., Blumenthal, J., Caspersen, C., Chaitman, B., Epstein, S., Falls, H., Sivarajan-Froelicher, E. S., Froelicher, V. F., & Pina, I. L. (1992). Statement on exercise: Benefits and recommendations for physical activity programs for all Americans. A statement for health professionals by the Committee on Exercise and Cardiac Rehabilitation of the Council on Clinical Cardiology, American Heart Association. *Circulation, 86*(1), 340–344.

The known benefits of regular aerobic exercise and recommendations for implementation of exercise programs are described with inactivity recognized as a risk factor for CAD. It is now known that healthy persons as well as many patients with cardiovascular disease can improve their exercise performance with training. Improvement comes about because of an increased ability to use oxygen to derive energy for work. Exercise training results in a decrease in myocardial oxygen demands for the same level of external work as is reflected in the product of heart rate by systolic arterial pressure. For women, as well as men the societal, cultural and personal factors that affect development or maintenance of lifelong patterns of physical activity must be identified and considered in strategies to promote exercise.

Marti, B., Tuomilehto, J., Salonen, J. T., Puska, P., & Nissinen, A. (1987). Relationship between leisure-time physical activity and risk factors for coronary heart disease in middle-aged Finnish women. *Acta Med Scand, 222*, 223–230.

Risk factors for CHD and leisure-time physical activity levels were examined in 4,059 women between 25 and 64 years of age. Findings revealed that while leisure-time physical activity predicted risk of CHD to some extent, age and BMI were the most important independent predictors of risk of CHD. Therefore, the benefits of leisure-time

physical activity in primary prevention of CHD in women is questioned by the findings of this study.

Schuler, G., Hambrecht, R., Schlierf, G., Niebauer, J., Hauer, K., Neumann, J., Hoberg, E., Drinkmann, A., Bacher, F., Grunze, M., & Kubler, W. (1992). Regular physical exercise and low-fat diet: Effects on progression of coronary artery disease. *Circulation, 86*(1), 1–11.

Following coronary angiography for stable angina, subjects were randomized into an intervention group and usual care groups. Over the course of 12 months, those in the intervention group followed a low-fat, low-cholesterol diet (American Heart Association recommendation phase 3), and received intensive physical exercise 2 hours per week supplemented with daily home exercise periods (20 min/day). Repeat coronary angiography at 12 months revealed that in the intervention group: progression of coronary lesions was noted in nine patients (23%), no change in 18 patients (45%) and regression in 13 patients (32%). In the control group, progression of coronary lesions was noted in 25 patients (48%), no change in 18 patients (45%) and regression in 9 patients (17%). These changes were significantly different from the intervention group. While no differentiation was made by gender, these findings are worth noting for women who undergo a program of exercise and follow a low-fat diet over a sustained time period.

Sedgwick, A. W., Taplin, R. E., Davidson, A. H., & Thomas, D. W. (1988). Effects of physical activity on risk factors for coronary heart disease in previously sedentary women: A five-year longitudinal study. *Aust NZ Med., 18*, 600–605.

Level of physical fitness, blood pressure, weight and blood lipids were measured in 290 women who initiated an exercise program. Five years later, over a third of these women remained physically active with the remainder again becoming sedentary. The net effect of remaining active over the five-year period was a decrease in weight by 1.9 kilograms, a decrease in diastolic blood pressure by 3 mmHg and a decrease in triglycerides by 0.15 mmol/L. Another important finding was the association between the maintenance of physical activity, the reduction in smoking, and the maintenance of stable weight. The present findings add credence to the notion that being physically active is an important factor in preventing the weight gain associated with smoking cessation.

Shangold, M. (1990). Exercise in the menopausal woman. *Obstetrics and Gynecology, 75*(4), Supplement 53S–58S.

The author highlights findings of several studies which have demonstrated the importance of exercise in the prevention and treatment of several health problems such as cardiovascular disease. It is a known fact that risk of cardiovascular disease increases after the menopause but that regular aerobic exercise may improve cardiorespiratory endurance and prevent the age-related increases in body fat. Based upon the findings of the cited studies, women should try to engage in regular physical activity to reduce their risk of heart disease.

Stress

Chesney, M. (1989). Women and work: Do new roles mean new risks? Women and Heart Disease Invitational Conference, American Heart Association, Washington D.C.

While women have always assumed multiple roles involving family and work, in previous times these roles were assumed sequentially rather than simultaneously as is occurring today. There are a number of issues associated with women assuming multiple roles. For example, there is evidence that multiple roles can have adverse cardiovascular consequences in women as manifested in the distinctly different patterns of cardiovascular arousal between men and women in the evening hours following the work day. Men, it seems, experience a decrease in arousal (unwinding) that begins when they arrive home while women experience an increase in arousal that extends well into the evening. Although the cause and long-term cardiovascular effects of this phenomenon require

further study, it would serve contemporary women well to examine how much of their lifestyles consist of self-induced unrealistic expectations.

Dixon, J. P., Dixon, J. K., & Spinner, J. C. (1991). Tensions between career and interpersonal commitments as a risk factor for cardiovascular disease among women. *Women & Health, 17*(3), 33–57.

It is clear that for professional women, the tension between career and interpersonal commitments results in conflict. This conflict translates into an important factor for increased risk of heart disease. Career and interpersonal sacrifice appear to play an important role in distinguishing women who will be at increased risk.

Frankenhaeuser, M., Lundberg, U., Fredrikson, M., Melin, B., Tuomisto, M., & Myrsten, A-L. (1989). Stress on and off the job as related to sex and occupational status in white-collar workers. *Journal of Organizational Behavior, 10,* 321–346.

In this study of 30 middle managers (15F;15M) and 30 clerical workers (15F;15M), cardiovascular and neuroendocrine responses were examined for 12 hours on a typical work day and for 12 hours on a typical day away from work. Findings revealed that in all groups, blood pressure and heart rate as well as epinephrine excretion were significantly elevated during the work day. In the male managers, blood pressure and norepinephrine excretion decreased after work indicating "rapid unwinding." In the female managers, however, their blood pressures remained elevated after work and their norepinephrine levels increased. The importance of these findings is that these investigators have identified the physiological correlates of the stress induced by the multiple roles women assume.

Kritz-Silverstein, D., Wingard, D. L., & Barrett-Connor, E. (1992). Employment status and heart disease risk factors in middle-aged women: The

Rancho Bernardo Study. *American Journal of Public Health, 82*(2), 215–219.

Based upon the responses of 242 women (40-to 59-years) who participated in the Rancho Bernardo Heart and Chronic Disease Survey (1984 to 1987), these investigators found that women who were employed smoked fewer cigarettes, drank less alcohol and exercised more than unemployed women. The primary implications include interventions to help employed women maintain and improve health with more intense interventions aimed toward women who are not actively employed to become cognizant of the need to practice good health habits.

LaRosa, J. (1988). Women, work, and health: Employment as a risk factor for coronary heart disease. *American Journal of Obstetrics and Gynecology, 158*(6), 1597–1602.

Currently, women represent 43 percent of the employed population and 73 percent work full-time. Most recent evidence suggests that employment is not a risk factor for CAD and it may even have a beneficial effect on health. Studies have shown that working women have better health than do homemakers and unemployed women. Health is better in single and married working women compared with divorced, separated or widowed women. Finally, multiple roles may enhance health although too much intensity in one role may diminish health. It is also believed that health is compromised among working women who perceive little control over their lives. These conclusions are based on a paucity of data and further studies are needed to substantiate these preliminary findings.

Murdaugh, C. (1986). Coronary heart disease in women. *Progress in Cardiovascular Nursing, 1,* 2–8.

This review article identifies that CHD is the leading cause of death in women. It has been previously noted, however, that men have a 2 to 4 times greater risk of heart disease possibly due to the difference in risk factors, physical and emotional hazards at work, and the lack of protective female sex hormones. Risk factors such as elevated serum cholesterol, high blood pressure, smoking, obesity, glucose intolerance, lack of exercise and stress have been reported to increase the risk of heart disease similarly in men and women. Studies have found that hormonal changes do increase the risk of heart disease in postmenopausal women. As more women enter the work force and are exposed to the same stressors and demands as men, the incidence of coronary disease may rise. Studies have shown an association between CHD and occupational stress in men. In working women, it has been reported that the presence of Type A behavior, smoking, hyperlipidemia and glucose intolerance increase the incidence of CHD. Employment itself, however, has not been found to increase risk of heart disease in women although further research is needed.

Penckofer, S., & Holm, K. (1990). Women undergoing coronary artery bypass surgery: Physiological and psychosocial perspectives. *Cardiovascular Nursing, 26*(3), 13–18.

This comprehensive review article on the physiological and psychosocial consequences of CABS as a treatment modality for women with CHD is unique in that the impact of women's multiple roles and the stressors these create following CABS are presented. Several theories regarding the impact of women's multiple roles on health and illness are also addressed. The authors clearly identify the need for further research in the areas of women's multiple roles and the consequences they may have on cardiovascular disease.

Yeung, A. C., Vekshtein, V. I., Krantz, D. S., Vita, J. A., Ryan, T. J., Ganz, P., & Selwyn, A. P. (1991). The effect of atherosclerosis on the vasomotor response of coronary arteries to mental stress. *The New England Journal of Medicine, 325*(22), 1551–1556.

During cardiac catherization, 26 patients were asked to perform mental arithmetic. Results varied from 38 percent constriction to 29 percent dilation whereas change in coronary blood flow varied from a decrease of 48 percent to an increase of 42 percent. The direction and magnitude of the change in coronary diameter were not predicted by the change in heart rate, blood pressure, or plasma norepinephrine. In patients with atherosclerosis paradoxical constriction occurred during mental stress, particularly at points of stenosis.

Menopause and Estrogen Replacement Therapy

Colditz, G., Willett, W., Stampfer, M., Rosner, B., Speizer, F., & Hennekens, C. (1987). Menopause and the risk of coronary heart disease in women. *New England Journal of Medicine, 316*(18), 1105–1110.

The effect of menopause on the development of CAD is controversial although numerous studies have documented increased rates of CAD following menopause. This study examined the effect of naturally occurring menopause and surgically induced menopause on risk of CHD. A cohort of 121,700 women aged 30 to 55 years were prospectively studied. Results revealed that after controlling for age and cigarette smoking, women who had a natural menopause and who had never taken estrogen replacement had no appreciable increased risk of CHD when compared with premenopausal women. Women who had a surgically induced menopause and were never on estrogen replacement following surgery were noted to have an increased risk for CHD when compared to those who received estrogen therapy postoperatively.

Cummings, S., Black, D., & Rubin, S. (1989). Lifetime risks of hip, colles', or vertebral fracture and coronary heart disease among white postmenopausal women. *Archives of Internal Medicine, 149*(11), 2445–2448.

Estimating and comparing lifetime risks of CAD, osteoporotic fractures, breast and endometrial cancer may dictate the need for estrogen replacement therapy. Lifetime risk is defined as the probability of developing a certain condition before death. Based on an analysis of incidence rates for CHD mortality and noncoronary heart disease mortality for 1983, a 50-year-old white woman was found to have a 31 percent risk of dying from CHD. This is 10 times greater than the risk for either hip fracture or cancer. Therefore, benefits of estrogen replacement therapy far outweigh the risks. For example, a 10 percent decrease in risk of death from CHD facilitated by estrogen replacement therapy would outweigh the potentially twofold increase in death associated with breast or endometrial cancer.

Gruchow, H. W., Anderson, A. J., Barboriak, J. J., & Sobocinski, K. A. (1988). Postmenopausal use of estrogen and occlusion of coronary arteries. *American Heart Journal, 115*(5), 954–963.

A majority of studies have shown that estrogen replacement therapy is protective against CHD in postmenopausal women. This study examined the difference in the extent of CAD between those who took estrogen replacement after menopause and those who did not. Of the 933 women investigated, only 154 were currently taking estrogen replacement. Coronary angiography results showed that postmenopausal estrogen users had lower coronary artery occlusion rates than those not taking estrogen replacement. Also, statistically significant differences were found between the two groups on HDLs. It was noted that the estrogen replacement group had significantly higher levels of HDL cholesterol. The investigators hypothesized that higher levels of HDL cholesterol, which are protective against CAD, may be the result of exogenous estrogen administration. Although other studies have found estrogen to be protective against CAD, postmenopausal estrogen use has declined over the years primarily due to its potential cancer risks.

Henderson, B., Paganini-Hill, A., & Ross, R. (1988). Estrogen replacement therapy and protection from acute myocardial infarction. *American Journal of Obstetrics and Gynecology, 159*(2), 312–317.

A longitudinal study was previously conducted to determine the effects of estrogen replacement therapy on the incidence of MI. This report further elaborates on the cohort investigated in that study. Women who used estrogen replacement therapy had a 41 percent reduction in mortality and a 29 percent reduction in morbidity due to acute MI compared to those women who did not take estrogen. Users of estrogen had a lower mortality rate from MI in the presence or absence of other risk factors such as hypertension, exercise, and BMI. This effect was not seen in women who were current cigarette smokers or with women with a late menopause. The cohort examined in this study, however, is only representative of a white, affluent population.

Lobo, R. (1990). Cardiovascular implications of estrogen replacement therapy. *Obstetrics & Gynecology, 73*(4), Supplement 18S–25S.

Cardiovascular disease affects more than 2 million women per year and is the leading cause of death today. The decrease in the level of estrogen following menopause has been associated with an increased risk for CHD. Although cardiovascular risk is not significantly increased in the first several years following a natural menopause, in those women who have a premature or surgically induced menopause the risk is significantly greater. As previously noted, estrogen increases HDL while decreasing LDL. It is now thought that the type of estrogen used in replacement therapy and the route of administration have a direct effect on the benefits observed. In addition, when prescribing estrogen therapy, side effects must also be considered. Therefore, in order for women to make informed decisions, they must be counselled on the benefits as well as the risks when considering estrogen replacement therapy.

McFarland, K., Boniface, M., Hornung, C. A., Earnhardt, W., & O'Neal Humphries, J. (1989). Risk factors and noncontraceptive estrogen use in women with and without coronary disease. *American Heart Journal, 117*(6), 1209–1214.

This study examined 208 women with angiographically normal coronary arteries and 137 women with severe CAD. Risk factors in addition to postmenopausal estrogen replacement were studied. Hypertension and obesity did not significantly increase the risk of CAD regardless of menopausal status while history of smoking, diabetes, elevated total cholesterol level and a positive family history were significant factors. Furthermore, the odds of CAD were reduced by one-half in those women on estrogen replacement therapy. Only 41 percent of this sample were currently on estrogen therapy which is similar to percentages identified in other studies. Therefore, although the cardioprotective effects of estrogen have been well documented, estrogen replacement therapy is still not being prescribed for a majority of women following menopause.

Nabulsi, A. A., Folsom, A. R., White, A., Patsch, W., Heiss, G., Wu, K. K., & Szklo, M., for the Atherosclerosis Risk in Communities Study Investigators. (1993). Association of hormone-replacement therapy with various cardiovascular risk factors in postmenopausal women. *New England Journal of Medicine, 328*(15), 1069–1075.

There have been a number of investigations suggesting that estrogen is protective against heart disease with current thinking emphasizing that combination therapy, namely estrogen with progestin may negate the positive effects of estrogen alone. In this study, current users of combination therapy had higher mean levels of HDLs and lower mean levels of LDLs. Current users of estrogen alone had higher triglyceride, factor VII and protein C levels than either nonusers or current users of estrogen in combination with progestin. These findings are based on cross-sectional data of 4,958 women who were assigned to one of four groups: current users of estrogen alone, current users of estrogen with progestin, nonusers who had formerly taken hormones, and nonusers who had never taken hormones. Note that the type of hormone therapy for former users could not be accurately determined. While findings suggest that combination therapy is associated with an improved lipid profile, a randomized clinical trial is needed to further elucidate outcomes of combination therapy.

Salonen, J., Nyyssonen, K., Korpela, H., Tuomilehto, J., Seppanan, R., & Salonen, R. (1992). High stored iron levels are associated with excess risk of myocardial infarction in Eastern Finnish men. *Circulation, 86*(3), 803–811.

Salonen and colleagues studied a random sample of 1,931 Eastern Finnish men aged 42, 48, 54 or 60 years at baseline who were enrolled in the Kuopio Ischaemic Heart Disease Risk Factor Study (KIHD) between 1984 and 1989. They excluded all men with prevalent heart disease (defined as history of MI or angina pectoris) from their analyses. Serum specimens were frozen for a period of one to five years at minus 20 degrees Celsius. Radioimmunoassay was used to measure serum ferritin levels. In addition, other serum levels included: blood leukocytes, serum lipoproteins (VLDL, LDL and HDL), triglycerides, serum copper and blood glucose. Cardiac risk factors such as age, smoking, systolic blood pressure, maximal oxygen uptake and ischemic EKG upon exercise testing were also measured. Using a BMDP Cox proportional hazards index, these risk factors and others were entered into a model. It was identified that men with serum ferritin concentrations greater than 200 mg/l had a 2.2 fold risk of acute MI as compared with men with lower serum ferritin levels after adjusting for all of the above stated variables. In addition, serum ferritin had significant positive linear correlations with blood glucose, serum triglycerides and systolic blood pressure. It was concluded that high stored iron levels were associated with greater cardiovascular risk. Whether the risk of cardiovascular disease associated with elevated serum ferritin found in men is consistent with that found in women is unknown.

Stampfer, M. J., Colditz, G. A., Willett, W. C., Manson, J. E., Rosner, B., Speizer, F. E., & Hennekens, C. H. (1991). Postmenopausal estrogen therapy and cardiovascular disease: Ten year follow-up from the Nurses' Health Study. *New England Journal of Medicine, 325*(11), 756–762.

During ten years of follow-up of the Nurses' Health Study cohort (n = 48,470; 337,854 person years), 224 strokes, 405 cases of nonfatal MI or deaths from coronary causes and 1,263 deaths from all causes were documented. Adjusting for age and other coronary risk factors, overall risk of major coronary disease in women currently taking estrogen (n = 45) was 0.56 (95% confidence interval, 0.40 to 0.80). No effect of duration of estrogen use independent of age was observed. These findings, while significant, must be considered in reference to the total number of women enrolled in the study as well as the number who were taking estrogen at the time of analysis, 48,470 and 45 respectively.

Tikkanen, M., & Nikkila, E. (1988). Menopause, estrogens and risk for coronary heart disease. *Acta Obstet Gynecol Scand Suppl*, 39–45.

In this review, the effect of menopause on levels of serum cholesterol and triglycerides as well as the effect of estrogen replacement therapy on lipoproteins are discussed. Various studies have shown that cholesterol and triglyceride levels are elevated in the postmenopausal woman and it is the LDLs that are responsible for this increase. Because menopause is the time when women lose the protective effect of estrogen, the incidence of CHD equilibrates between men and women. Although menopause is associated with a decrease in the levels of HDLs, women consistently have higher levels of HDLs when compared to men even after menopause. Therefore, the primary benefit of estrogen replacement therapy is the reduction of LDL which are responsible for the increase in triglycerides and cholesterol levels observed in the postmenopausal period.

Witteman, J., Grobbee, D., Kok, F., Hofman, A., & Valkenburg, H. (1989). Increased risk of atherosclerosis in women after menopause. *British Medical Journal, 298*, 642–644.

Few studies address the association between the menopausal state and the presence of atherosclerosis. This study examined premenopausal ($n = 294$) and postmenopausal women ($n = 315$) aged 45 to 55 for evidence of calcification in the abdominal aorta by radiography. Atherosclerosis was present in only 3 percent ($n = 8$) of the premenopausal women, however, 12 percent ($n = 38$) of the postmenopausal women had the disease. Women with natural menopause had a 3 to 4 times greater risk of atherosclerosis than premenopausal women while those with a surgically induced menopause had a 5 times greater risk of atherosclerosis. Of the postmenopausal women, 5 percent ($n = 17$) were currently taking an estrogen replacement and atherosclerosis was present in only one of these women. The increased risk of cardiovascular disease in postmenopausal women is once again demonstrated by the results of this study.

Chapter 10

Sexually Transmitted Diseases

Catherine Ingram Fogel

INTRODUCTION

In the last century, many infectious diseases in the United States largely have been conquered. In stark contrast and despite the United States Surgeon General targeting sexually transmitted diseases (STDs) as a priority for prevention and control efforts, STDs are among the most common health problems in the United States today. STDs are a direct cause of tremendous human suffering, place heavy demands on health care services and cost hundreds of millions of dollars to treat. Twenty-three STDs and a dozen STD syndromes affect more than 12 million women and men in the United States every year (Donovan, 1993). At current rates it is estimated that at least one in four—and maybe as many as one in two—Americans will contract an STD at some point during their lifetime (CDC, 1993). No sexually active person is without risk of infection. More than one in five Americans (at least 56 million people) are thought to be infected with a viral STD other than AIDS.

Traditionally public health efforts were aimed at the control of gonorrhea and syphilis; however, more recently concern has focused on the bacterial and viral syndromes associated with Chlamydia trachomatic, herpes simplex virus (HSV), human papilloma virus (HPV) and the human immunodeficiency virus (HIV). Unfortunately this does not mean that gonorrhea and syphilis are no longer of concern. In the United States, syphilis infections are at their highest levels in 40 years and gonorrhea is the most commonly reported communicable disease (CDC, 1993). The total cost for care of patients with STDs exceeds 2 billion dollars annually (McGregor, French & Spencer, 1988). The direct and indirect costs for pelvic inflammatory disease (PID) are estimated at more than 2.5 billion every year (Sullivan, 1988).

The epidemic problems of STD are especially serious for women. STDs have a disproportionate effect on women because they are more easily transmitted to and more difficult to diagnose in women than in men (Aral & Guinan, 1984). Health complications caused by STDs tend to be more frequent and more severe in women than men. These include infertility, numerous perinatal infections, chronic disease, genital tract neoplasia and death from ectopic pregnancy, ruptured tubo-ovarian abscess, and hepatitis B virus infections. Their children and fetuses are frequently placed at risk of morbidity and mortality, experiencing congenital anomalies, mental retardation and death (Fogel, 1990). STDs are most common in young women between the ages of 15 and 24 and it is these women who suffer inordinately from PID, increased risks of ectopic pregnancy and its associated mortality, subfertility and chronic pelvic pain. Women also experience a greater share of the burden of suffering from STDs for another reason. Women constitute the majority of women at or below the poverty level in the United States today (Wilson, 1988). Poor women, due to limited access to adequate medical care, are impacted most heavily by the complications of sexually transmitted diseases (McBarnette, 1988). Further the impact of STDs on poor women extends beyond their own personal health to their children.

Societal attitudes influence public and individual responses to sexually transmitted diseases and have a critical impact on behavior. Without an understanding of societal attitudes and how they impact behavior, strategies to prevent transmission of sexually transmitted diseases cannot be developed or practiced. The meanings associated with a diagnosis of sexually transmitted disease were discussed in an earlier volume (Fogel, 1990); however, societal views have not altered in a few years and women continue to express feelings of fear, disbelief, anger, victimization and guilt. These feelings may prevent a woman from seeking health care for an infection. The stigma attached to receiving a diagnosis of sexually transmitted disease remains and has intensified with the increasing threat of acquired immunodeficiency syndrome (AIDS). The behaviors involved in contracting STDs (sexual intercourse and possible drug use) are often labeled "deviant" and thus carry the social construct of stigma and "spoiled identity" (Goffman, 1963). Women are more vulnerable to stigmatization and labeling of their behavior as deviant because of the prevailing double standard applied to women's behavior. Societal views that women should be pure and chaste persist largely due to women's general social subordination and relatively poor power position. Societal reactions to women who contract a sexually transmitted disease are generally more punitive than are those toward men perhaps due in part to differential standards regarding acceptable sexual behavior for the sexes. These standards also operate to control the sexual behavior of women. Victorian mores that associate sex with sin and sexually transmitted diseases with punishment for past transgressions persist in our society. Women who contract a sexually transmitted disease may be viewed as promiscuous and a reservoir of disease. In the minds of many, sexually transmitted diseases are equated with promiscuous behavior, immorality and low social station.

The emergence of AIDS as an increasingly larger health threat to women has highlighted issues concerning women's sexuality, relationships with men, and reproductive rights that potentially can influence a woman's ability to practice preventive behaviors, shape public policy and influence health care provider attitudes. Worldwide women at greatest risk for HIV infection and STD infection are, in general, disadvantaged and disenfranchised. Gender role expectations regarding female dependency may prevent women from initiating sexual behavior changes to protect themselves (Fullilove, Fullilove, Haynes & Gross, 1989). Further, it is the youngest women who are at greatest risk for sexually transmitted diseases and these are also the women who may have the greatest difficulty in negotiating sexual practices. In a society that commonly views a woman who carries a condom as over-prepared, possibly oversexed and willing to have sex with any man (Hankins, 1990), expecting her to insist on the use of condoms in a sexual encounter is unrealistic. As long as women remain unequal partners in relationships and society, they will find it difficult to act as autonomous beings with a right to and responsibility for self-determination (Hankins, 1990). The feminization of poverty also impacts on the ability of women to assume autonomous responsibility for protection against sexual transmission of disease. Programs aimed at prevention through empowerment of women to initiate behavior change will be largely unsuccessful until political and economic empowerment of women occurs.

Sexuality may be the only way some women have of attaining intimacy. Other women may fear rejection and abandonment, conflict, potential violence or loss of economic support. All of these reasons may constrain a women's ability to require partners to follow safe sex practices.

Because the majority of children are infected perinatally, knowledge of a woman's HIV status prior to conception would seem desirable. However, not all women take or have control over conception and many pregnancies are unintended. Nor do all pregnant women know prior to conception that they are HIV positive. Further, motherhood is fostered by many cultures and is often critical to a woman's self-esteem. Childbearing for some women is a cultural imperative and thus they may risk their own infection with a sexually transmitted disease such as AIDs or consider the 25–50 percent chance of having an HIV-infected child an acceptable risk (Campbell, 1990). Women may also risk infection and/or not opt for abortion due to religious beliefs and/or family or partner pressure to have a child.

A central issue in reproductive rights continues to be the right of a woman to become pregnant and to maintain a pregnancy. However, as more child-bearing women become HIV positive and give birth to infected children, childbearing could come under state surveillance (Campbell, 1990). Women of childbearing age could become the first group to experience mandatory testing. It is possible that the state's traditional interest in protecting and preserving the rights of the fetus could shift to an interest in protecting society from another person infected with AIDS.

Three years later, there continues to be little hope for a curative medical strategy in the near future for viral STDs and the expanding number of drug-resistant strains of gonorrhea. The rising number of cases of syphilis suggests that the belief that diseases once considered to be a major health risk are no longer a threat is erroneous. Education of women who are health care professionals and who are the recipients of health care services continues to be critical. Many of the issues and concerns raised in this introduction can be more effectively addressed through increased understanding and knowledge. An important focus of health care must be prevention of or decreased exposure to sexually transmitted diseases. Increased understanding of transmission and subsequent alteration of at-risk behaviors is essential in prevention.

The following guidelines were employed in selecting articles for this chapter from the enormous number published in the past three years. First, does the article contribute to the reader's understanding of a particular STD in terms of incidence, prevention and/or treatment? Second, does the article enrich the reader's understanding of societal influences and responses to STDs? Third, does the article add to information presented in previous reviews of literature on women's health perspectives? Only articles directly relevant to women were included in the review. While the focus is primarily on the health literature, attention was given to psychological and sociological references. Four themes emerged on sexually transmitted diseases. There has been a significant increase in articles dealing with AIDS and women. This is both a reflection of the increasing number of women who are HIV positive and who have AIDS and a recognition of the desperate need for information specific to women and AIDS. The literature identifies numerous controversies and conflicting results regarding occurrence and treatment of STDs. Finally, there are research studies that advance the treatment of STDs by supporting and/or refuting current clinical practices. A greater proportion of the articles selected for abstraction in this chapter address HIV/AIDs in women. This reflects the growing awareness and concern and the ever increasing numbers of women who are infected.

While specific diseases have changed and, in some cases, cycled over time, STDs have caused enormous misery, morbidity and mortality for women and their offspring and will continue to do so for the foreseeable future. Providing information for individual women to use in making informed decisions regarding sexual behavior, and obtaining health care can decrease the adverse consequences of STDs. Understanding how societal attitudes influence personal behavior, delivery of health care and acquisition of research knowledge will enable women to work more effectively to improve outcomes.

REFERENCES

Aral, S. O., & Guinan, M. E. (1984). Women and sexually transmitted diseases. In K. K. Holmes et al. (Eds.), *Sexually Transmitted Diseases*, 85–89. New York: McGraw-Hill.

Campbell, C. I. (1990). Women and AIDS. *Social Science Medicine, 30*, 407–415.

Centers for Disease Control. (1993). Division of STD/HIV Prevention 1992 Annual Report, CDC, Atlanta: CDC.

Donovan, P. (1993). *Testing Positive: Sexually Transmitted Disease and the Public Health Response.* New York: Alan Guttmacher Institute.

Fogel, C. I. (1990). Sexually transmitted diseases. *Women's Health Perspectives, Vol. 3*, 122–139.

Fullilove, M., Fullilove, R., Haynes, K., & Gross, S. A. (1989). Gender roles as barriers to risk reduction in black women. Paper presented at Fifth International Meeting on AIDS, Montreal.

Goffman, E. (1963). *Stigma.* Englewood Cliffs, NJ: Prentice-Hall.

Hankins, C. I. (1990). Issues involving women, children, and AIDS primarily in the developed world. *Journal of Acquired Immune Deficiency Syndromes, 3,* 443–448.

McBarnette, L. (1988). Women and poverty: The effects on reproductive status. *Women and Health,* 55–81.

McGregor, J. A., French, J. I., & Spencer, N. E. (1988). Prevention of sexually transmitted diseases in women. *Journal of Reproductive Medicine, 33,* 109–118.

Sullivan, M. L. (1988). Infectious diseases. *Women's Health, News and Features from NIH, 88,* 3–8.

Wilson, J. B. (1988). Women and poverty: A demographic overview. *Women and Health,* 21–40.

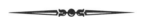

BOOKS AND ARTICLES

Alexander, L. L. (1992). Sexually transmitted diseases: Perspectives on this growing epidemic. *Nurse Practitioner, 17,* 31, 34, 37–38, 41–42.

Alexander summarizes eight major STDs for the nurse clinician, providing information on pathogens, symptoms, diagnosis, and treatment. Issues surrounding the provision of care to clients with STDs are discussed including the problems of constrained public resources and deficient public awareness. An overview of counseling is provided and a checklist for STD counseling given. Behavioral counseling messages are delineated.

Aral, S. O., & Cates, W. (1989). The multiple dimensions of sexual behavior as risk factors for sexually transmitted diseases: The sexually experienced are not necessarily sexually active. *Sexually Transmitted Diseases, 10*(4), 173–177.

A crucial risk factor for sexually transmitted diseases is sexual behavior and thus modification of such behavior has emerged as a key intervention for STD prevention. Currently no population-based distribution of sexual behavior in the United States is available. Existing information is based on specific population groups such as adolescents and women in their twenties. Although sexual behavior encompasses a number of variables including current and lifetime number of sex partners, age at first intercourse, frequency of intercourse, consistency of sexual activity, mode of recruitment of sexual partners, and duration of sexual unions, previous studies have operationalized the concept as only sexual experience (a person's ever having had sexual intercourse). Analyzing data from a nationally representative sample of reproductive aged women, the authors generated estimates of exposure to STD risk based on multiple measures of sexual experience. They found that 86 percent of women aged 15 to 45 were sexually experienced and that adolescents were the least experienced and least sexually active of all reproductive women. While sexual experience increased with age, sexual activity had a curvilinear pattern: it increased up to age 35 and decreased slightly between ages 35 and 44. Teenagers had the least consistent sexual activity and the highest level of sexual abstinence. The researchers also found that, except for the

teen years, women of other races were less sexually active and less consistently sexually active than white women. These findings suggest
that levels of sexual activity may not explain
the higher STD rates among teenagers and non-
whites. Based on this data, relatively higher
levels of sexual activity of all members of these
groups is not the explanation. Rather, the authors contend that subsets of these groups account for a large proportion of STD morbidity, a
finding that is consistent with the "core group"
hypothesis of STD transmission. They suggest
that the answer then seems to be either that
the existing high STD prevalence in these
groups makes each sexual encounter carry a
higher risk or that the nature of the sexual activity (number of partners or choice of partners
or both) place the woman at greater risk. The
findings demonstrate that sexual experience as
a measure of sexual behavior is an inadequate
estimate of the population at risk for STD. Further, the findings suggest that clinicians
should not arbitrarily screen for STD on the basis of race or age alone.

Aral, S. O., & Holmes, K. K. (1991). Sexually
transmitted diseases in the AIDS era. *Scientific
American, 264,* 62–69.

In almost all of the industrialized nations,
gonorrhea, syphilis, and chancroid have disap-
peared. In shocking contrast, these STDs are increasing at epidemic rates in minority populations in the United States. Further complicating
the problem is the rise of drug-resistant strains of
sexually transmitted bacterial infections and the
rapid spread of incurable viral STDs. The authors
review available data on incidence of STDs and
detail the social, political, and economic forces
that seem to be fueling the epidemic. They suggest that in the United States there is increasing
homogeneity within social groups, a widening
gap between these groups, and a growing under-
class, the results of which are social problems
such as poor education, joblessness, homelessness, family dissolution, drug abuse, homicide,
and other crimes particularly in inner city neigh-
borhoods. The authors assert that STDs and many
other health problems also follow this pattern

and that the risk factors for individual cases of
specific STDs in specific subgroups may be less
important than the overriding social forces. This
article, by placing the epidemic of STDs in a population rather than individual focus, forces the
reader to conclude that in the 1990s the solution
to the STD crisis cannot rest solely on preventing
high-risk behaviors in individuals.

Binkin, N. J., & Koplan, J. P. (1989). The higher
cost and low efficacy of weekly viral cultures for
pregnant women with recurrent genital herpes:
A reappraisal. *Medical Decision Making, 9*(4),
225–230.

Transmission of herpetic infections at time
of delivery can have disastrous consequences
for the neonate; nearly 20 percent of infected infants will die and 25 percent will have some disability. Most infectious lesions are symptomatic
and women at risk for transmitting the virus can
be readily identified by history and examination.
In these instances, neonatal transmission largely
may be prevented through cesarean section delivery. A more difficult dilemma occurs when the
pregnant woman has a history of recurrent genital herpes but no signs and symptoms at or near
term. Reducing the risks of neonatal infection for
these women also means increasing the risk of
maternal morbidity and mortality associated
with cesarean deliveries. Formerly, in an attempt
to reduce the number of neonatal herpes cases
while minimizing adverse maternal consequences, screening for herpes virus four to eight
weeks prior to delivery was recommended for all
pregnant women with histories of genital herpes,
for those with active disease during the pregnancy, and for those whose sexual partners have
proven histories of genital herpes. In recent years
the cost-effectiveness of weekly cultures has
been questioned. In this study, the authors analyzed recent national data to evaluate current recommendations for treatment of pregnant women
with histories of genital herpes. Their findings reveal that weekly screening of pregnant women
with recurrent genital herpes is costly and may
cause more deaths than it prevents. Further, only
two cases of neonatal herpes would be prevented
each year and for every infant death averted there

would be two excess maternal deaths. This study supports new screening strategies proposed by the American College of Obstetrics and Gynecology which recommends abandoning weekly prenatal cultures for women with histories of genital herpes. For women with no lesions at time of delivery, vaginal deliveries would be acceptable. For women with genital lesions at the time of delivery, a cesarean section would be indicated even when the membranes have ruptured. This study is important in that it challenges existing clinical practice and the findings support the abandonment of practices that have a high cost and low effectiveness rate.

Buckley, H. B. (1992). Syphilis: A review and update of the 'new' infection of the '90s. *Nurse Practitioner, 17*, 25, 29–32.

Recognized as a clinical entity since the 16th century, reported cases of primary, secondary, and congenital syphilis have reached epidemic proportions in the United States. This clinical article presents essential information pertinent to the care of women with syphilis by reviewing the pathogenesis, clinical stages and presentation, serological testing, treatment, and pertinent patient education for syphilis. Recommendations for identification and prevention are provided. The information is easily accessible, concise, and accurate.

Butterfield, C. R., Schockley, M., San Miguel, G., & Rosa, C. (1990). Routine screening for Hepatitis B in an obstetric population. *Obstetrics & Gynecology, 76*(1), 25–27.

The transmission of the hepatitis B virus (HBV) from mother to fetus at the time of delivery has serious health implications for the newborn. It is estimated that 85–90 percent of newborns who acquire perinatal HBV infection will become carriers of hepatitis B surface antigen and have over a 25 percent probability of dying from primary hepatocellular carcinoma or cirrhosis of the liver. Until recently the Centers for Disease Control (CDC) recommended pregnant women at high risk for hepatitis B be screened to identify carriers for the hepatitis B

surface antigen. This prospective study evaluated the efficacy of the CDC recommendation. At their initial prenatal visit, 1,466 women were screened for hepatitis B surface antigen and interviewed regarding the presence of any risk factors (ethnicity or history of STD, blood transfusion, hepatitis exposure, occupational exposure, drug abuse, liver disease). Twelve women tested positive for the hepatitis B surface antigen. Historic risk factors were identified in six of these. Thus, if screening had been conducted in accordance with CDC recommendations, half of the hepatitis B surface antigen carriers would not have been detected. This study highlights the limitations of the use of historic factors as a screening method for this problem and provides support for the CDC's recently updated (1988) recommendation for routine hepatitis B surface antigen testing for all pregnant women at their initial prenatal visit.

Campbell, C. A. (1990). Women and AIDS. *Social Science and Medicine, 30*(4), 407–415.

In this excellent article, the author describes the epidemiology of acquired immunodeficiency syndrome (AIDS) in women in the United States illustrating the inadequacy of current data collection procedures and lack of attention paid to female AIDS cases. At the present time, a heterosexual woman in the United States has a greater risk of becoming infected with HIV through sexual intercourse than does a heterosexual man. Yet, as the author points out educational efforts have not targeted women as much as men despite women's vulnerability to infection. Reproductive issues surrounding AIDS are thoughtfully examined including artificial insemination transmission, prenatal testing, contraception and reproductive rights. Some of the special problems women with AIDS face such as the issues of single parenthood, IV-drug use and prostitution and the need for special family care facilities are discussed. The lack of responsiveness of health care providers is illustrated. Women's role as nurturer and caregiver for persons with AIDS is examined and the way in which AIDS is associated with the traditional female role is explored. This article is required reading for any health care professional providing services to women.

Chow, J. M., Yonekura, M. L., Richwald, G. A., Greenland, S., Sweet, R. L., & Schachter, J. (1990). The association between Chlamydia trachomatis and ectopic pregnancy. *Journal of the American Medical Association, 263*(23).

Ectopic pregnancy is a major health problem and a leading cause of maternal mortality. There is an urgent need to identify the most effective means of reducing ectopic pregnancy rates. Thus, identifying factors associated with ectopic pregnancy is essential. A case-control study of 306 patients with an ectopic pregnancy (cases) and 266 pregnant patients (controls) suggested that, after adjusting for age at first intercourse, total lifetime partners, douching, history of infertility and parity, past chlamydial infection is associated with a greater than twofold risk of ectopic pregnancy. Another important finding was that current douching remained an independent risk factor after controlling for chlamydial exposure. It should be noted however, that the study sample was not representative of the United States population since approximately 69 percent of the cases were relatively poor, white, Hispanic women and socioeconomic class impacts the rates of STDs and douching behavior. The odds ratio for chlamydial seropositivity and ectopic pregnancy were similar to those reported in other studies. The results stress the importance of controlling chlamydial infections and discussing douching practices with clients.

Cohen, I., Veille, J-C., & Calkins, B. M. (1990). Improved pregnancy outcome following successful treatment of chlamydial infection. *Journal of the American Medical Association, 263*(23), 3160–3163.

As the previous article by Chow et al. demonstrates chlamydial infections are increasingly being recognized as a problem in obstetrics. Certain factors place pregnant women at increased risk (2–3 times greater) for chlamydial infections including age less than 20, low socioeconomic status, multiple sex partners and single marital status.

In this study, a retrospective analysis of pregnancy outcomes in 244 women successfully treated for cervical chlamydial infection were compared with 79 chlamydia-positive pregnant women who did not respond to treatment and 244 chlamydia-free pregnant women who were not treated. All three groups were at high risk for infection. The successfully treated patients had more favorable pregnancy outcomes than did the pregnant women who remained chlamydia-positive throughout pregnancy. The frequencies of premature rupture of the membranes, premature contractions, and small-for-gestational-age infants were significantly lower in the successfully treated women when compared to the chlamydia-positive women and were not significantly different from the control women. The authors suggest that their findings indicate that in a high-risk pregnant population, repeated prenatal chlamydial testing, plus successful treatment can significantly reduce some adverse effects on pregnancy outcomes. Clinicians caring for pregnant women with factors that place them at risk for chlamydial infections and/or women who are at high risk for premature delivery would do well to consider these recommendations.

Crane, M. J. (1992). The diagnosis and management of maternal and congenital syphilis. *Journal of Nurse-Midwifery, 37,* 4–16.

Syphilis is reemerging as an endemic disease in minority heterosexual populations in the United States; the dramatic increases in primary and secondary syphilis in women has resulted in a dramatic rise in congenital syphilis. Unfortunately, most nurse clinicians know very little about a disease only recently thought to no longer be a problem. This clinical update of maternal and congenital syphilis is both timely and necessary. The epidemiology of the disease is given and modes of transmission discussed. The four stages of syphilis and their presentation are reviewed. Methods of diagnostic testing and screening for maternal syphilis are given. Treatment and management of maternal and congenital syphilis is discussed in depth. The author emphasizes that the key to prevention of syphilitic stillbirths and congenitally infected infants is early diagnosis and treatment of infected pregnant women.

Donovan, P. (1993). *Testing Positive: Sexually Transmitted Disease and the Public Health Response.* New York: Alan Guttmacher Institute.

The number of articles, books, and pamphlets being published on STDs is staggering. Often what is needed is an overview/review of the problem. This publication meets this need satisfactorily. The scope of the problem in the United States is summarized and specific information about women provided. The risk factors for acquiring an STD are reviewed, again with special attention to women. The governmental response to the epidemic of STDs in America is outlined including funding and surveillance and changes in priorities that are needed. Issues involved in changing governmental priorities and response are discussed.

Debuono, B. A., Zinner, S. H., Daamen, M., & McCormack, W. M. (1990). Sexual behavior of college women in 1975, 1986 and 1989. *New England Journal of Medicine, 322*(12), 821–825.

The purpose of the study reported by Debuono and associates was to compare sexual practices in college women before and after the start of the current epidemics of chlamydia, genital herpes, and HIV. The authors surveyed 486 college women who consulted gynecologists at a student health service in 1975, 161 in 1986, and 132 in 1989 at the same university. There were no statistically significant differences in age, age at menarche, or reason for visiting the physician in the three groups. The percentages of sexually experienced women in the groups were the same (87%). Little change in sexual practices in response to new and serious epidemics of STDs were found. In the three years studied, an equal proportion of women had six or more male partners. Also, these women had three or more male partners in the year prior to the study. Similarly, the proportion of women who engaged in oral and anal sex, though low, was unchanged. There was a significant decrease in use of oral contraceptives from 1975 to 1989. One encouraging

observation was an increase in regular use of condoms from 12 percent in 1975 to 41 percent in 1989. An additional sample of 189 women who did not consult the health service were surveyed in 1989 and similar sexual behavior was reported by those who were sexually experienced (65%). This study adds important information regarding sexual behaviors in a population group at high risk for STDs.

Deitch, K. V., & Smith, J. E. (1990). Symptoms of chronic vaginal infection and microscopic condyloma in women. *Journal of Obstetrical, Gynecological and Neonatal Nursing, 19*(2), 133–138.

Genital tract human papilloma virus infections are a significant public health problem. These infections are the fourth most common sexually transmitted disease in the United States, treatment is difficult and not 100 percent effective, and the neoplastic potential of the disease is alarming. The purpose of this study was to determine if women who self-reported symptoms of chronic vaginal infection might be at risk for microscopic condyloma, and thus need colposcopic examinations. A sample of 30 women selected from a private gynecological practice were interviewed regarding infection symptoms, examination and laboratory results, number of office visits and treatment used in past year. Additional information collected included colposcopy examination, Papanicolaou smear results, vulvar biopsy results and information about male partners. Findings demonstrated that women who report yeast-type symptom chronicity and who had yeast-negative laboratory studies had a significant incidence of microscopic vulvar condyloma. While the study did not have a control group and the sample size was small, the investigators suggest that results support the conclusion that there is a need to broaden the use of the colposcope to detect condyloma in women with chronic yeast-like symptoms. These findings should alert clinicians to the need for indepth questioning about symptoms of vaginal discomfort and alertness to statements implying chronic symptoms, symptoms unrelieved by treatment, or symptoms that seem to recur after treatment.

Dorfman, L. E., Derish, P. A., & Cohen, J. B. (1992). Hey girlfriend: An evaluation of AIDS prevention among women in the sex industry. *Health Education Quarterly, 19,* 25–40.

This article describes a process and outcome evaluation of an AIDS prevention program for sex workers (*n* = 181). Both qualitative and quantitative methods including questionnaires, open-ended interviews, and ethnographic field notes were used to overcome problems inherent when doing research involving street-based populations. Findings showed that sex workers felt at risk for AIDS, usually from clients rather than from partners. Thus they used condoms more often with clients than with steady partners. Most participants demonstrated a clear understanding of HIV transmission as well as intention to avoid infection. This study provides much needed information about a population that is often "invisible" yet at high-risk for contracting STDs. The authors suggest ways in which the findings can be used to reach sex workers with effective AIDS risk reduction messages.

Flaskerud, J. H., & Nyamathi, A. M. (1989). Black and Latina women's AIDS related knowledge, attitudes, and practices. *Research in Nursing and Health, 12,* 339–346.

Flaskerud, J., & Rush, C. E. (1989). AIDS and traditional health beliefs and practices of black women. *Nursing Research, 38*(4), 210–215.

Both of the analyses reported in these articles utilize data drawn from a study designed to provide an AIDS education and prevention program for low-income black and Latina women. The first article describes a pilot study designed to gather baseline data on black (51) and Latina (56) women's' AIDS related knowledge, attitudes, and practices and to test an instrument that would measure these variables. Differences in sociodemographic variables, knowledge, and attitudes were identified between the two groups. In general, black women had more knowledge of and more positive attitudes towards AIDS than did Latina women. No differences in practices were found with both groups denying drug use and multiple sexual partners. The findings suggest that there is a need for separate, culturally relevant education and prevention programs for Latina women and for black women. The second analysis examines whether traditional health beliefs and practices of black Americans previously reported in the literature were consistent with those of low-income black women in California and describes how traditional classifications of illness and healing practices were related to an understanding of AIDS. Findings revealed that AIDS had been integrated into the traditional conceptualizations of illness, health practices, and healing. Findings suggest that AIDS education, prevention and, treatment programs should be within the context of the traditional health belief system of black Americans. Both of these articles emphasize the need for culturally relevant and specific education programs and health care. Further, they call attention to the importance of considering race differences in health and illness beliefs if appropriate and effective care is to be provided.

Flaskerud, J., & Thompson, J. (1991). Beliefs about AIDS, health, and illness in low-income white women. *Nursing Research, 40,* 266–271.

Using a focus group format, the authors investigated the lay beliefs of 42 low-income white women about AIDS and its treatment and whether these beliefs were related to their general beliefs about illness and treatment. The women were knowledgeable about the major modes of transmission of HIV. Causes and treatment of AIDS were categorized as professional sector, popular sector, and traditional sector health care beliefs. Professional sector beliefs included cause and major modes of transmission and prevention identified by the biomedical system and public health service. Popular sector misconceptions included beliefs about casual transmission and immunizations. Traditional sector beliefs concerned causes such as contamination and impurities and remedies such as diet and herbs. Subjects had also integrated their biomedical, popular, and traditional explanations for the cause and treatment of AIDS into their understanding of the immune system. The research findings reported provide additional knowledge necessary for designing programs that will be effective in communicating information and motivating behavioral change.

Fullilove, M. T., Fullilove, R. E., Haynes, K., & Gross, S. (1990). Black women and AIDS prevention: A view towards understanding the gender rules. *The Journal of Sex Research, 27,* 47–64.

This paper presents the results of intensive group discussion with 28 lower-income black women and adolescent females. Women were asked about sexual practices, use of drugs with sex, current and past relationships, history of STDs; individual responses and group interaction were recorded. Analysis suggests that traditional sex roles permitting men to have sexual freedom, but censuring women for the same activities, still operate in the black community. A major problem identified was the lack of effective communication about sexual practices, particularly condom use when partners are not mutually monogamous. Communication difficulties were aggravated by imbalance of power between men and women; older women reported that with experience they became clearer about what was acceptable and what was not. Respondents also identified the dramatic increase in male unemployment and decline of stable adult relationships as factors adversely affecting communication difficulties. This study provides valuable knowledge on sexual communication between black women and men—information that is essential if health professionals are to develop culturally appropriate interventions to reduce risk of STDs including HIV.

Goldberg, L. H., et al. (1993). Long-term suppression of recurrent genital herpes with acyclovir. *Archives of Dermatology, 129,* 582–587.

Acyclovir is highly effective against herpes viruses. The safety and efficacy of oral and intravenous acyclovir in decreasing morbidity associated with both first-episode and recurrent genital herpes has been demonstrated. In this study, results are reported of a multicenter trial (19 sites) begun in 1984 to assess long-term safety and efficacy. Mean annual number of recurrences per patient declined from 1.7 during the

first year to 0.8 during the fifth year of suppressive therapy. More than 20 percent of the patients receiving suppressive therapy for 5 years were recurrence free the entire time. Therapy was well tolerated and acyclovir usage was not associated with serious side effects or cumulative toxicity. This study further validates the safety and efficacy of long-term oral acyclovir use over 5 years.

Grodstein, F., Goldman, M. B., & Cramer, D. W. (1993). Relation of tubal infertility to history of sexually transmitted diseases. *American Journal of Epidemiology, 137,* 577–84.

Tubal occlusion and adhesions are estimated to account for approximately 20 percent of infertility in developed countries. STDs are among the factors implicated in infertility through their relation with pelvic inflammatory disease. The researchers studied the history of 283 nulliparous women diagnosed with infertility due to tubal adhesions or occlusion and 3,833 women admitted for delivery. Women who reported prior infection with gonorrhea were at a significantly higher risk of tubal infertility. Additionally, risk of tubal infertility was almost twice as high in women reporting previous trichomoniasis infection compared with women without such infection. The researchers also found a trend of increasing risk with an increasing number of episodes of gonorrhea or trichomoniasis. A significant limitation of this study is the lack of information on previous chlamydial infections in the subjects.

Hankins, C. A. (1990). Issues involving women, children, and AIDS primarily in the developed world. *Journal of Acquired Immune Deficiency Syndromes, 3*(4), 443–448.

The author presents an excellent overview of the problems poor women face regarding AIDS. AIDS prevention is placed in the social context in which women live and the point made that prevention of sexual transmission of HIV to women is made more difficult in part by the reticence of decision-makers to seriously examine the conditions that foster HIV transmission to women. Hankins believes that standard models of intervention based on empowerment concepts that urge women to take control, to avoid unprotected intercourse and to insist that sexual activity be conditional on condom use do not take into account that the vast majority of women at greatest risk for HIV acquisition have no power within their sexual relationships. She stresses that, while some women may have control over some situations, most do not have sufficient power with which to negotiate a change in rules within sexual relationships. A significant point made in this article is that empowerment as a prevention strategy must be considered within the individual woman's social and political context. If this is not done prevention efforts are likely to be unsuccessful. Hankins advocates for efforts directed at improving the economic circumstances of women based on the belief that without economic equality women will not be in a position to fully protect themselves from HIV infection. Specific strategies to be considered are universal comprehensive maternity care, pay equity, and an equitable distribution of care-giving responsibilities.

Jemmott, L. S., & Jemmott, J. B. (1992). Increasing condom-use intentions among sexually active black adolescent women. *Nursing Research, 41*, 273–279.

Because AIDS disproportionately affects low-income women of color, it is imperative that interventions to reduce risk of HIV infection be developed. In this article the researchers report the results of a study to test the effects of a social cognitive AIDS prevention intervention designed to increase intention to use condoms among 109 sexually active inner-city black adolescent women. The intervention, designed to increase self-efficacy regarding the ability to use condoms, increase knowledge of AIDS, and increase expectancies regarding use of condoms to prevent sexually transmitted HIV infection, consisted of 3 small group sessions. Content included information of the cause, transmission, and prevention of AIDS and risks faced by black women of childbearing age; expectancies regarding partner reactions and effects of condom use

on sexual pleasure; and skill-building and self-efficacy to use condoms. Analyses demonstrated that the women scored higher on intention to use condoms, AIDS knowledge, outcome expectancies regarding condom use, and self-efficacy to use condoms after the intervention than before the intervention. These findings support the value of culturally sensitive social cognitive AIDS risk-reduction interventions for women at high-risk for HIV infection. Further, the present study supports the effectiveness of social cognition theory as a framework for designing interventions to reduce HIV risk.

Karan, L. D. (1989). AIDS prevention and chemical dependence treatment needs of women and their children. *Journal of Psychoactive Drugs, 21*(4), 395–399.

In this paper, Karan addresses the special needs of female drug abusers and pays special attention to sexually transmitted diseases in general and HIV infection in particular. Factors associated with the drug abuser's increased risk of acquiring, transmitting, and experiencing a rapid progression of disease are considered. These include needle-sharing, the immunosuppressive features of alcohol and other drugs, associated poor health and inadequate nutrition, higher incidence of anorexia and bulimia, poor sanitary habits, using sex to procure drugs and delayed seeking of care and diminished compliance. The inadequacies of chemical dependence outreach and treatment programs are detailed including their inability to address issues of contraception, pregnancy, motherhood, childrearing, and prevention of STDs. Karan points out that most chemically dependent women infected with HIV are in their childbearing years and experience grief due to loss of health, body image, sexuality and childbearing potential. Further, these women are isolated and lack support they might otherwise have from family members and friends. This article presents a compelling review of the problems associated with childbearing in the HIV-infected, chemically dependent woman.

Kelley, K. F., Galbraith, M. A., & Vermund, S. H. (1992). Genital human papillomavirus infection in women. *JOGNN, 21,* 503–514.

This review article provides information on genital HPV infections in women for nurse clinicians. Information on definitions, prevalence, transmission, risk factors, and natural history of the virus is given. Diagnosis and screening methods, including indirect and direct analysis, and recommendations for screening are discussed. Treatment measures are reviewed. The authors review nursing roles and suggest areas of needed nursing research. This article is a comprehensive review of HPV that clinicians will find very useful.

Koretz, R. L. (1989). Universal prenatal hepatitis B testing: Is it cost effective? *Obstetrics & Gynecology, 74*(5), 808–814.

Citing problems inherent in screening procedures, the lower rates of hepatitis B surface antigen and hepatitis B E antigen positivity in the population without risk factors, and the expense of maternal testing, Koretz does not feel that universal prenatal testing for hepatitis B virus is cost effective. According to Koretz, the cost to prevent a clinically important case of hepatitis B in the neonates of mothers with no risk factors is $180,000, which is 15 times the cost of preventing a case in neonates of mothers with risk factors. He believes that screening should be limited to only those women with risk factors because it is too costly to prevent the remaining cases. This recommendation is in direct contrast to the previously cited Butterfield et al. (1990) study. These two widely divergent views point up the need for health professionals and individual women to be aware that controversies continue to exist in STD health care. Further, all women, be they professional or patient, should be wary of blanket acceptance of medical recommendations.

Lawrance, L., Levy, S. R., & Rubinson, L. (1990). Self-efficacy and AIDS prevention for pregnant teens. *Journal of School Health, 60*(1), 19–24.

AIDS represents a serious health threat for teenagers. The researchers suggest that self-efficacy is a construct that can measure the likelihood preventative behaviors will be performed and thus can be used to identify specific areas where AIDS education should be improved for adolescents. In this study, the self perceived ability of pregnant teenagers to participate in preventive behavior and avoid at-risk behaviors for AIDS was examined. The researchers found four areas of greatest vulnerability for the 58 pregnant, mostly black adolescents attending an alternative school in a large, midwestern city who participated in the study. These were using condoms, discussing previous homosexual activity, discussing previous bisexual activity and telling a partner about a previous bisexual experience. The last three situations resulted from an inability to discuss a partner's past sexual history. The researchers suggest that these difficulties stem in part from the fact that the young woman may be in a lesser position of power in her relationships with males, find it difficult to assert herself, and thus decrease high risk behaviors.

Lewis, D. K., Watters, J. K., & Case, P. (1990). The prevalence of high-risk sexual behaviors in male intravenous drug users with steady female partners. *American Journal of Public Health, 80*(4), 465–466.

A sample of 149 (70 white, 79 black) male intravenous drug users with steady female partners were interviewed about their sexual practices in the past 5 years. Eighty-three percent had multiple partners, 15 percent reported male contact, 38 percent reported heterosexual anal intercourse and 73 percent never used condoms. While the focus of this study was males, the findings are important for women's health in that it points out the risk of exposure to STDs in women. The male subjects in this study, all of whom had on-going, stable relationships with a woman, also participated in numerous high risk behaviors.

Marcus, A. C., Crane, L. A., Kaplan, C. P., Goodman, K. J., Savage, E., & Gunning, J. (1990).

Screening for cervical cancer in emergency centers and sexually transmitted disease clinics. *Obstetrics & Gynecology, 75*(3), 453–455.

Low-income women are at increased risk for developing cervical cancer compared with middle- and upper-income women. Yet these women are more difficult to reach for screening. Observing that a high percentage of the unscreened population has received some form of health care in the past 5 years, often in an emergency room or STD clinic, the authors suggest that these health care facilities represent potential resources for cervical cancer screening. However, in a survey of 19 hospitals with a high proportion of low-income patients, they found only five reported conducting cervical cancer screening in their emergency rooms. Of the 11 STD clinics surveyed, less than 5 percent of the female patients seen had a Papanicolaou smear taken even though virtually all had received a pelvic examination. Based on these findings, the researchers recommend that cancer prevention programs be improved by using emergency rooms and STD clinics for screening.

Nyamathi, A. M., Leake, B., Flaskerud, J., Lewis, C., & Bennett, C. (1993). Outcomes of specialized and traditional AIDS counseling programs for impoverished women of color. *Research in Nursing and Health, 16,* 11–21.

The researchers investigated the efficacy and differential effects of specialized and traditional AIDS education programs on cognitive, behavioral, and psychological outcomes. The Comprehensive Health Seeking and Coping Paradigm was used as the framework to guide this study of nursing interventions directed toward 858 homeless, drug-addicted women of color. Subjects were divided into two groups: traditional and specialized. At baseline, women in the traditional group reported significantly higher distress, greater knowledge of AIDS and less problem-focused coping. Significant improvements were seen in participants of both groups following the 2-week intervention period for appraisal of threat, concerns, knowledge, and attitudes about AIDS, emotion-focused coping, number of sexual partners,

IV and non-IV drug use, depression and distress. Multivariate analysis revealed that the traditional group had slightly better posttest scores on concerns, emotional-focused coping, knowledge of AIDS, and number of partners than did the specialized group. The specialized group reported greater problem-focused coping. The researchers concluded that these differences reinforce the conclusion that one type of program was not more effective than the other. The results also support recent findings that basic, culturally relevant information alone may be sufficient to reduce a substantial number of high risk activities such as unprotected sexual exposure and use of IV- and non-IV drug use. This article is important both for the reported findings which add to a growing body of literature testing nursing interventions to decrease the risk of STDs and for the description of the development of the interventions and the interventions themselves.

Oh, M. K., Feinstein, R. A., Soileau, E. J., Cloud, G. A., & Pass, R. F. (1989). Chlamydia trachomatis cervical infection and oral contraceptive use among adolescent girls. *Journal of Adolescent Health Care, 10*(5), 376–381.

Chlamydial infections are the most common STD among adolescents and young women of child-bearing age. About 50 percent of acute pelvic inflammatory disease is associated with chlamydial infections and it is a major cause of perinatal morbidity. In this study, the relationship between oral contraceptive use and C. trachomatis infection were investigated in 73 girls with chlamydial infection and 303 girls who were infection free. Use of an oral contraceptive for 6 months or longer was associated with chlamydial infection. This association continued after possible confounding variables were controlled for. The authors state that these findings suggest that oral contraceptive use may promote chlamydial infection of the cervix or enhance the detection of the infection. These findings should be compared with those of Wolner-Hassen and associates (1990) who found that oral contraceptive use protects against symptomatic PID among women infected with C. trachomatis.

Rotmensch, S., Rosenzweig, B. A., & Phillippe, M. (1989). The impact of the acquired immunodeficiency syndrome epidemic on the philosophy of childbirth. *American Journal of Obstetrics and Gynecology, 161*(4), 855–856.

In this thoughtful opinion piece, the authors point out that the guidelines for universal infection precautions developed to minimize the risk of HIV transmission are mutually exclusive to currently popular childbirth practices. In addition to the physical barriers imposed, universal infection precautions create psychological barriers between the laboring woman and her health care providers. The fear of infection is a powerful psychological barrier that can erode the woman's sense of trust. Additionally, anxiety and the need for physical isolation are a poor basis for an empathetic human relationship. The authors challenge health professionals to develop strategies for maintaining a sensitive, child-centered approach in the AIDS era.

Schaffer, S. D., & Philput, C. B. (1992). Predictors of abnormal cytology: Statistical analysis of human papillomavirus and cofactors. *Nurse Practitioner, 17*, 46–48, 50.

Carcinoma of the cervix is the third most common malignancy in women in the United States. In the past decade, extensive research has documented the continuum of abnormal cellular changes that ultimately lead to cervical cancer and substantiates the oncological contribution of human papillomavirus (HPV). Reported increases in the incidence of HPV have lead to the speculation that cervical cytology abnormalities may also be increasing. The purpose of this study was to develop and compare cohort profiles for cervical-cytology smears from 1977 to 1989 at the student health center in a large southeastern university. The 10-year retrospective study of cervical cytology in 2,919 college women revealed a significant increase in the frequency and severity of cervical-cytology abnormalities. The peak year for abnormal cervical cytology coincided with the peak year for overt HPV infection. These concurrent increases in HPV infection and cervical-cytology severity point to an association that requires further study. Women with HPV, women with genital herpes, and those who smoked had mean cervical cytology severity scores significantly worse than those with none of these factors.

Shanis, B. S., Check, J. H., & Baker, A. F. (1989). Transmission of sexually transmitted diseases by donor semen. *Archives of Andrology, 23*, 249–257.

Therapeutic insemination by donor (TID) is used with increasing frequency today. Because many diseases can be transmitted through semen, the American Fertility Society has established guidelines for use of donor sperm. These are discussed in this article as are current recommendations for HIV testing. The necessity for using frozen samples rather than fresh is stressed and new techniques of cryopreservation discussed. In light of the recent reports of HIV transmission by artificial insemination in Australia, the information presented in this article is essential reading for health professionals caring for women in their childbearing years.

Smeltzer, S. C., & Whipple, B. (1991). Women and HIV infection. *IMAGE, 23*, 249–255.

This "State of the Science" article comprehensively reviews what was known about HIV infection and AIDS in women through September 1991. Particular attention is paid to the special issues concerning women and AIDS. Issues addressed include problems associated with the CDC case definition of AIDS, disproportionate representation of minority women affected with AIDS, view of women as vectors, transmitters, or infectors of AIDS to their offspring, and risk group status versus risk behaviors. The authors evaluate current research on AIDS knowledge, attitudes, and beliefs and suggest how nurses can use this information in their practice. The research on female specific symptoms including candida infections and sexually transmitted diseases is reviewed. HIV and pregnancy is examined from the perspective of the woman and her offspring. The article concludes with a discussion of the contribution nursing can make in the provision of women infected with HIV. This thoughtful, comprehensive, and challenging article should be read by all nurses who care for women.

Stein, Z. A. (1990). HIV prevention: The need for methods women can use. *American Journal of Public Health, 80,* 460–462.

Currently the condom is the sole physical barrier promoted for the prevention of sexual transmission of HIV infection from men to women. Condom usage can be accomplished only with active male cooperation and requires the woman to assert dominance in the sexual act. For many, if not most women, this is not the traditional mode of interaction with men. Stein asserts that empowerment of women is crucial for the prevention of HIV transmission of women. She also reminds the reader that while men control condom usage, women control the use of diaphragms and can control use of topical virucides. It may be that these methods, while less efficacious than condoms, may be more effective in the long run, if consistently and widely used. She also points out that initial HIV educational and prevention efforts were developed for and aimed at men. These same programs are now being used to inform women. They may not be appropriate or effective for women. Stein suggests that health care providers could use the knowledge gained from years of family planning research to design more effective educational programs for women. Finally, she recommends that tactics which interrupt transmission of the virus should be considered in their own right and separated from pregnancy prevention methods.

Williams, A. B. (1990). Reproductive concerns of women at risk for HIV infection. *Journal of Nurse-Midwifery, 35,* 292–298.

Williams, A. B. (1991). Women at risk: An AIDS educational needs assessment. *IMAGE, 23,* 208–213.

Both of the analyses reported in these articles utilize data drawn from a qualitative, exploratory study of 21 women at risk for AIDS

through their IV-drug use or as partners of IV-drug users. In-depth interviews utilizing open-ended questions were conducted to assess educational needs. Perception of AIDS as a serious and personal health risk motivated the women to practice safe sex and safe drug use. However, they did not always believe that condom use was completely effective in preventing HIV transmission. Further, they identified specific costs including rejection of potential sexual partners and risk of disrupting established sexual relationships. Balance between motivation for sexually self-protective behaviors and perception of associated risks was influenced by specific contextual factors, specifically knowledge of HIV antibody status. Those who knew that they or a potential partner were HIV-positive were more likely to use condoms or abstain. Contextual themes which ran throughout the interviews and reflected the context in which the women had experienced the AIDS epidemic were fear of AIDS and isolation. Another analysis of the data identified additional contextual factors: fear of HIV antibody testing, a belief that perinatal HIV transmission is inevitable, support for pregnancy termination in the event of HIV-associated pregnancy, strong desire for children, pride in mothering behavior, and guilt over possible transmission of HIV to unborn children. The author concludes that AIDS education and counseling will be most effective if these contextual factors are considered when planning interventions.

Wolner-Hassen, P., Eschenbach, D. A., Paavonen, J., Stevens, C. E., Kiviat, N. B., Critchlow, C., DeRouen, T., Koutsky, L., & Holmes, K. K. (1990). Association between vaginal douching and acute pelvic inflammatory disease. *Journal of the American Medical Association, 263*(14), 1936–1941.

The vaginal douching practices of 100 hospitalized women with pelvic inflammatory disease (cases) were compared with those of 762 randomly selected control and 119 women thought to have PID but in whom diagnosis was not confirmed (internal controls). Among current douchers (any douching in the past 2 months), PID was significantly related to frequency of douching. After adjustments for demographic, behavioral, and other possible confounding variables, this relationship remained. These results suggest that vaginal douching may be a risk factor for PID and have important client assessment and educational implications.

Worth, D. (1989). Sexual decision-making and AIDS: Why condom promotion among vulnerable women is likely to fail. *Studies in Family Planning, 20,* 297–307.

This article examines the reasons for resistance among high-risk women in AIDS prevention programs. Data were collected from women attending the Women's AIDS Program ($n = > 1,000$) and the Women's Center program ($n = 121$) through behavioral observation, structured questionnaires, participant observation, process ethnography, focus groups, and in-depth individual interviews. Findings indicate that an important focus for these vulnerable women is to concentrate on addressing more immediate risks in their lives: poverty, homelessness, and the frequent disruption of socioeconomic support systems. The process by which decisions regarding condom usage were made involved a complex mixture of social, economic, and cultural influences that promote motherhood for women even when they know they might be infected with HIV. Imbalances in power in their relationships with their male partners were reported. Women expressed anger at being made to feel responsible for men's sexual behavior. Worth's findings underline the fact that women most vulnerable to HIV infection are those who have the least control over sexual decision-making whether because of drug use, lack of economic power, culturally sanctioned gender-role behavior, racism or sexism. The studies reported in this article have a wealth of information regarding why many women are unable to use condoms in their sexual relationships.

Chapter 11

Acute Care of Women

Patricia A. Geary

INTRODUCTION

Women do not fare well in acute care settings. The information which is beginning to surface regarding cardiovascular disease in women gives factual support to the concern that the acute health care of women suffers from as much of a gender bias as women have faced in the work place. While women have more contact with physicians and form the majority of client populations in hospitals in the United States, little attention is paid to them as a clinical group. That women as a group, are hospitalized longer than men should foster more research to investigate the causes of this discrepancy and to change the outcome.

Hospitals are organized generally by medical specialties. Women's health care, in practice, is often simply reproductive track care without serious attention to women as a special population with physiologic differences which can affect their diseases and their response to treatment. Moreover, women are under represented in clinical trials, yet treated according to the results of those trials. The medical specialties with their focus on systems have resulted in a research bias which limits access to useful information on the acute care of women.

Although cardiovascular disease is a major killer of women, it has until just recently been considered a male disease. The articles reviewed here demonstrate just how little is known about the diagnosis and treatment of women with cardiovascular disease. Women have greater operative mortality and risk of death from myocardial infarction, and their chest pain is more likely to be seen as non-cardiac. The choice and dose of drugs used in women who are older, have less body mass, and a different hormonal status, are based on studies done on middle-aged men.

Women die from cancer as frequently as men, (Taeuber, 1991), yet even breast cancer, a "woman's" disease, has received nowhere near the research attention received by cardiovascular disease. The articles on risk factors show that the cause of breast cancer is not yet known and only a quarter of the women diagnosed with breast cancer are in risk groups. Breast cancer treatment has remained stable despite the gains represented by lumpectomy and radiation and the setback of a rising incidence. Prevention by administration of hormones, resulting in the manipulation of women's physiology so that women too easily become afraid of their own bodies is being discussed (Bernstein, Ross, & Henderson, 1990). Women die more often than men from lung cancer (Taeuber, 1991) and the incidence is rising in women. However, little can be found in the literature on prevention and treatment of women with lung cancer.

What should be the standard of care for women in acute facilities? How do we begin to ensure that a woman admitted to a hospital has adequate health care, including screening examinations, a history which reviews for major risks, health education based on a specialized knowledge of women, and treatment which is based on knowledge of risks, diseases, age, body mass, and hormonal influence? One way is to re-look at the distribution of resources and provide specialists in women's health for inpatient women. It is not enough to mandate the inclusion of women in research as the U.S. Congress has done. It is also necessary to re-look at the use of resources to change the care being given to women. Women receiving acute care whether in major medical centers or community hospitals must be the beneficiaries of what is known about care of women. There is a need to inform all professionals and specialties about what is known so that specialized clinical approaches and preventive care can be provided. Control and choice for women with acute health problems is undercut by the lack of an adequate information base.

REFERENCES

Bernstein, L., Ross, R. K., & Henderson, B. E. (1992). Prospects for the primary prevention of breast cancer. *American Journal of Epidemiology, 135,* 142–152.

Taeuber, C. M. (1991). Health aspects. In *Statistical Handbook on Women in America.* Phoenix: Oryx Press.

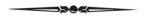

BOOKS AND ARTICLES

Ayanian, J. Z., & Epstein, A. M. (1991). Differences in the use of procedures between women and men hospitalized for coronary heart disease. *The New England Journal of Medicine, 325,* 221–225.

The authors present findings from discharge data of patients hospitalized with known or suspected coronary artery disease. Generally, women were older, their diagnosis was more likely to be unstable anginal chest pain and less likely to have diagnoses of myocardial infarction or chronic atherosclerotic heart disease. Men were more likely to have had coronary angiograms and revascularization procedures. An excellent discussion of the potential meaning of the findings is included. Anyone interested in the acute care of women should read this study.

It is, of course, a possibility that women should not undergo as much invasive medical treatment as men and that women are actually receiving a better standard of care. However, this study certainly does point out that the experience of women in acute care is different from that of men and raises the unanswered question: why do women receive fewer cardiac procedures than men?

Badwe, R. A., Gregory, W. M., Chaudar, Y. M. A., Richards, M. A., Bentley, A. E., Rubens, R. D., & Fentinman, I. S. (1991). Timing of surgery during menstrual cycle and survival of premenopausal women with operable breast cancer. *The Lancet, 337,* 1261–1264.

McGuire, W. L., Hilsenbeck, S., & Clark, G. M. (1992). Optional mastectomy timing. *Journal of the National Cancer Institute, 84,* 346–348.

The outcomes of 249 patients who underwent surgery for breast cancer were studied in relationship to their menstrual cycle at the time of surgery. Women were divided into two groups by last menstrual cycle. The first group had surgery 3–12 days after their last menstrual period and the second group 0–2 or 13–32 days after their last menstrual period. The survival of statistics for the second group were significantly better over a 10-year period. Primary treatment and tumor size were subjected to multivariate analysis. The authors suggest that surgery for breast cancer should be timed in relation to the patient's menstrual cycle. The article raises issues seldom considered in the timing of surgery and identifies issues that should be considered in this acute condition of women.

Becker, R. C. (1990). Coronary thrombolysis in women. *Cardiology, 77,* 110–123.

Corrao, J. M., Becker, R. C., Ockene, I. S., & Hamilton, G. A. (1990). Coronary heart disease risk factors in women. *Cardiology, 77,* 8–24.

Hamilton, G. A. (1990). Recovery from acute myocardial infarction in women. *Cardiology, 77,* 58–70.

Hendel, R. C. (1990). Myocardial infarction in women. *Cardiology, 77,* 41–57.

Taylor, P., & Becker, R. C. (1990). Noninvasive diagnosis of coronary heart disease in women. *Cardiology, 77,* 91–98.

(All above studies appear in supplement 2 titled "Cardiovascular Disease of Women.")

That women fare differently than men when they have cardiac disease is clearly demonstrated in this excellent series of review studies. Each study demonstrates how little is actually known about cardiovascular disease in women when compared with what is known about the problem in men. The authors conclude that further research is necessary. We know that cardiovascular disease is one of the primary killers of women, that women develop it later in life, and that they become sicker. What we do not know is how to maximize treatment outcomes for women or even

to successfully predict cardiovascular disease from risk factors. Additionally, diagnosis may be different. This excellent, thought-provoking series illustrates the lack of attention to the acute problems women suffer.

Bernstein, L., Ross, R. K., & Henderson, B. E. (1992). Prospects for the primary prevention of breast cancer. *American Journal of Epidemiology. 135,* 142–152.

The authors review studies to present three means of hormonal intervention to prevent breast cancer: tamoxifen, luteinizing hormone, and the reduction of estrogens through physical activity. Dietary changes as a preventive mechanism are also discussed as a mediator due to dietary effect on age at menarche. Much attention has been focused on changing a women's hormonal environment through administration of exogenous hormones—emphasizing, in a sense, that a women's own body is her own initmate enemy. This article is refreshing in its inclusion of physical activity as a potential intervention which can reduce the risk of breast cancer. Physical activity, as well, is an intervention which women can control.

Harris, R. B., & Weissfeld, L. A. (1991). Gender differences in the reliability of reporting symptoms of angina pectoris. *Journal of Clinical Epidemiology, 44,* 1071–1078.

The results of using a structured questionnaire, the Rose Questionnaire, to determine its short-term reliability in reporting angina in men and women are reported. Women had a higher prevalence of angina when measured with a single questionnaire. There were differences in the younger groups by gender with women under 50 having four times the prevalence of angina. Use of the Rose Questionnaire in research is discussed. The study demonstrates some of the problems in recognizing angina in women and emphasizes the need for further research in the area.

Healy, B. (1991). The yentl syndrome. *The New England Journal of Medicine, 325,* 274–276.

This editorial suggests that in current practice a woman must be "more like a man" before her coronary artery disease is recognized, taken seriously, and treated. Women are treated aggressively once they have had a myocardial infarction, but not if they present with angina. This differentiation in treatment occurs despite the fact that myocardial infarction is one of the major causes of death among women in the United States. Women have more chronic problems than men and their quality of life, in the approximately seven years that they live longer than men, may be burdened by chronic disease.

The editorial mentions the Women's Health Initiative, a major multidisciplinary intervention study for women and suggests that it may provide information useful to the treatment of women. Providing a medical perspective on the gaps in women's health care, this editorial is worth reading.

Mesko, T. W., Dunlap, J. N., & Sutherland, C. M. (1990). Risk factors for breast cancer. *Comprehensive Therapy, 16,* 3–9.

The authors review the various risk factors which have been attached to the development of breast cancer. Very few factors demonstrate a clear association with the development of breast cancer. The authors do identify factors which have relatively little association with the disease. The authors also indentify this significant point: only a quarter of the cases of breast cancer are found in women identified at risk.

Raymond, C. (1991). Recognition of the gender differences in mental illness and its treatment prompts a call for more health research on problems specific to women. *The Chronicle of Higher Education, 37,* A5(2).

In this brief report, individuals in the mental health field are interviewed. Interviewees note in various ways that women's physiology results in difference in their responses to various substances including alcohol and nicotine. Because such responses have been poorly studied, potentially inadequate treatment is currently being offered to women. Illnesses more common

in women are cited and the case is made for more research in this area.

Sclafani, L. (1991). Management of the high-risk patient. *Seminars in Surgical Oncology, 7,* 261–266.

The author describes a program for women at high risk of development of breast cancer maintained at Memorial Sloan Kettering and Cancer Center in New York. What is known about risk factors for breast cancer is discussed as well as the screening and follow-up utilized with women at high risk. The study is valuable for its summary of risk factors for breast cancer and contains information which can be useful in working with women in acute care institutions, including referral for follow-up if they are at high risk.

Steingart, R. M., Packer, M., Hamm, P., Coglianese, M. E., Gersh, B., Geltman, E. M., Sollano, J., Katz, S., Moyé, L., Basta, L. L., Lewis, S. J., Gottleib, S. S., Bernstein, V., McEwan, P., Jacobson, K., Brown, E. J., Kukin, M. L., Kantrowitz, N. E., & Pfeffer, M. A. (1991). Sex differences in the management of coronary artery disease. *The New England Journal of Medicine, 325,* 226–230.

Treatment of men and women who were enrolled in a larger study after acute myocardial infarction was studied. The authors collected data prospectively using systematic and uniform procedures for data collection in a multicenter study. Data were collected for each patient including coronary risk factors, numbers of hospitalizations, cardiac catherization, angioplasty or bypass surgery, angina, functional status, and medications. Both men and women gave similar histories of angina and had been placed on similar drugs. However, women were more likely to state that they had some type of disability from their angina. Despite diagnoses, catherization and bypass surgery was done on men more frequently than on women. Multiregression analysis showed that differentiation in cardiac catherization and bypass surgery by sex occurred independently of other variables. Although men were twice as likely to undergo catherization and bypass surgery, once women did have a cardiac catherization the differences in treatment were less. This can be considered a watershed study as it demonstrates the differences in acute treatment of men and women and suggests that if such differences exist in a common health problem, coronary disease, other less common illnesses may demonstrate treatment discrepancies.

Taeuber, C. M. (1991). Health aspects. In *Statistical Handbook on Women in America*, 220–246. Phoenix: Oryx Press.

This handbook is an excellent reference for evaluating the condition of women in America and worth the perusal of those who are involved in women's health. The chapter on health aspects gives an overview of health conditions of women including institutionalization, individual health practices, mental health, chronic disease, individuals from whom women get their health care both outside the household and within the household, and acute conditions. Anyone who questions whether the foci of research and of funding in health care addresses areas of common problems, should review this chapter.

Wood, C. (1989) The reality of women's health. *Nursing Times*, 85, 54–55.

This brief review of women's health problems focusing on mental health, depression, and coronary artery disease is well worth reading. It points out that women's problems are often undetected, poorly treated, and reflect a lack of control over their life's work. The article is brief, succinct, and thought provoking.

Other Books of Interest from NLN Press

Book Title	Pub. No.	Price	NLN Member Price
☐ Critique, Resistance, and Action: Working Papers in the Politics of Nursing *Edited by Janice L. Thompson, David G. Allen, and Lorraine Rodrigues-Fisher*	14-2504	38.95	34.95
☐ On Nursing: A Literary Celebration *By Margretta Styles & Patricia Moccia*	14-2512	29.95	26.95
☐ On Nursing: A Literary Celebration *Collectors' Leatherette-Bound Edition*	14-2513	54.95	49.95
☐ The Hidden Dimension of Illness: Human Suffering *Edited by Patricia L. Starck and John P. McGovern*	15-2461	32.95	29.95
☐ Nursing As Caring: A Model for Transforming Practice *By Anne Boykin & Savina Schoenhofer*	15-2549	35.95	30.95
☐ Living a Caring-Based Program *Edited by Anne Boykin*	14-2536	27.95	24.95
☐ A Global Agenda for Caring *Edited by Delores A. Gaut*	15-2518	34.95	30.95

DATE DUE

GAYLORD			PRINTED IN U.S.A.